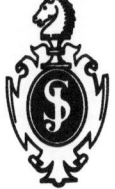

Clinical Practice in Urology
Series Editor: Geoffrey D. Chisholm

Titles in the series already published

Urinary Diversion
Edited by Michael Handley Ashken

The Pharmacology of the Urinary Tract
Edited by M. Caine

Bladder Cancer
Edited by E.J. Zingg and D.M.A. Wallace

Percutaneous and Interventional Urology and Radiology
Edited by Erich K. Lang

Adenocarcinoma of the Prostate
Edited by Andrew W. Bruce and John Trachtenberg

Controversies and Innovations in Urological Surgery
Edited by Clive Gingell and Paul Abrams

Combination Therapy in Urological Malignancy
Edited by Philip H. Smith

Current Perspectives in Paediatric Urology
Edited by Robert H. Whitaker

Practical Urology in Spinal Cord Injury
Edited by Keith F. Parsons and John M. Fitzpatrick

Forthcoming titles in the series

Male Infertility (Second Edition)
Edited by T.B. Hargreave

Urodynamics (Second Edition)
Paul Abrams, Roger Feneley and Michael Torrens

Urological Prostheses, Appliances and Catheters

Edited by
John P. Pryor

With 111 Figures

Springer-Verlag
London Berlin Heidelberg New York
Paris Tokyo Hong Kong
Barcelona Budapest

John P. Pryor, MS, FRCS
Consultant Urologist, King's College and St. Peter's Hospitals,
London, UK

Series Editor

Geoffrey D. Chisholm, ChM, FRCS, FRCSEd
Professor of Surgery, University of Edinburgh; and Consultant
Urological Surgeon, Western General Hospital, Edinburgh, Scotland

Cover illustration: Ch. 3, Fig. 8b. From Mardis HK et al. (1979) Double pigtail uretal
stent. Urology 14:23–26.

ISBN-13:978-1-4471-1463-5   e-ISBN-13:978-1-4471-1461-1
DOI: 10.1007/978-1-4471-1461-1

British Library Cataloguing in Publication Data
Pryor, J. P. (John P)
  Urological prostheses, appliances and catheters.-
  (Clinical practice in urology)
  I. Title II. Series
  616.6
ISBN-13:978-1-4471-1463-5

Library of Congress Cataloging-in-Publication Data
Urological prostheses, appliances, and catheters / edited by John P.
  Pryor.
    p. cm. — (Clinical practice in urology)
  Includes index.
  ISBN-13:978-1-4471-1463-5

  1. Urological prostheses. I. Pryor, J. P. (John P.) II. Series.
  [DNLM: 1. Prosthesis. 2. Urogenital Diseases—surgery.
3. Urology—instrumentation. WJ 168 U78]
RD571.U756 1991
617.4′60592—dc20
DNLM/DLC
                                                    91–5158
for Library of Congress   CIP

Typeset by Best-set Typesetter Ltd., Hong Kong
28/3830-543210 Printed on acid-free paper

Series Editor's Foreword

The title of this book gives a clear indication of the changes in emphasis that are occurring in urology. Is it possible that prostheses, appliances and catheters represent such a significant part of urology that they require a book devoted to them? The answer is most certainly "yes", mainly because there are now so many aspects to this theme and yet it is difficult to find a ready reference source.

Urology has always been a subject that dealt with "plumbing and tubes": historically this was a major part of urology. Now many urological problems can be treated by a range of procedures many of which require the implantation of manufactured devices. The range of materials currently available for these devices has led to further developments in the prostheses and appliances available for urological care.

Until now the knowledge on these topics has been covert: articles here and there, lectures mentioning some developments, commercial companies pressing their new products on the profession, etc. Hard facts on the merits of these developments were difficult to obtain. Often, just when a device is becoming accepted and experience gained, along comes another modification. The facts can only be obtained from the experience of those with special interests in these matters. I have been and remain a strong supporter of the controlled clinical trial, but the evaluation of surgical procedures and prostheses is not easily applicable to this discipline. We must therefore rely on the accumulated experience of acknowledged experts. This book brings together such expertise in a variety of situations that are constant problems for the urologist. The aim of this Series is to bring to the reader the best possible opinions in the clinical practice of urology. Mr. Pryor and his well-selected colleagues have easily achieved this aim.

Edinburgh   Geoffrey D. Chisholm
November 1991

Preface

This volume is intended to collect together those aspects of urology which depend upon manufactured articles that are inserted in or attached to patients. They are of relevance to every urologist and range from the mundane to the highly specialised.

Urological practice has changed a great deal during the past decade or so and this is reflected in the current volume. In some areas, the innovations are rapidly succeeded by newer techniques and fade to oblivion. The increased pace of change is the result of manufacturers and urologists working together to take advantage of the new technologies and materials that have been developed. Some manufacturers have a major commitment to genitourinary surgery and this financial investment is to the benefit of our patients. Such is the speed of change that it is impossible to be up-to-date in all areas. Nevertheless, it is to be hoped that the current volume provides a sound basis for clinical urologists.

The original concept was to divide the book into the different aspects of the title but on reflection it seemed better to group the chapters on a more functional and anatomical basis.

Institute of Urology, London   John P. Pryor
February 1991

Contents

List of Contributors   xi

Editorial: Synthetic Soft Tissue Substitutes
J.P. Pryor   xiii

Chapter 1
Open Nephrostomy
J.W.A. Ramsay   1

Chapter 2
Percutaneous Nephrostomy
R.A. Miller   19

Chapter 3
Ureteric Stents
R.P. Finney and S.C. Hopkins   33

Chapter 4
Urethral and Suprapubic Catheters
M.C. Bishop and R.J. Lemberger   73

Chapter 5
Implantable Incontinence Devices
P.H.L. Worth   109

Chapter 6
Urinary Incontinence Appliances, Aids and Equipment
R.N.P. Carroll   133

Chapter 7
Prosthetic Urethral Substitution
P.J.R. Shaw   167

Chapter 8
Urostomy Appliances
R.N.P. Carroll 175

Chapter 9
Penile Prostheses
J.P. Pryor 197

Chapter 10
Vas Deferens Prostheses
S.S. Schmidt 229

Chapter 11
Alloplastic Spermatocele (Sperm Reservoirs)
A. Kelâmi 239

Chapter 12
Testicular Prostheses
J.P. Pryor 247

Chapter 13
Vascular Access
C.J. Rudge 257

Chapter 14
Antibiotic Therapy
W.R. Gransden and P.M. Thompson 269

Subject Index 283

Contributors

M.C. Bishop, MD, MRCP, FRCS
Consultant Urological Surgeon, City Hospital, Nottingham, UK

R.N.P. Carroll, MB, BCh, BAO, BSc, FRCS, FRCS(Ed)
Consultant Urologist, Manchester Royal Infirmary and St. Mary's
Hospital, Manchester, UK

R.P. Finney, MD, FACS
Professor of Surgery, Division of Urology, University of South
Florida Medical College and James A Haley Veterans Hospital,
Tampa, Florida, USA

W.R. Gransden, MRCPath
Senior Lecturer, Department of Medical Microbiology, United
Medical and Dental School of Guy's, St. Peter's and St. Thomas's
Hospitals, London, UK

S.C. Hopkins, MD, FRCS(C)
Assistant Professor of Surgery, Division of Urology, University
of South Florida Medical College and James A Haley Veterans
Hospital, Tampa, Florida, USA

A. Kelâmi, MD
Consultant Urologist, Brahmsstrasse 32, D-1000 Berlin 45, Germany

R.J. Lemberger, FRCS
Consultant Urological Surgeon, Mansfield Hospitals and City
Hospital, Nottingham, UK

R.A. Miller, MS, MB, FRCS
Consultant Urologist, Whittington Hospital, London, UK

J.P. Pryor, MS, FRCS
Consultant Urologist, King's College and St. Peter's Hospitals,
London, UK

J.W.A. Ramsay, MS, FRCS
Consultant Urologist, Charing Cross and West Middlesex Hospitals,
London, UK

C.J. Rudge, FRCS
Consultant Transplant Surgeon, St. Peter's Hospitals, London, UK

S.S. Schmidt, MD
Consultant Urologist, Department of Urology, University of
California School of Medicine, San Francisco, California, USA

P.J.R. Shaw, FRCS
Senior Lecturer and Honorary Consultant Urologist, St. Peter's
Hospitals, London, UK

P.M. Thompson, FRCS
Consultant Urologist, Joyce Green Hospital, Dartford, Kent, UK

P.H.L. Worth, FRCS
Consultant Urologist, St. Peter's Hospitals, London, UK

Editorial: Synthetic Soft Tissue Substitutes

Materials must feature in any book about prostheses, appliances and catheters and this introduction attempts to summarise some of the basic considerations that are relevant to clinicians and common to all prostheses.

In 1953 Professor John Scales of the Institute of Orthopaedics, London, listed the ideal characteristics of synthetic soft tissue substitutes. These are worth repeating as they remain relevant today. He stated that they should:

1. not be physically modified by body fluids
2. be chemically inert
3. not incite inflammatory or foreign body cell response in the tissues
4. not be carcinogenic
5. not produce a state of allergy or hypersensitivity
6. resist mechanical strains
7. be capable of manufacture in the desired form
8. be capable of being sterilised

In addition, synthetics should also be cheap to manufacture. An additional quality that is necessary for catheters is that they should not be subject to encrustation.

Rubin et al. (1971) reviewed a 20-year experience with synthetic plastics and found that polyethylene was suitable for use in the head and neck region. Beheri (1966) reported the implantation of paired polyethylene prostheses into the penis in 600 men, but the mechanical qualities of the prosthesis were unsatisfactory. It was not until medical grade silicones were developed that a suitable material was found for the manufacture of flexible soft tissue prosthetic use. Frisch (1983) reviewed the technology of silicones and these form the basis of most urological prostheses and of many catheters.

Silicones are not entirely inert and Habal (1984) reviewed the clinical aspects of their use. Silicone particles may enter the bloodstream to cause granulomatous hepatitis or pancytopenia (Ellenbogen et al. 1975; Bommer and Ritz 1981) or lymphadenopathy (Travis et al. 1985). Such findings have not been observed after urological procedures.

The occurrence of neoplasia after the insertion of silicone has been described (Digby and Wells 1981) but is usually related to the development of breast cancer (Bowers and Radlauer 1969; de Cholnoky 1970; Johnson and Lloyd 1974; Zafiracopoulos and Rouskas 1974; Dalal et al. 1980). Such a relationship may be no more than happenstance.

Silicone prostheses are not rejected by the body and the major problem is the prevention of infection and it is for this reason that the topic merits a separate chapter. The pathobiology of infection in prosthetic devices was reviewed by Dougherty (1988) and all authors advocate the use of prophylactic antibiotics. The impregnation of a prosthesis with antibiotics (Olanoff et al. 1979) or antiseptics (Habal 1984) has not entered urological practice although the soaking of the prosthesis in antibiotics at the time of implantation is not uncommon.

It is interesting to read the chapter headings in an earlier book entitled Genitourinary Reconstruction and Prostheses (Wagenknecht et al.) which was published in 1981. This book contained the results of much experimental work and background information about the early development of ureteric stents and incontinence and penile prostheses. However ureteric, bladder and urethral prosthetic replacement remains experimental and has not passed into clinical usage. It is impossible to include everything and omissions occur not only as a result of developing practice but due to an overlap in practice. The use of transluminal balloon catheters is a good example of this. Some of these aspects are discussed in *Percutaneous and Interventional Urology* (Lang 1986). Balloon dilatation of the renal artery (Zeitler 1986) or occlusion of the testicular veins (Barth 1986) were included, as was balloon dilatation of ureteric strictures (Bigongiari 1986). Balloon dilatation for the prostate has received more recent interest (Burhenne et al. 1984; Gill et al. 1989; Dowd and Smith 1990) as have other non-operative techniques for treatment of benign prostatic obstruction.

The technological revolution has just begun to impinge upon urology and our clinical practice is likely to change even more in the next decade.

References

Barth KH (1986) Balloon embolization for the treatment of primary varicocele. In: Lang EK (ed) Percutaneous and interventional urology and radiology. Springer Verlag, Berlin, pp 211–216

Beheri GE (1966) Surgical treatment of impotence. J Plast Reconstr Surg 38:92–97

Bigongiari LR (1986) Transluminal dilatation of ureteric strictures. In: Lang EK (ed) Percutaneous and interventional urology and radiology. Springer Verlag, Berlin, pp 113–118

Bommer J, Ritz E (1981) Safety and silicone. Lancet 2:419

Bowers DG, Radlauer CB (1969) Breast cancer after prophylactic subcutaneous mastectomies and reconstruction with silastic prostheses. Plast Reconstr Surg 4: 541–544

Burhenne HJ, Chisolm RJ, Quenville NF (1984) Prostatic hyperplasia: radiologic intervention. Radiology 152:655–657

Dalal JJ, Winterbottam T, West RR, Henderson AH (1980) Implanted pacemakers and breast cancer. Lancet 2:311

de Cholnoky T (1970) Augmentation mammoplasty; survey of complications in 10,941 patients by 265 surgeons. Plast Reconstr Surg 45:573–577

Digby JM, Wells AL (1981) Malignant lymphoma with intranodal refractile particles after insertion of silicone prostheses. Lancet 2:580

Dougherty SH (1988) Pathobiology of infection in prosthetic devices. Rev Infect Dis 10:1102–1117

Dowd JB, Smith JJ (1990) Balloon dilatation of the prostate. Urol Clin North Am 15:671–677

Ellenbogen R, Ellenbogen R, Rubin L (1975) Injectable fluid silicone: human morbidity and mortality. JAMA 234:308–309

Frisch EE (1983) Technology of silicones in biomedical applications. In: Rubin L (ed) Biomaterials in reconstructive surgery. CV Mosby, St Louis, pp 73–91

Gill KP, Machan S, Allison DJ, Williams G (1989) Bladder outflow tract obstruction and urinary retention from benign prostatic hypertrophy treated by balloon dilatation. Br J Urol 64:618–622

Habal MG (1984) The biologic basis for the clinical application of the silicones. Arch Surg 119:843–848

Johnson M, Lloyd HED (1974) Bilateral breast cancer 10 years after an augmentation mammoplasty. Plast Reconstr Surg 53:88–90

Lang EK (ed) (1986) Percutaneous and interventional urology and radiology. Springer Verlag, Berlin

Olanoff LS, Anderson JM, Jones RD (1979) Sustained release of gentamicin from prosthetic heart valves. Trans Am Artif Intern Organs 25:334–338

Rubin LR, Bromberg BE, Walden RH (1971) Long term human reaction to synthetic plastics. Surg Gynec Obstet 132:603–608

Scales JT (1953) Tissue reactions to synthetic materials. Proc R Soc Med 46:647–652

Travis WD, Balogh K, Abraham JC (1985) Silicone granulomas. Hum Pathol 16: 19–27

Wagenknecht LV, Furlow WL, Auvert J (1981) Genitourinary reconstruction with prostheses. George Thieme Verlag, Stuttgart

Zafiracopoulos P, Rouskas A (1974) Breast cancer at site of implantation of pacemaker generator. Lancet 1:1114

Zeitler E (1986) Technique and results of percutaneous renal artery dilatation. In: Lang EK (ed) Percutaneous and interventional urology and radiology. Springer Verlag, Berlin, pp 233–249

Chapter 1

Open Nephrostomy

J.W.A. Ramsay

Introduction

The need for nephrostomy drainage at open surgery has significantly diminished since the advent of successful percutaneous techniques. However, there remain occasional indicators for nephrostomy drainage at open surgery and familiarity with this form of urinary diversion remains essential for every surgeon.

Long experience with various types of plastics in the urinary tract allows a sensible choice of materials, whilst specific designs of tube are indicated in different clinical situations.

Indications for Nephrostomy Drainage in Malignant Disease

To Do or Not To Do?

Central to this question is the wisdom of relieving ureteric obstruction in cancer patients. Most of the reviews of this subject have referred to longterm replacable loop nephrostomies rather than percutaneous drainage tubes which may suffice to drain the kidney during other therapy to relieve the cause of the obstruction. Although the percutaneous procedure is undeniably better tolerated in terms of morbidity and mortality, the real point at issue is whether life with a nephrostomy tube with little hope of survival beyond 6 months, even with therapy, is a reasonable proposition. The benefit of nephrostomy drainage in malignant obstructive uropathy is difficult to establish. The decision whether or not to operate involves emotional and moral issues. Often the patients are referred by colleagues with an unduly optimistic view of the natural history of the underlying pathology. However, comprehensive reviews of large numbers of patients have been reported.

Table 1.1.   Quality of life following nephrostomy

	No. of patients
Activity	
Full or mildly limited	9
Marked limitation	6
Invalid	3
Post-operative death	1
Pain	
No complaints	7
Relieved with analgesics	9
Severe, unrelieved	3

McNamara and Buktus (1980) reviewed the effect of nephrostomy on renal function and blood pressure in a group of patients with obstructive nephropathy due to non-urological malignant disease. They showed significant objective improvement in blood urea nitrogen (BUN), serum creatinine and blood pressure. They were only able to record a patient mean survival of 6.7 months following nephrostomy drainage.

Kohler et al. (1980) achieved some objectivity in assessing the quality of life after loop nephrostomy in patients with advanced pelvic malignancy. Twenty patients with a mean survival of 5.3 months following operation were placed in one of three categories: (1) never left hospital or went home to die: (2) went home but had limited activities and frequent readmissions: (3) went home with moderately limited activity or returned to full function. Complaints of post-operative pain were similarly grouped as shown in Table 1.1. The most important point to emerge from this survey was the not-unexpected inability of nephrostomy drainage to relieve the severe pain of malignant disease. Such pain may represent a contra-indication to nephrostomy. Despite these attempts at objectivity the authors reasonably concluded that individual assessment of each patient remains the basis on which the decision for urinary diversion by nephrostomy is made. Survival following nephrostomy may be related to the type of obstructing malignancy.

Fallon et al. (1980) reviewed a 10-year experience of 100 patients who underwent nephrostomy for invasive, incurable cancer. From the many statistics from this large survey two important points stand out. Patients with prostatic and cervical cancer generally fared better and this observation is supported by other series (Brun et al. 1975; Grabstald and McPhee 1973; Khan and Utz 1975). Patients for whom effective therapy was still available had a more favourable prognosis. This was particularly true of carcinoma of the prostate which responded to bilateral orchidectomy in 65% of those with obstructive uropathy. Interestingly, the age of the patients at the time of operation was not found to be a useful prognostic indicator.

In a further attempt to define the most satisfactory group of patients for nephrostomy diversion, Holden et al. (1979) reviewed 218 consecutive cases of open diversion with a minimum 4-year-period of follow up. These patients were divided into groups according to an arbitrary system of staging their disease according to its spread rather than to its organ of origin. Notable survival figures were only achieved in the Stage A patients, 88% of whom were alive 2 years following nephrostomy. This is a highly selected group which could only be segregated in such a large series, but it serves to highlight the importance of patient selection.

Another indicator for the usefulness of nephrostomy was described by Meyer et al. (1980) who found that in patients with cervical cancer an interval between diagnosis and ureteric obstruction of less than 2 years was associated with a poor post-nephrostomy survival of less than 6 months. However, these patients had all received definitive therapy before they were diverted.

Finally, the decision to perform nephrostomy may rely on factors which defy any form of clinical measurement. Some patients may desire or even require a short prolongation of life, even when availed of the inevitably short prognosis.

From these series it is possible to define a group of relatively favourable prognostic indicators for nephrostomy drainage in patients with malignant ureteric obstruction.

1. Malignant disease confined to the organ of origin
2. Untreated cancer of prostate or cervix
3. Planned further treatment of proven benefit

No specific comment has been made about transitional cell carcinoma of the bladder. In most series the results of nephrostomy drainage are extremely poor. However, the valid point was made by Ortlipp and Fraley (1982) that temporary urinary diversion may be of benefit in patients who respond favourably to nephrotoxic chemotherapeutic agents.

The placement of percutaneous palliative nephrostomy must represent considerable immediate advantage, but at the present time, there is no information about large series of cancer patients treated in this way. However, it can be predicted that operative mortality should be reduced and that morbidity in terms of sepsis, haemorrhage and prolonged ileus – often associated with the need for reoperation – should significantly improve. Holden et al. (1979) reported life-threatening complications of 45% and it is difficult to imagine that percutaneous nephrostomy could be associated with such a complication rate even in patients weakened by malignant disease. It is also reasonable to predict that an increasing number of cancer patients will be suitable for nephrostomy as the scope of cancer therapy extends. The only possible disadvantage of percutaneous nephrostomy in cancer patients is that it removes one element of selection, that is the ability to survive open surgery. Doubtless, the considerable preoperative mortality of open nephrostomy has deterred many from embarking on palliation in the most hopeless cases, but there now exists a means of diversion which can more frequently be performed in cases of malignant disease refractory to treatment.

The Role of Nephrostomy in Pyonephrosis

Albarran (1909) was the first to describe the treatment of pyonephrosis by preliminary nephrostomy and elective nephrectomy. More recent reports (Jimenez et al. 1978; Androulakakis 1982; Harrison 1983) advocate primary nephrectomy in up to 80% of cases with excellent results. The advent of radioisotope-imaging with ^{99m}Tc-DMSA has done much to help in the selection of kidneys whose function is beyond the point of recovery. In Harrison's (1983) series, most of the patients in the conservative group had complicated stone disease; nephrostomy was used to preserve as much renal function as possible in the post-operative phase. None of the patients thus managed subsequently required nephrectomy. Treatment by nephrostomy alone was reserved for those patients who were severely ill, or in those in whom the potential for recovery of function was thought to be dubious. When one kidney was deemed to be damaged beyond the point of recovery, primary nephrectomy was the procedure of choice. In cases of urolithiasis when kidney function was reasonable as delineated by depth of cortex on ultrasonography, DMSA scanning and urographic appearances, the treatment was by pyelolithotomy and nephrostomy.

Nephron preservation is of paramount importance. At present there are imperfections in the measurement of function in a diseased kidney and even more uncertainty about the prediction for the recovery of function. As technical skill in these areas improves, it is likely that more patients will be treated conservatively by initial nephrostomy drainage. Under these circumstances, percutaneous nephrostomy should be the procedure of first choice. The theoretical objection of blockage of small-calibre percutaneous nephrostomy tubes is already being overcome and the percutaneous placement of ring nephrostomy tubes has recently been described (Reddy and Smith 1982).

The Role of Nephrostomy in Ureteric Injury

The place of urinary diversion in ureteric repair has been a subject of intense debate and prodigious research since the classic paper on intubated ureterotomy by Davis in 1943. The history of the treatment of ureteric injury does much to explain the controversies which exist in this important area of reconstructive urology.

After the first report of ureteroureterostomy (Schopf 1886) the operation attracted much adverse comment. Despite early recognition of the concepts of proximal urinary diversion (Iselin 1928) and indwelling stents (Boari 1900) the results of ureteric surgery were generally poor. In 1929 Marion published a review of 84 cases of ureteric anastomoses: the conclusion was that "the operation was usually attended by stricture and hydronephrosis". It is unlikely that anastomotic techniques were solely to blame. Bovée (1897) described techniques of elliptical anastomosis designed to avoid stricture formation which are still in common use. A high rate of infection and the absence of suitable means of controlling it were probably largely responsible for earlier poor results of ureteric surgery. As recently as 1954, Moore advised against ureteroureterostomy as a stricture would be inevitable in the majority of the patients.

Proximal urinary diversion was the basis of Davis' work and this was the first paper to describe consistently acceptable results from ureteric surgery. Davis' clinical cases were well documented and the severity of the pathology successfully treated was impressive. He described the regeneration of a 12-cm length of upper ureter divided longitudinally for stricture such that two-thirds of its circumference could be applied to a T-tube. Extensive experimental work has since confirmed the propensity of the ureter to regenerate under suitable clinical circumstances. Weaver (1958) defined the limits of ureteric regeneration and his work constitutes the principles of repair upon which reconstructive attempts can be based.

1. Long segments of ureter will regenerate provided that a narrow strip of undisturbed ureteric wall remains; the process is complete at six weeks
2. Despite haphazard regeneration of smooth muscle, drainage from the kidney above the area of repair is usually adequate
3. Small calibre stents cause less periureteric fibrosis provided that they enhance drainage through the damaged segment

The exact nature of regeneration of ureteric smooth muscle remains obscure. Studies with radioactive-tritium-labelled thymidine in dogs (Ross et al. 1966) failed to confirm the apparent clinical capacity for the ureter to regenerate. Recent experimental studies in the pig (Dalley et al. 1976) suggested that smooth muscle hyperplasia was the principal means of repair in partial defects and that wound contracture alone did not account for the replacement of the length of the defect created. Attempts to assess ureteric repair by electomyographic means (Verreecken et al. 1975) reaffirmed that normal peristalsis across the anastomosis returned between the fourth and seventh post-operative week. Transverse anastomoses showed a delay in return to normality which occurred pari passu with smooth muscle regeneration. This basis of ureteric repair has not changed. Recent long series of ureteric injuries can now be studied to define the role of proximal urinary diversion in ureteric repair.

The potential for ureteric injury has increased over the past two decades. The advent of high velocity weapons in civil and military violence has significantly increased the understanding and treatment of soft tissue injury. Major retroperitoneal dissection for vascular reconstruction and the extirpation of massive tumour bulk has increased the risk of iatrogenic ureteric damage. The absolute need for nephron preservation in cases of ureteric damage associated with bilateral pathology – particularly calculous disease and retroperitoneal fibrosis – has caused a more conservative and exacting approach in cases which would previously have been treated by nephrectomy.

The indicators for urinary diversion either by stent or nephrostomy depend upon the degree of ureteric damage. In cases of post-operative trauma the decision is influenced by the nature of the pathology and by the interval between injury and diagnosis. If ureteric injury is evident within 48 h of otherwise uncomplicated surgery, there is a good case for immediate repair. However, if, as is often the case, diagnosis is delayed beyond 7 days or if sepsis, irradiation, or uraemia is complicating the injury, temporary diversion by nephrostomy or stent may be indicated (Zinman et al. 1978). Three means of diversion under these circumstances are possible. These are percutaneous nephrostomy, percutaneous antegrade insertion of a "double-J" or similar stent and retrograde insertion of double-J stent.

In cases of traumatic ureteric damage there is general agreement on the policies to be followed (Carlton et al. 1971; Parker 1971; Stutzman 1977). Where possible, a water-tight elliptical anastomosis must be achieved. This may be impossible where there is extensive damage such as occurs with high velocity missile injuries in which the degree of tissue disruption exceeds the macroscopic appearances of trauma. Adequate debridement of the remaining ureteric parts then results in an anastomosis under tension. In this situation proximal nephrostomy, including an indwelling stent to bridge the anastomosis, is suggested. These series have also revealed an absolute need for nephrostomy diversion in cases of multiple trauma involving other intra-abdominal organs, particularly pancreas, colon and major vessels.

Diversion is aimed at the avoidance of leakage at the anastomosis particularly in the presence of infection and contamination. In this context Turner Warwick (1976) has stressed the importance of a stent with multiple fenestrations to allow adequate drainage of exudate from the surrounding tissues and to minimise periureteric fibrosis. A Cummings tube is designed to bridge the ureteroplasty and drain the kidney in many series of upper ureteric reconstructions. Turner Warwick et al. (1967) strongly recommend the use of an omental wrap to support the repair of damaged ureters and this procedure is now well established (Turner Warwick 1976).

> I believe we can conclude that the splinting–no splinting debate will end as so many others have ended, that is, with the realisation that there was right on both sides (Davis 1958).

Nephrostomy in Open Renal Surgery

The indications for intrarenal drainage following open renal surgery depend upon the same principles of urothelial healing as previously described. The indications for nephrostomy drainage depend upon the continence of the pelvic and pelviureteric anastomosis and the state of the surrounding tissues. If drainage is the only way to achieve continence at the suture line, thus minimising perinephric and periureteric fibrosis, then it is the correct procedure. Occasionally it may be necessary to leave a nephrostomy tube in the kidney to allow further treatment with stone-dissolving solutions or to allow future percutaneous access to the kidney.

Pyeloplasty

There is much controversy over the use of intrarenal drainage and splints following dismembered pyeloplasty (Anderson and Hynes 1949). The trend is away from drainage. Thomas et al. (1982) reviewed 117 patients who underwent 135 pyeloplasties. Nephrostomy drainage was reserved for 35 kidneys whose anastomoses seemed compromised by oedema at the time of surgery.

Rickwood and Phadke (1978) commented that nephrostomy drainage seemed to be advantageous in children under 2 years of age. At the far end of the spectrum Persky et al. (1977) reported prolonged urinary drainage in only four of a series of 109 non-intubated, non-splinted Anderson–Hynes pyeloplasties. A small Cummings tube with multiple fenestrations is a popular design in this operation, but equally satisfactory is a small 6F or 8F "Neoplex" nephrosotomy tube of the type made by Porges, once again with multiple side-holes which can be fashioned at the time of positioning. A silicone nephrostomy tube, equipped with a maleable probe, after the design of Gil-Vernet is particularly useful following pyeloplasty.

After pyelocalycostomy (Turner Warwick 1968; Stephenson et al. 1976) which involves a long anastomosis, a small fenestrated nephrostomy tube lead into the upper ureter is a wise precaution. Ureterocalycostomy is an alternative to pyeloplasty when previous surgery, long-standing pelviureteric junction obstruction or stone disease have so damaged the pelvis and upper ureter that the use of the pelvis for anastomosis is impossible. As in pyelocalycostomy a long anastomosis in difficult conditions is best protected by nephrostomy tube drainage.

When ileal substitution of the ureter is indicated, a long, wide nephrostomy tube should pass through the full length of the ileal segment into the bladder. Partial nephrectomy for calculous disease would seem to have little prophylactic benefit (Rose and Fellows 1977). However, partial nephrectomy for tumour is advocated by Wickham (1975) and is clearly the operation of choice in those with solitary kidneys despite the two main complications of haemorrhage and urinary fistula. Should the ureter become obstructed by clot in the immediate post-operative period (Maddern 1967) the remaining nephron function is severely at risk. Adequate nephrostomy drainage is thus of great importance in this operation.

Calculous Disease

Open stone surgery is often complicated by distorted anatomy and infection. Under these circumstances the principles of urinary diversion and urothelial healing apply and the pyelotomy or nephrotomy can be protected by a nephrostomy. Despite many recent advances in open stone surgery, particularly those of inosine perfusion and external cooling (Wickham et al. 1974) fragments of calculi are either impossible to remove or are inadvertently left behind. The object of any operation for renal lithiasis must be to rid the kidney of all calculi, as is supported by Williams' (1963) large survey which showed that 47% of those with retained stones required further operation. For this reason chemolysis via a large nephrostomy tube has found favour in recent years (Table 1.2). The most satisfactory agent, a 10% solution of hemiacidrin (marketed as Renacidin) is not universally accepted as being entirely safe. Since Mulvaney (1959) introduced this solvent, several hazards of its use have been described. Urothelial ulceration (Cunningham et al. 1973) and hypermagnesaemia (Cato and Tulloch 1974) seem to be infrequent and are reversible. However, infection and obstruction are difficult to avoid. Renacidin is effective in dissolving struvite stones (Blaivis et al. 1975) but its use is restricted in the USA for "therapy or preventative therapy above the ureterovesical junction". Stamey and Nemoy (1971) described useful guidelines for the use of Renacidin as a nephrostomy irrigant. A post-operative nephrostogram should indicate free flow of contrast without extravasation before commencing irrigation. The patient should be afebrile and the urine from the bladder and kidney would be sterile. Back pain during infusion may indicate obstruction, extravasation or infection and irrigation should be discontinued. When this policy was followed

Table 1.2. Solutions for chemolysis of renal calculi

Stone	Solution	pH	Composition
Triple phosphate	Renacidin	3.6	10% soln of gluconic and citric acid
Uric acid	Sodium bicarbonate	8.5	132 Meq sodium bicarbonate per 1.5 l of normal saline

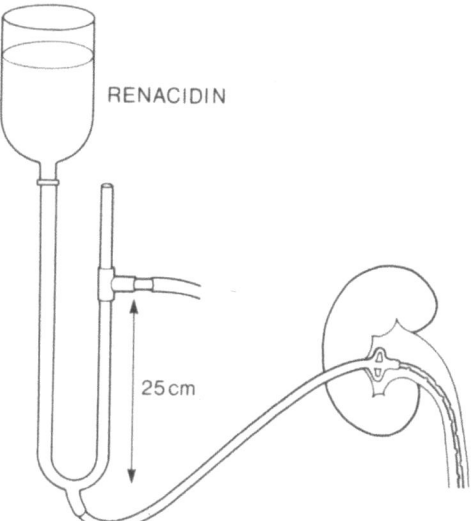

Fig. 1.1. Irrigating system via nephrostomy.

by Blaivas (1975) for 10 post-operative days in a series of 10 patients, a 75% stone dissolution rate was achieved. Several methods for irrigation have been described but safety depends upon a secure nephrostomy tube and a healed collecting system. If a straight nephrostomy tube of Foley or Malecot design is to be used, an irrigating system as shown in Fig. 1.1 (after Blaivas 1975) is desirable. The manometer allows decompression to occur when intrapelvic pressure exceeds that exerted by a 25-cm column of irrigant. However, the Foley balloon may cause obstruction and uneven irrigation of the pelvis. A loop nephrostomy used for irrigation has the advantage of providing continuous decompression of the renal pelvis with little risk of obstruction. The problem of partial displacement with consequent perinephric extravasation is illustrated in Fig. 1.2. This risk of displacement is difficult to overcome by secure skin fixation alone; there are many descriptions of methods of anchoring the centre of the loop in the renal pelvis. Gillenwater (1977) records the use of a Cummings tube as a loop nephrostomy (Fig. 1.3). The mushroom serves to prevent the fenestrated part of the tube slipping into the perinephric tissues. Finney and Sharpe (1977) introduced a silastic loop nephrostomy tube through a Foley catheter so that the Foley balloon would prevent displacement. The most sensible design of irrigating nephrostomy tube has been introduced for percutaneous use by Hare and McOmish (1982). It consists of a loosely fit-

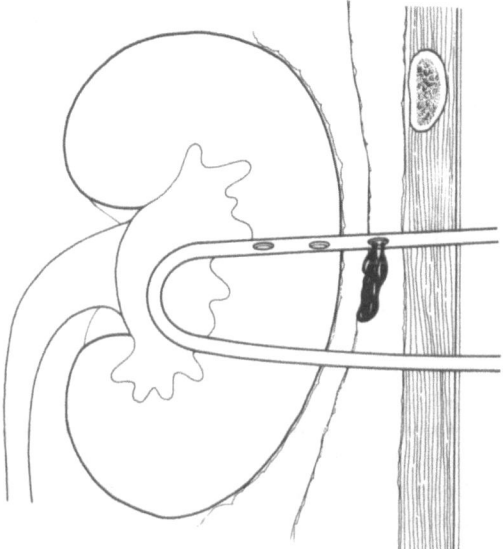

Fig. 1.2. Extravasation from displaced loop nephrostomy.

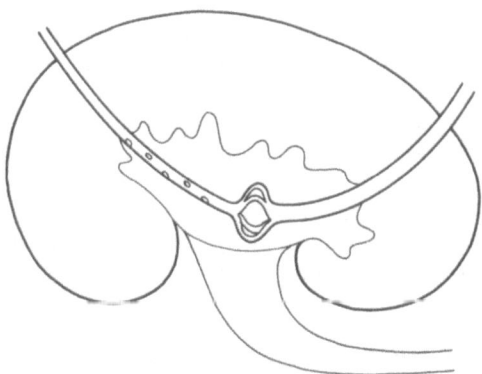

Fig. 1.3. Cumming's tube loop nephrostomy.

ting coaxial arrangement of an outer 14F-PTFE sheath with an inner 8.3F polythene pigtail catheter. The advantage of the dirigable pigtail is that it can be closely placed to a stone within a calyx and thus deliver the chemolytic agent in the most effective way. Synchronous drainage during irrigation is achieved by the gap between the two catheters and this protects against an increase in intrapelvic pressure.

The technique of extracorporeal shock-wave lithotripsy (ESWL) either alone or in combination with percutaneous surgery has reduced the incidence of open surgical procedures which previously required longterm nephrostomy drainage. However, there still remains a hard core of complicated cases requiring open surgery, drainage and occasional irrigation. Cases requiring a combination of percutaneous and extracorporeal stone treatment may also require prolonged nephrostomy drainage to protect the kidney from obstruction and to aid the passage of stone fragments. Recent research has shown that most nephrostomy tubes are not destroyed by ESWL (McNicholas et al. 1986)

Materials and Designs of Nephrostomy Tubes

The following polymers are available in configurations suitable for nephrostomy drains: polyethylene, polyurethrane, polyvinyl chloride, polyamide (nylon), polydimethylsiloxane (silicone), latex rubber.

Polyethylene, polyurethrane and polyamide tend to be more rigid and have achieved popularity for percutaneous use. Polyvinyl chloride is more flexible, and is available in several formulations both as nephrostomy tubes and ureteric splints. The silicone rubbers have been used both as coatings for urological prostheses and for the complete moulding of many different designs of tubing. Latex rubber has been implicated in urethral stricture formation, (Graham et al. 1983) and there have been suggestions that plasticisers used in the manufacture of latex have leached from the tubing to a variable extent (Wilksch et al. 1983). Correlation of direct cell cytotoxicity and the occurrence of clinical stricturing has not been definitive.

Although there is at present no clinical evidence of upper tract stricturing consequent on the use of potentially cytotoxic prostheses, Drake (1962) found that rubber prostheses induced more ureteric fibrosis in an experimental model. When Ramsay et al. (1985) compared various upper urinary tract prostheses in experimental surgery, they found that the urothelium of the ureter underwent a form of metaplasia with mucous production which progressed in a similar manner for polyethylene, polyurethrane and silicone tubes. This phenonmenon has been confirmed in clinical practice, but the relationship of these histological changes to the longterm healing of the upper urinary tract is the subject of continuing research.

In considering biomaterials for use in the urinary tract the usual concept of biocompatibility must be extended. For most implanted surgical devices, biocompatibility infers minimal local or general tissue reaction throughout the requisite period of implantation. For nonbiodegradable prostheses, the practical consideration is the effect of the graft on the host tissue which can be assessed by the degree of the acute and/or chronic inflammatory process in the tissues surrounding the implant. In the urinary tract three further considerations are of importance:

1. The effect of urine on the implant (Degradation: Fragility)
2. The effect of the implant on urine (Encrustation)
3. The effect of the implant on epithelial surfaces

It is only with the recent use of longterm, indwelling upper urinary tract prostheses that these particular features have become more relevant.

An ideal nephrostomy tube must possess physical and chemical properties resulting in: (1) high biotolerance, (2) no biodegradation, (3) ease of placement, (4) ease of removal, and (5) adequate and prolonged drainage capacity. These features rely upon the basic structure of a polymer, but particularly on the subsequent chemical and physical treatment of that polymer. By way of example, the handling properties and biocompatability of two different polymers, polyurethane and polyvinylchloride, can be rendered almost indistinguishable by various manufacturing processes. Because such polymers are sold by trade name, the user cannot easily relate any chemical difference to the type of polymer that he is handling.

In conclusion, polyethylene, polyvinyl chloride, and polyurethrane are suitable for kidney drainage post-operatively. Silicone tubes should be used for longer periods or when infection is likely. Encrustation of nephrostomy tubes is to be avoided; the use of antibiotics and urinary antiseptics may help to reduce this phenomenon. Loop nephrostomies are easier to change should encrustation and infection supervene but percutaneous placement of straight nephrostomy tubes is reducing the need for exchangeable devices.

The various patterns of nephrostomy tubing are illustrated in Fig. 1.4. The simplest polyvinylchloride for general use is manufactured without fenestrations or tapes and can be cut to the appropriate shape and length. Foley and Malecot designs have the advantage of being self-retaining, with the proviso that the Foley balloon may actually impair proper drainage from a small pelvis. In the past, loop nephrostomies have been adapted from all kinds of silicone-coated tubes, abdominal drains and dialysis tubing. It is probably best to choose an appropriate diameter from the range of level non-fenestrated tubes and fashion an appropriate number of side holes to fit the renal pelvis and allow some leeway for slipping and displacement. Some tubes are supplied with a radio-opaque filament which allows easier visualisation should displacement

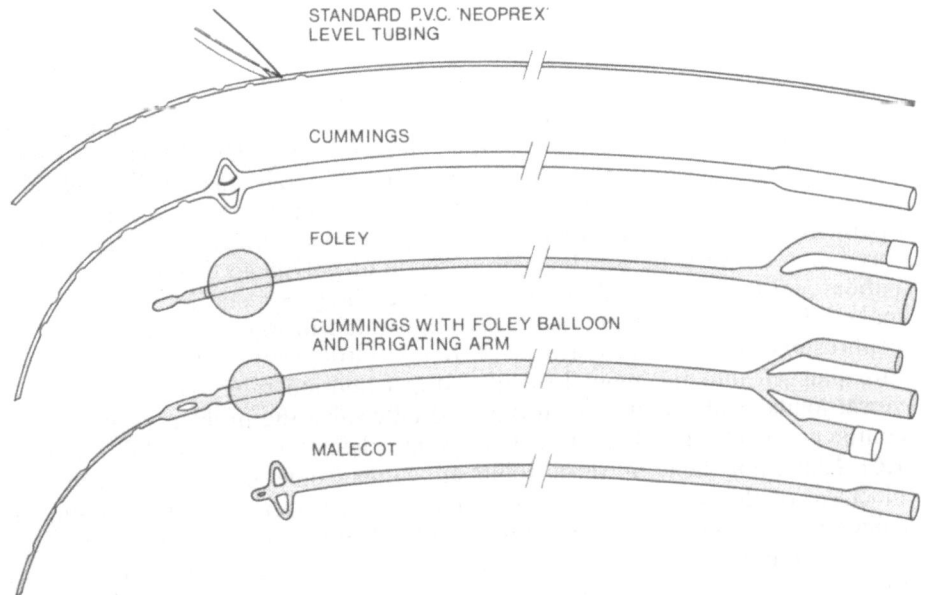

STANDARD P.V.C. 'NEOPREX'
LEVEL TUBING

CUMMINGS

FOLEY

CUMMINGS WITH FOLEY BALLOON
AND IRRIGATING ARM

MALECOT

Fig. 1.4. Patterns of nephrostomy tubes.

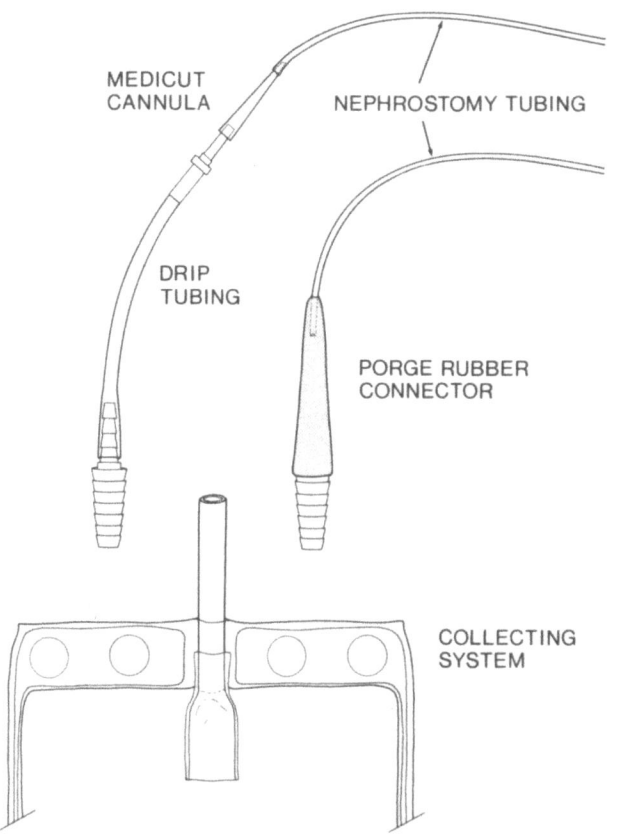

MEDICUT
CANNULA   NEPHROSTOMY TUBING

DRIP
TUBING

PORGE RUBBER
CONNECTOR

COLLECTING
SYSTEM

Fig. 1.5. Methods of connecting nephrostomy tubes to drainage systems.

occur. In practice a nephrostogram will be necessary to define displacement and extravasation. The Cummings tube, incorporating the self-retaining features of the malecot with a fenestrated and fine tapering tail is ideal for nephrostomy drainage following complicated pyelolithotomy or reconstructive operation. A problem common to all nephrostomy drains is an unsatisfactory union between the small-calibre silicone or polythene emerging from the patient and the larger-calibre tubing of the drainage system. Most often some makeshift device has to be employed. Illustrated in Fig. 1.5 is an 8F Porge nephrostomy tube connected to a shortened intravenous cannula which is in turn plugged into the inner lock of a drip extension tube. The various universal joints available at present only partially solve the problem of providing continence between tubes of such disparate diameters and flexibilities (Fig. 1.6). Rigid, polythene universal joints are cumbersome and cause kinking and blockage of the nephrostomy tube if not properly secured to the patient or splinted. The more flexible soft joints – rather like the end of a latex catheter – are not entirely leak-proof (Fig. 1.5). Careful arrangement and care of these tubes is necessary to prevent the extravasation and complications which they were designed to avoid.

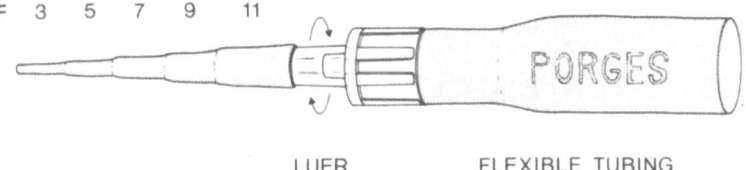

F   3   5   7   9   11

LUER   FLEXIBLE TUBING

Fig. 1.6. Adaptable nephrostomy tube connector.

The Technique of Nephrostomy Tube Placement at Open Surgery

If performed as a definitive procedure a formal exposure of the kidney e.g., the twelfth rib incision or lumbotomy will be required. For the correct positioning of a loop nephrostomy full mobilisation of the kidney is necessary to allow proper access to the upper and lower poles. The temptation to introduce any tube through a nephrostomy is to be avoided. The first step is to open the renal pelvis between stay sutures and select a suitable calyx through which to introduce the tube. Most descriptions, including Tresidder's (1957) original paper on loop nephrostomy, involve the passage of a forceps through the cortex from within an upper or lower pole calyx. The forceps then have to be opened to grasp the tube and drag it back through the renal substance into the pelvis. For a loop nephrostomy the procedure is repeated and a second tube is drawn into the pelvis, sutured to the end of the first, which is thus extracted from the kidney to complete the loop. These manoeuvres are awkward, damaging to renal tissue and can provoke considerable haemorrhage. Trauma to the kidney can be reduced by using a blunt-ended malleable probe which can be directed precisely through the cortex from within a calyx. The nephrostomy tube can be made to fit snugly to the end of the probe and is thus drawn into position rather as a suction drain introducer is used. Such an instrument has been devised by Gil-Vernet and is marketed by Porges (Fig. 1.7). The nephrostomy tube that fits the probe is equipped with a specially pliable distal segment which, while gripping the introducer, does not form a damaging ridge which would traumatise the kidney as the instrument is pulled through the cortex. The tubing is made of pure silicone and is supplied with multiple fenestrations.

Other descriptions (McLoughlin and Jeffs 1977) are derived from the same principle but employ the standard silver malleable sinus probe with a flattened end, equipped with a small hole. The drainage end of the chosen nephrostomy tube can be tapered and the eye of the probe stitched to it, so that the device presents an elliptical profile for atraumatic traction through the kidney. Kim and Fjeldborg (1975) have used a uterine sound in a similar manner. Tunner (1973) described a malleable sound which could be directed through the calyx allowing a malecot catheter to be drawn into the kidney from without. In summary, the ideal introducer should be maleable, of variable diameter and allow attachment of the drainage end of a nephrostomy tube so that it can be drawn through the kidney from within outwards. Gil-Vernet's instrument conforms to these requirements and is currently available.

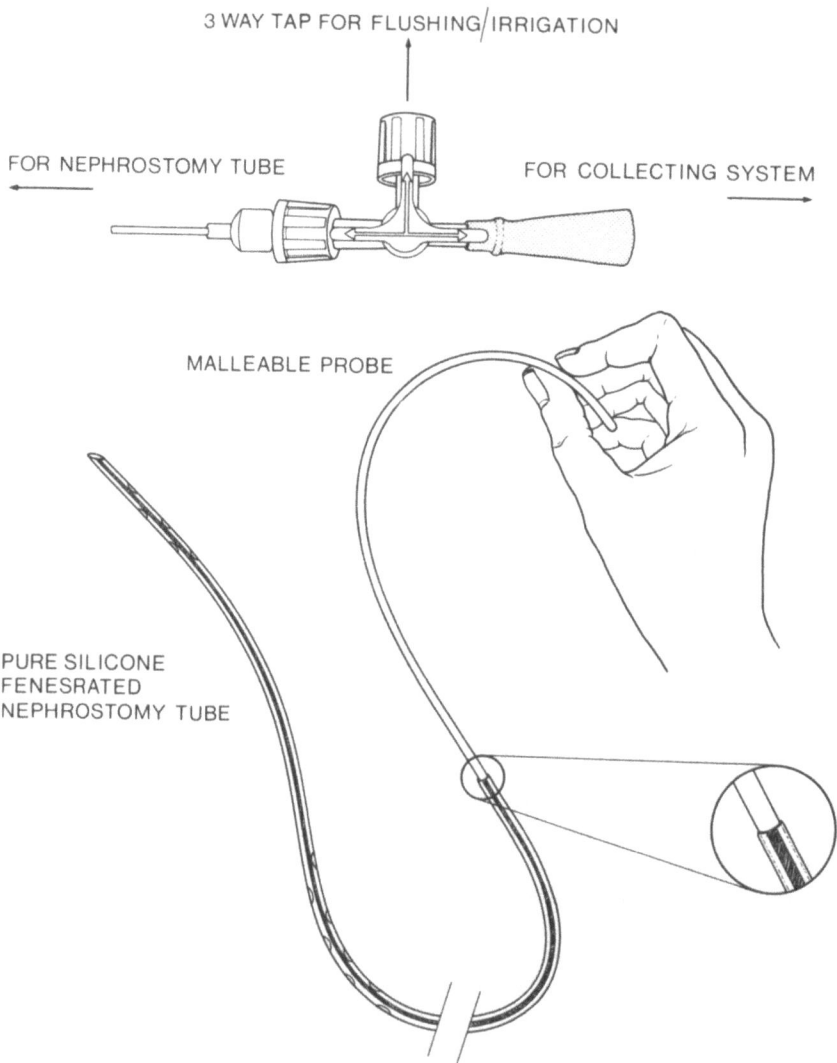

3 WAY TAP FOR FLUSHING/IRRIGATION

FOR NEPHROSTOMY TUBE

FOR COLLECTING SYSTEM

MALLEABLE PROBE

PURE SILICONE
FENESRATED
NEPHROSTOMY TUBE

Fig. 1.7. Nephrostomy tube introducer (Gil-Vernet).

Complications of Open Nephrostomy

Holden et al. (1979) reported a 45% incidence of life-threatening complications following open nephrostomy (Table 1.3). Though this figure is higher than might be expected, careful placement of the tube with atraumatic instruments will significantly reduce the risk of haemorrhage. Alagaratnam and Leong (1975) report a case of false aneurysm of the kidney following nephrostomy; they comment that incision of the renal cortex and introduction of the malecot catheter from without inwards may have been responsible for this complica-

Table 1.3. Complications of open nephrostomy

Haemorrhage (pseudo-aneurysm)
Infection (septicaemia)
Encrustation (stone formation)
Blockage
Extravasation
Displacement
Anaesthetic risk

tion. As a guideline for the treatment of continued bleeding following percutaneous nephrostomy, Cope and Zeit (1982) advised irrigation of the nephrostomy
tube with cold saline as a preliminary measure. If the bleeding continues for
4 days, immediate angiography with a view to selective embolisation was
recommended.

Displacement may be a problem in ring nephrostomies when irrigation is in
progress. The infusion should be discontinued and a nephrostogram performed. It should be possible to resite or replace the tube under X-ray control.
Blockage of nephrostomy tubes is a not-infrequent occurrence. Often the
method of joining the tubing is to blame and this should be inspected first.
Other causes of obstruction such as blood clot or pus can usually be irrigated
away. If a nephrostomy tube suddenly ceases to drain in the early post-operative
phase, a nephrostogram may reveal extravasation and, depending upon the
clinical situation and the original pathology, re-exploration may be necessary.

Infection and encrustation have been reduced by the use of silicone-coated
tubes and antibiotics. It should be possible to continue nephrostomy drainage
for months or years without significant encrustation. Infection may still be
difficult to eliminate in the presence of residual stones and any manipulation of
the tube should be covered by antibiotics appropriate to the bladder and
nephrostomy urine cultures.

Conclusion

"Permanent nephrostomy is an affliction seldom offered to any patient today"
(Blandy 1978). Even with the enormous advantages of percutaneous techniques this statement is still true. Nephrostomy should, therefore, be viewed as
a temporary procedure for use as an adjunct to conservative surgery or while
further therapy resolves the obstructing lesion. Although the indicators for all
forms of open nephrostomy have diminished, it remains an invaluable option
for the difficult case or where there are limitations in available resources.
Advances in technology have been described and there will doubtless be many
more in the wake of the advances in percutaneous surgery.

References

Alagaratnam TT, Leong CH (1975) An iatrogenic complication of nephrostomy. J Urol 113: 286–287

Albarran J (1909) Medecine operatoires des voies urinaires. Masson, Paris, p 171

Anderson JC, Hynes W (1949) Retrocaval ureter. A case diagnosed preoperatively and treated successfully by a plastic operation. Br J Urol 21:209–213

Androulakakis PA (1982) Pyonephrosis: a critical review of 131 cases. Br J Urol 54:89–92

Blaivas JG, Pais VM, Spellman RM (1975) Chemolysis of residual stone fragments after extensive surgery for staghorn calculi. Urology 6:680–686

Blandy JP (1978) Operative urology. Blackwell, London

Boari A (1990) Chirugia dell' ureter XIV. Roma

Bovée JW (1897) Uretero-ureteral anastomosis. Ann Surg 25:52–79

Brun EN, Schiff MJ, Weiss RM (1975) Palliative urinary diversion for pelvic malignancy. J Urol 113:619–622

Carlton CE, Scott R, Guthrie AG (1971) The initial management of ureteral infections: a report of 78 cases. J Urol 105:335–340

Cato AR, Tulloch AGS (1974) Hypermagnesaemia in a uraemic patient during renal pelvis irrigation with Renacidin. Urology 3:312–313

Cope C, Zeit RM (1982) Pseudonaneurysms after nephrostomy. Am J Radiol 139:255–261

Cunningham JJ, Friedland GW, Stamey TA (1973). Radiological changes in the urothelium during Renacidin irrigation. J Urol 109:556–558

Dalley BK, Bartone FF, Gardner PJ (1976) Smooth muscle regeneration in swine ureters. Invest Urol 14:104–110

Davis DM (1943) Intubated ureterotomy. Surg Gynecol Obstet 76:513–523

Davis DM (1958) The process of ureteral repair; a recapitulation of the splinting question. J Urol 79:215–223

Drake WM, Carroll J, Bartone F, Caltone RN, Kazal HL, Sumerai S, Felter TR (1962) Evaluation of materials used as ureteral splints. Surg Gynecol Obstet 114:47–51

Fallon B, Olney L, Culp DA (1980) Nephrostomy in cancer patients: To do or not to do? Br J Urol 52:237–242

Finney RP, Sharpe JR (1977) Loop nephrostomy with the Cummings catheter. J Urol 117:641–642

Gillenwater JI (1977) Loop nephrostomy with the Cummings catheter. J Urol 117:641–642

Grabstald H, McPhee M (1973) Nephrostomy and the cancer patient. South Med J 66:217–220

Graham DT, Mark GE, Pomery AR (1983) Cellular toxicity of urinary catheters. Med J Aust 1:456–459

Hare WSC, McOmish D (1982) Nephrostomy lavage set for dissolving renal stones. Radiology 144:932

Harrison GSM (1983) The management of pyonephrosis. Ann R Coll Surg Eng 65:126–127

Holden S, McPhee M, Grabstald H (1979) The rationale of urinary diversion in cancer patients. J Urol 121:19–24

Iselin M (1928) Recherches experimentales sur. la suture de l'uretere. Bulletin et memoures Societe Nationale de Chirugerie 54:650–667

Jimenez JF, Lopez Pacios MA, Llamazares G, Gonejero J, Sole Bacellas F (1978) The treatment of pyonephrosis: a comparative study. J Urol 120:287–289

Khan AU, Utz DC (1975) An easy and safe technique for nephrostomy. Surg Gynecol Obstet 141:95

Kim C, Fjeldborg OC (1975) An easy and safe technique for nephrostomy. Surg Gynecol Obstet 141:95

Kohler JP, Lyon ES, Schoenberg HW (1980) Reassessment of circle tube nephrostomy in advanced pelvic malignancy. J Urol 123:17–18

McLoughlin GC (1977) Nephrostomy. Br J Urol 29:130–134

McLoughlin MG, Jeffs RD (1977) Safe placement of nephrostomy tube. Urology 9:184

McNamara TE, Buktus DE (1980) Nephrostomy in patients with ureteral obstruction secondary to non urologic malignancy. Arch Int Med 140:494–497

McNicholas TA, Ramsay JWA, Crocker PR, Wett DR, Wickham JEA (1986) The effects of extracorporeal shock ware lithotropsy in urological prostheses and endoprostheses. Urol Res 14:309–313

Maddern JP (1967) Surgery of the staghorn calculus. Br J Urol 39:237–275

Marion H (1929) Etude eritique et experimentale des plaies transvessales de l'uretere. Deductions chirugicales et therapeutiques. J Urol Nephrol 27:273, 369

Meyer JE, Green TH Jr, Yatsubashi M (1980) Palliative urinary diversion in carcinoma of cervix. Obstet Gynecol 55:95–98

Moore TD (1954) Surgery of the ureter. In: Campbell M (ed) Urology. WB Saunders and Co, Philadelphia, pp 1843–1889

Mulvaney WP (1959) A new solvent for certain urinary calculi. A preliminary report. J Urol 82:546–548

Ortlipp SA, Fraley EE (1982) Indications for palliative urinary diversion in patients with cancer. Urol Clin North Am 9:79–83

Parker JM (1971) Re emphasising the importance of urinary tract diversion and splinting in injuries of the upper third of the ureter. J Urol 106:368–370

Persky L, Krausse JR, Boltuck RL (1977) Initial complications and late results dismembered pyeloplasty. J Urol 118:162–165

Ramsay JWA, Payne SR, Gosling PT, Whirfield HN, Wickham JEP, Levison DA (1985) The effects of Double J stenting on unobstructed ureters. An experimental and clinical study. Br J Urol 57:630–634

Reddy P, Smith AD (1982) Circle tube nephrostomy and nephroureterostomy. Urol Clin North Am 9:69–73

Rickwood AMK, Phadke D (1978) Pyeloplasty in infants and children with particular reference to the method of drainage post operatively. Br J Urol 50:217–221

Rose OA, Fellows OJ (1977) Partial nephrostomy for stone disease. Br J Urol 49:605–610

Ross G, Thompson IM, Bynum WR, Thompson EP (1966) The role of smooth muscle and regeneration in urinary tract repair. J Urol 95:541–548

Schopf F (1886) Untra ligamentare orariencyste ovariotomie. Durchtrenning des ureters unol vereiningung durch die naht. Allg Wien Med Ztg 31:374–380

Stamey TA, Nemoy NJ (1971) Surgical, bacteriological and biochemical management of infection stones. JAMA 215:1470–1476

Stephenson TP, Bauer S, Hargreave TB, Turner Warwick RT (1976) The technique and results of pyelocalycostomy for staghorn calculi. Br J Urol 47:751–758

Stutzman RE (1977) Ballistics and the management of ureteral injuries from high velocity missiles. J Urol 118:947–949

Thomas DFM, Agrawal M, Laidin Az, Eckstein HB (1982) Pelviureteric obstruction in infancy and childhood. A review of 117 patients. Br J Urol 54:204–208

Tunner WS (1973) A malleable nephrostomy sound and a technique for its use. J Urol 109: 775–776

Turner Warwick RT, Wynne EJC, Handley Ashken M (1967) The use of omental pedicle graft in repair and reconstruction of the urinary tract. Br J Surg 54:849–853

Turner Warwick RT (1968) Renal calculi. Diagnosis and management. Br J Urol 47:17–24

Turner Warwick RT (1976) The use of omental pedicle graft in urinary tract reconstruction. J Urol 116:341–347

Tressidder GC (1957) Nephrostomy. Br J Urol 29:130–134

Vereecken RL, De Jaegher K, Van Damme B (1975) Urinary transport in transected and reanastomosed ureters of dogs. Acta Urol Belg 43:282–291

Weaver RG (1958) Ureteral regeneration: experimental and clinical. Part III. J Urol 79:31–40

Wickham JEA, Coe N, Ward JP (1974) One hundred cases of nephrolithotomy under hypothermia. J Urol 112:701–705

Wickham JEA (1975) Conservative renal surgery for adenocarcinoma: the place of bench surgery. Br J Urol 47:25–36

Wilksch J, Vernon-Roberts B, Garrett R, Smith K (1983) The role of catheter surface morphology and extractable cytotoxic material in tissue reactions to ureteral catheters. Br J Urol 55:48–52

Williams RE (1963) Long term survey of 538 patients with upper urinary tract stones. Br J Urol 35:416–425

Zinman LM, Libertino JA, Roth RA (1978) Management of operative ureteral injury. Urology 12:290–303

Chapter 2

Percutaneous Nephrostomy

R.A. Miller

Introduction

The indications for open nephrostomy have been discussed in the previous section. While there will always be a need for nephrostomy tubes following open renal surgical procedures, there is no doubt that percutaneous placement has superseded "open" placement of such tubes in almost every other situation. The percutaneous placement of nephrostomy tubes does, however, require special radiological expertise and equipment which is not available in every centre. In this chapter I shall describe the technique of placement, the equipment available and the possibilities that such access provides.

The requirement for antegrade renal access is now so fundamental to urology that in many centres it is the urologist himself who performs the procedure. Whether the technique is performed by the radiologist or urologist is of little consequence. It is, however, essential that the two disciplines work in close cooperation, especially if complex theraputic procedures such as nephrolithotomy are contemplated. The urologist embarking on percutaneous placement of nephrostomy tubes will have a great deal to learn from his radiological colleagues and in particular will have to become aware of the risks of radiation exposure, especially to the eyes and hands.

Anatomical Considerations

A firm understanding of dynamic renal anatomy is fundamental to success in all percutaneous renal procedures (Miller 1983a). The kidneys are highly mobile. Not only do they move with respiration (amplitude 3–6 cm) but they also move in the anteroposterior plane. Renal movements are accentuated by general anaesthesia as a result of abdominal wall relaxation. The control of respiration either by verbal command or by cessation of respiration during anaesthesia is thus of extreme importance.

There are three possible positions for percutaneous access. Prone (Bartley et al. 1965), prone oblique (Kellett et al. 1983) and anterior ipsilateral oblique

(Barbaric and Wood 1977). Of these we prefer the prone oblique position. A bolster is wedged between the hypochondrium and the iliac fossa of the side which is to be punctured and the X-ray table. Pressure from the padding pushes the convex lateral border of the kidney posteriorly and limits the degree of movement of that organ. The posterior calyces are thus presented for direct puncture.

The site of puncture is usually below the 12th rib and lies in a triangle with the following borders: superiorly the 12th rib, medially the lateral border of the erector spinae muscle group and finally inferiorly a horizontal line 5–8 cm below the 12th rib which meets the tip of the 12th rib laterally.

The pleura dips below the 12th rib at the point where the lateral border of the erector spinae crosses the 12th rib. Supra 12 punctures are thus hazardous, but providing the track remains lateral to this point, can be performed with reasonable safety and provide good access to the middle and superior calyces in selected cases.

The lower calyces lie below the 12th rib in 75%–80% of the cases. They are thus often the only available calyceal group which can be reached via an infra 12 puncture using a vertical approach with vertical beam fluoroscopy. Access to the middle calyx, which is desirable if ureteric instrumentation is contemplated or when calculi are present in that location, either requires upward angulation of the needle or a supra 12 lateral approach.

The lateral borders of the kidneys are related to the liver, spleen and colon. Anteriorly the kidney is intimately related to the intra-abdominal viscera, especially the duodenum and colon. The depth to which needles are pushed is thus critical, as it is very easy to advance a needle too far anteriorly and thus perforate the colon or duodenum. Lateral puncture has a tendency to endanger the colon (Fernstrom 1983).

The kidney itself lies in a fascial envelope, the fascia of Gerota, and is surrounded by perirenal fat. It possesses a true connective tissue capsule which is richly innervated. Puncture of the capsule or dilatation causes pain which is conveyed via the coeliac plexus and the lesser splanchnic nerves to T10–T12.

The collecting system of the kidney is notoriously variable. The pelvis may be intra- or extra-renal. There are usually three calyceal groups, upper, middle and lower. These have minor calyces disposed in the anterior and posterior planes, the polar calyces usually having a third minor calyx pointing towards the upper and lower poles respectively. The posterior calyces are disposed at 60°–70° to the coronal plane and thus usually lie in a straight line corresponding to Brödel's plane of avascularity. On a radiograph these calyces are seen end on and lie medial to their anterior counterparts.

The segmental arrangement of the renal arteries is well known (Graves 1954). Of particular importance is that the lower pole of the kidney (the most frequent site of puncture) is supplied solely by the lower segmental branch of the anterior division of the renal artery. Damage to this vessel will result in a segmental infarct. The calyceal necks are surrounded by a dense venous plexus which is frequently the cause of bleeding during percutaneous manipulations. The intercalyceal spaces contain major vascular tributaries and are to be avoided if at all possible. Direct end-on puncture of the calyceal infundibulum is optimal from the point of view of bleeding.

Direct puncture of the pelvis, pyelostomy, would theoretically seem to be ideal as it avoids the risk of haemorrhage and structural renal damage. Experience, however, has shown that nephropyelostomy is to be preferred as the transparenchymal passage of the track stabilises the nephrostomy tubes, seals the track when the tube is withdrawn and greatly facilitates endoscopic manoeuvres should these be required.

Anaesthesia

Needle puncture of the collecting system can usually be achieved with local anaesthesia (2% lignocaine) and in the case of excessively nervous patients, intravenous Midazolam and pethidine. An intramuscular premedication with the latter agents is highly desirable. We recommend antibiotic cover with an intravenous aminoglycoside at the time of puncture to obviate the likelihood of gram-negative septicaemia.

Dilatation of tracks beyond 12F becomes extremely uncomfortable, and heavy intravenous sedation is usually required for tracks in the region of 26–30F. Under such circumstances we find neurolept anaesthesia useful. An initial premedication of oral lorazepam, and droperidol together with intramuscular gentamicin is followed by intravenous droperidol and phenoperidine administered during the actual manipulation. General anaesthesia is useful for children and is ideal for one-stage percutaneous nephrolithotomy. It is important that the intravenous fluids are somewhat restricted immediately prior to puncture of the collecting system or there will be inadequate opacification of the calyces, the dye being washed out by the intravenous fluid load.

Needle Puncture

This is the most critical part of the procedure. Several factors should be taken into consideration: the track should be straight and direct, the proposed exit site for the nephrostomy tube should be placed in such a manner that the patient can lie comfortably in the supine position without occluding drainage and the point of renal entry, optimal for any therapeutic manoeuvres (stone manipulation etc.). We use undercouch screening on a standard Siemen's angiographic X-ray table. Such a table will expose the operator to the minimum amount of radiation. Biplanar fluoroscopy is helpful when available. A standard C-arm which is commonly available in the operating theatre may also be used to good effect and has the advantage of being able to provide biplanar information. A freeze-frame facility on X-ray equipment is very useful. High-resolution fluoroscopy is essential in order to provide sufficient information to allow accurate puncture of selected calyces for therapeutic access. In many centres ultrasonic scanning (Baron et al. 1981, Pederson et al. 1976, Saitoh et al. 1979) is used as an adjunct to fluoroscopy or in some cases has totally replaced fluoroscopy. This has the advantage that there is no risk of irradiation (particularly in pregnancy) and it is ideal when renal opacification is not possible (severe obstruction, renal failure). There is, however, little doubt that fluoroscopy provides greater resolution and is a more familiar modality to the majority of clinicians. Ultrasound is particularly useful in very dilated systems. There are a number of different ways in which ultrasound may be used. It can simply be used to determine the exact depth of the pelvi-calyceal system. It may be used prior to fluoroscopy to determine a direct path to the collecting system. The skin can then be marked and needle puncture be performed under X-ray control. Alternatively, a real-time ultrasound scanner with a biopsy attachment may be used to puncture the collecting system under ultrasound control alone. Using such a system the needle either passes through the centre of the transducer or is passed through the ultrasonic beam at an angle. A fine 22-gauge needle can be used for such a procedure. The collecting system once breached can then be opacified with dilute contrast medium. The use of the larger 18-gauge needles and ultrasonic guidance requires considerable expertise and cannot be recommended for those embarking on such a procedure for the first time. Computed axial tomography (CT) (Haga et al. 1977) is of little importance to needle puncture as it is expensive and time-consuming. However, it can play a vital role in nephrostomy for stone removal. Not only can complications such as haematomata and fluid collections be rapidly identified but non-opaque calculi can also often be visualised. The CT scanner may also be used to determine the exact position of a stone relative the nephrostomy tube in difficult cases where the anteroposterior orientation of the calyces is difficult to interpret.

In our institution we do not restrict fluid to our patients prior to puncture and under normal circumstances give a double dose (2 ml/kg) of X-ray contrast (Urografin). The severely obstructed or uraemic patient poses a special problem. In these cases excretion will be severely delayed and this factor should be taken into account. Under such circumstances when the collecting system does not opacify (Goodwin et al. 1955), "blind" puncture is often recommended. This involves an approximate landmark level to L1, 4 fingers breadth lateral to the lumbar spine and 2 fingers breadth to the 12th rib. Careful tomography and ultrasound scanning are invaluable in these patients and have reduced the need for truely blind puncture to a minimum. In patients with a non-dilated collecting system about to undergo percutaneous stone removal, a ureteric catheter can be passed and contrast may be injected into the collecting system to facilitate accurate puncture. Such a manoeuvre is only rarely used by our radiologist but we have found it particularly useful in one-stage percutaneous nephrolithotomy where previous difficulty has been experienced in gaining access to the system.

There are many different approaches to actual puncture equipment and nephrostomy tube placement. The earlier papers favoured a trocar method. This involved puncturing the collecting system with a large-bore needle and feeding a polythene or ureteric catheter down the centre of the needle (Goodwin et al. 1955, Saxton et al. 1969). Alternatively, a trocar needle is inserted into the collecting system and not unlike a supra pubic catheter, a cannula is passed over the perforating trocar. (Almgard and Fernström 1974; Levy et al. 1979; Raz 1971). The Pfister Trocar Cannula Unit (Pfister et al. 1983) is rather different. The Trocar Cannula Unit has a specially designed distal tip which separates rather than cuts the parenchymal vessels, and a small side hole which allows urine to be aspirated. Once in position the trocar is drawn and a drainage tube is inserted. The walls of the cannula sheath can then

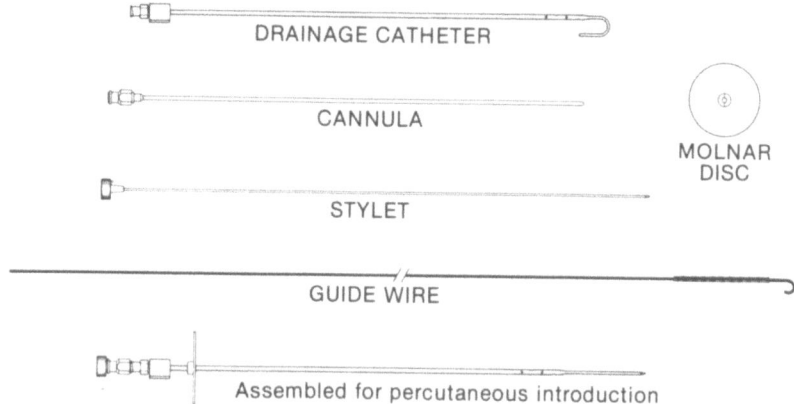

DRAINAGE CATHETER

CANNULA

MOLNAR
DISC

STYLET

GUIDE WIRE

Assembled for percutaneous introduction

Fig. 2.1. Trocar type nephrostomy set. (Courtesy of William Cook, Europe.)

Fig. 2.2. 18-gauge needle for percutaneous puncture: metal stylet, metal sheath. (Courtesy of Vance Products.)

be disrupted and separated by pulling the two tags which are attached to the proximal portion. The trocar method is only really suitable for providing drainage tubes up to 12F in diameter (Fig. 2.1). The main disadvantage is the possibility of seriously damaging the contralateral wall of the collecting system.

Angiographic techniques have replaced other methods in the majority of centres, especially where large-bore tracks are required. These are all based on the Seldinger technique (Seldinger 1953). Two different types of needle are available, metal trocar, metal sheath (Fig. 2.2) and metal trocar, PTFE sheath. Our preference is for the Becton and Dickinson Longdwell translumbar aortogram needle (metal trocar, PTFE sheath). This is not only less traumatic but has the additional advantage that the PTFE sheath can be passed well into the collecting system, over a coaxial guidewire should a check contrast film be required during puncture. This also facilitates the exchange of soft guidewires for more rigid ones.

In our experience, three types of guidewire have been useful: Floppy J, Straight and the Lunderquist wire (Fig. 2.3) which has a floppy distal end (long and short) but a rigid proximal end. The Floppy J is the least traumatic and is

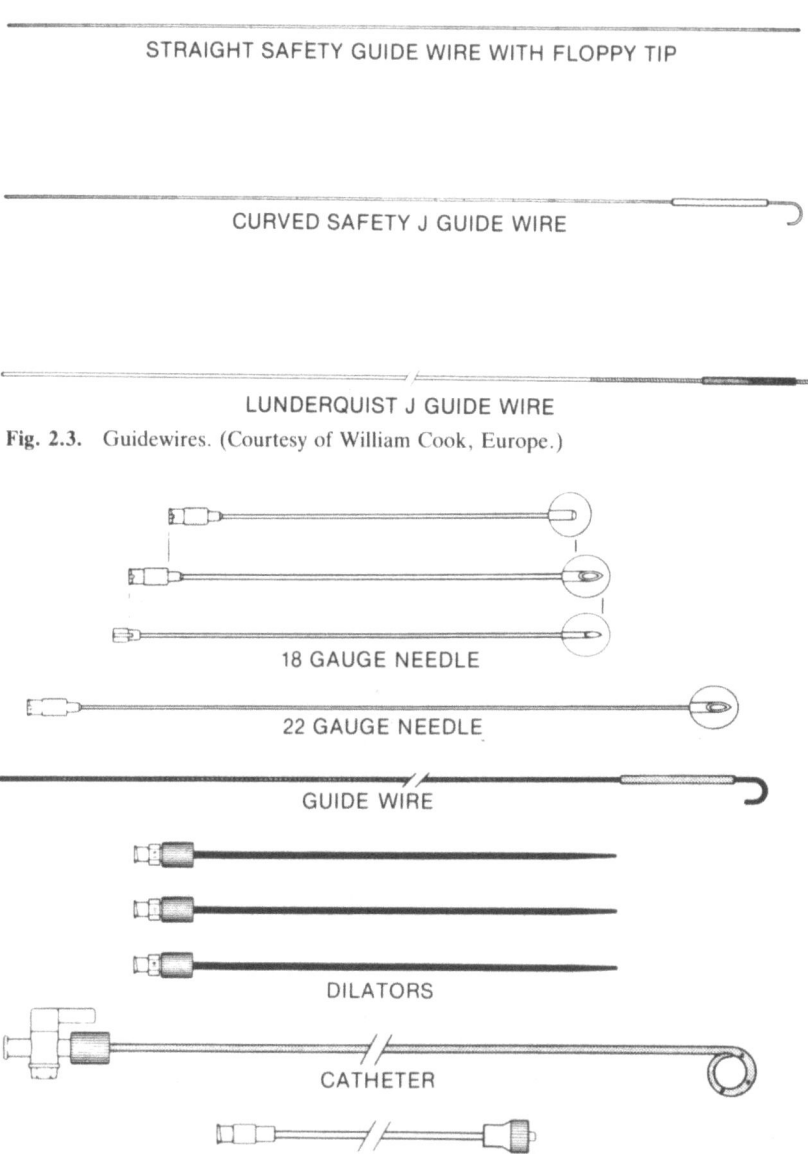

STRAIGHT SAFETY GUIDE WIRE WITH FLOPPY TIP

CURVED SAFETY J GUIDE WIRE

LUNDERQUIST J GUIDE WIRE

Fig. 2.3. Guidewires. (Courtesy of William Cook, Europe.)

18 GAUGE NEEDLE

22 GAUGE NEEDLE

GUIDE WIRE

DILATORS

CATHETER

CONNECTING TUBES

Fig. 2.4. Typical pigtail nephrostomy set. (Courtesy of William Cook, Europe.)

ideal for initial insertion but is liable to kink. The Floppy Straight wire can be useful for by-passing calyceal stones and tight calyceal necks. Once the exact position of the wire has been established it can be exchanged for the rigid Lunderquist wire which is liable to be more traumatic but is ideal for the passage of serial facial dilators and is less liable to kink.

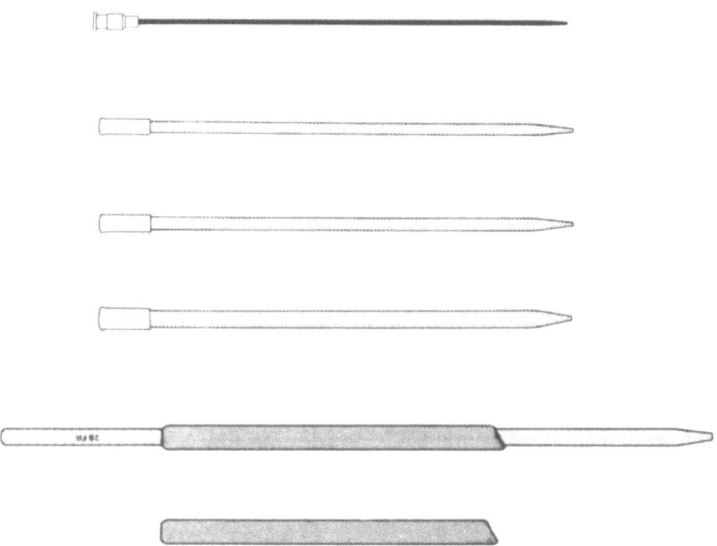

Fig. 2.5. Fascial dilator set. (Courtesy of William Cook.)

Before passing any large-bore needle or trocar (18 gauge or less) it is a wise precaution to attempt puncture using a 22-gauge needle (Skinny, Chiba, Lumbar puncture needle). In this way, multiple transparenchymal stabs can be made if necessary with the minimum amount of renal trauma. The collecting system is opacified and the definitive needle placed alongside the thin 22-gauge needle. A modification of this technique is the Günter system (Günter et al. 1979). The definitive needle assembly is placed into the perirenal tissues with the aid of a central stylet. A thin needle is then advanced into the collecting system and if correctly situated acts as a guide for the working needle assembly which is now advanced over the thin needle. A further option is the passage of a fine 0.25 guidewire through a 22F needle. This is then used to guide the definitive needle assembly into position. A typical pigtail nephrostomy set is shown in Fig. 2.4.

Methods of Dilatation

There are currently three methods of track dilatation over a guidewire. The serial passage of tapered fascial bougies (Fig. 2.5) is our current preference. Such dilators come in sizes which range from 3F to 32F. They are made of polyethylene, metal or PTFE. PTFE dilators, although expensive, are to be preferred as they slide better in the tissues. The metal dilators have fallen out of favour and are now little used. They tend to be difficult to pass through tissues but they have the advantage that they may be autoclaved and are long-lasting. The PTFE and plastic bougies can usually be re-used following ethylene oxide sterilisation, although they do have a limited life.

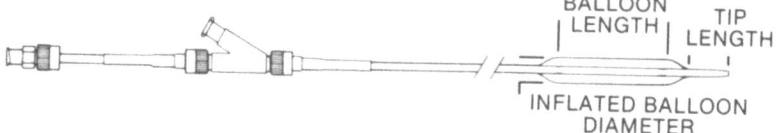

Fig. 2.6. Balloon dilator. (Courtesy of William Cook.)

Balloon dilatation is the second method. This is used for the placement of large-diameter tubes. An angioplasty balloon (Fig. 2.6) (Grunzig et al. 1973) may be used but suffers from the disadvantage that it is frequently 'nipped" by the lumbar fascia and scar tissue, resulting in failure of the balloon to inflate and thus track narrowing. This problem has been overcome with a newer reinforced balloon which will withstand colossal pressures (Clayman 1983). This type of balloon can be back-loaded with endoscopic accessories. Balloons are expensive and although re-sterilisable in ethylene oxide have a limited life. They should always be inflated with contrast so that inflation can be monitored radiographically.

The third method which has become popular especially in the United States and Germany is the Alken telescopic bougie (Alken 1981). This resembles a car aerial in construction. It consists of a central metal tube with a bulbous distal projection over which fit a series of coaxial metal cylinders which are distally coned onto the metal projection of the central stem. Having attained the required dilatation an endoscope sheath or catheter slide (Storz $\frac{1}{2}$ sheath) can be passed over the outer circumference of the bougie. The central metal stem is now withdrawn taking with it the cylindrical dilators but leaving in place the outer sheath or catheter slide which has been passed over the bougie. Such a system is said to tamponade the track continuously during dilatation, an advantage over an exchange system.

Types of Nephrostomy Tubes

A great variety of different tubes are in existence. These vary in material, diameter and design. Initially ureteric catheters and simple polyethelene tubes were used (3–8F). These had a tendency to become displaced and/or kinked. As a result the pigtail catheters were developed. These vary in size (from 6–12F) and can all be passed over guide wires. They have multiple side holes and are less liable (Fig. 2.7) to become displaced than are their straight counterparts. The ability to dilate tracts to virtually any size allowed the use of balloon catheters (Foley), malecot catheters and catheters with retaining wings. It is essential to be able to pass such catheters over a coaxial guide-wire system and it is for this reason that Vance have developed a catheter punch (Fig. 2.8) which will convert a standard Foley catheter for coaxial guide-wire application. For temporary drainage of urine a 6–8F pigtail is sufficient. For longer term drainage a 12F pigtail is better. For nephrolithotomy we use a Porges Whistle Tip Nephrostomy Catheter (26–30F). Similar intermediate sizes have been used for drainage of pyonephroses. All catheters should be sewn to the skin

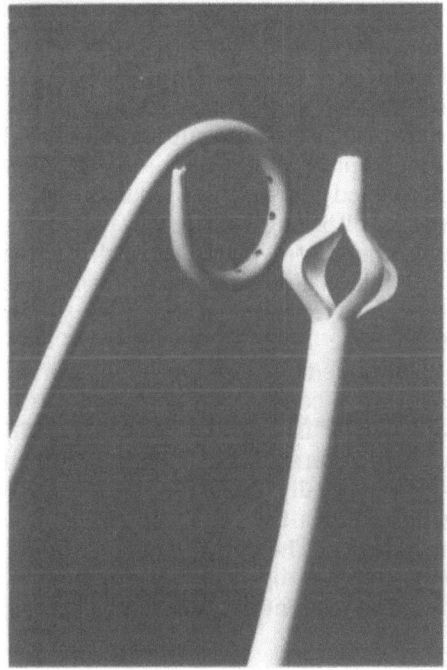

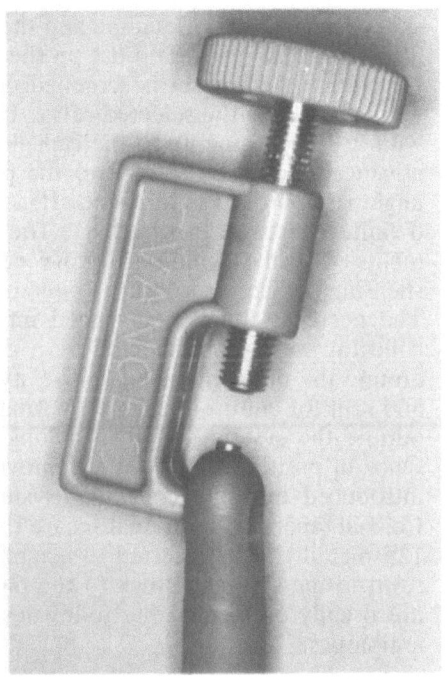

Fig. 2.7. Pigtail and malecot pattern catheters. (Courtesy of Vance Products.)

Fig. 2.8. Vance catheter punch. (Courtesy of Vance Products.)

with non-absorbable sutures and carefully stuck in a comfortable position with adequate quantities of adhesive tape. If this is done with care, displacement is very rare. Some sets have a plastic disc through which the catheter passes, which can be useful to aid retention. It should be sutured to the skin.

Institute of Urology Technique of Percutaneous Nephrostomy Tube Placement

Having talked about the basic equipment, the ensuing paragraphs will briefly describe the radiological techniques which have been developed under Dr. Kellett's direction at the Institute of Urology.

Puncture of the Obstructed System for Temporary or Longterm Drainage

The collecting system is opacified with contrast, the patient placed in the prone oblique position and the following landmarks are drawn onto the patient's back. The 12th rib, lateral border of erector spinae muscle and iliac crest. The skin is cleaned with Betadine and the area draped with sterile towels. A pair of artery forceps is now laid flat on the skin with the tip at the estimated point of puncture. The patient is screened and the clip is adjusted so that its tip lies vertically above the selected calyx. Using a spinal needle the track is infiltrated with 2% lignocaine up to the capsule of the kidney. A 22-gauge needle is now advanced along the track into the perirenal space and is then screened. The angle of approach is adjusted. It is now passed through the renal capsule (a definite resistance can be felt). The needle will swing with respiratory movements. Usually a mid-respiratory point is chosen for puncture as this avoids shearing, which may occur if puncture is made at the extremes of respiration. The needle is further advanced into the collecting system. Puncture of the collecting system is detected by a definite "give". Screening shows a "halo" around the tip of the needle. The stylet is now removed and urine is aspirated and sent for culture/cytology. A small amount of contrast is injected to further outline the system and then a longdwell needle is passed in the same way. Once in position the stylet is removed, urine aspirated and a floppy J-wire is introduced into the collecting system. This usually curls up in the pelvis. Coaxial tapered Teflon dilators are then passed over the guidewire and a 6.5 or 12F pigtail can be inserted to establish drainage. The pigtail is then carefully sewn to the skin and stuck to the patient. Definite diagnostic nephrostograms are usually performed the following day. The patient is always covered with antibiotics.

Nephrostomy for Elective Percutaneous Nephrolithotomy and Endoscopic Access to the Intra-renal Collecting System

This differs in several important aspects from nephrostomy for drainage. Firstly the collecting system is not dilated in at least 60% of our cases, secondly the puncture track must be accurately targeted onto the stone and, finally, wide-calibre tracks are required (26–32F). Puncture is carried out in much the same way as indicated above; double strength intravenous contrast greatly helps to outline the collecting system to facilitate accurate puncture. Once the longdwell needle is in the collecting system the stylet is withdrawn and urine is aspirated with a 10-ml syringe. A J guidewire is now passed alongside the stone. It is not necessary to have this passing into the ureter but it certainly helps if it does. Preformed angiocatheters can assist in placing the tip of the guide wire in the required location. It is quite essential that the guide wire remains straight during dilatation and it neither moves in nor out. Dr. Kellett has developed a method of placing (Kellett et al. 1983) the PTFE dilators which depends on feel rather than continuous X-ray monitoring. We call this the "cross-over feel technique". The elbow of the left arm rests on the patient's back and the left hand holds the proximal end of the guide wire straight in a fixed position. The dilators are then passed over the wire by the right hand (cross-over technique) and are screwed into the kidney. When the guidewire reaches the J tip of the wire, the left hand experiences a slight tug which indicates that the required depth has been attained. At this point, and not before, X-ray screening will confirm the correct position. Thus radiation is reduced to about 5-min screening time per patient. Whenever possible the X-ray field should be coned.

The Kellett triad – catching, kinking and cutting – summarises guidewire problems. The dilator may catch on the 12th rib, scar tissue or the contralateral side of the collecting system. All these situations can be clarified by screening. Kinking of the wire results from allowing the wire to be slack; if the operator persists in the passage of his dilator it will "cut". The PTFE tapered tip will then become dented and the track will be unsuitable as a false passage will develop.

To aid the passage of fascial dilators, it is helpful to exchange the floppy J for a Lunderquist wire when the position of the J has been confirmed as ideal. This manoeuvre involves advancing the plastic sheath of the longdwell needle to the tip of the J wire which is then removed and exchanged for the Lunderquist wire. This cannot be done with a needle assembly which includes a needle with a metal sheath. The floppy portion of the Lunderquist will lie in the collecting system, the rigid portion in the nephrocutaneous track being ideal for dilatation. The "cross-over feel" technique is again used. Care must, however, be taken to ensure that the junction of floppy and rigid parts of the wire is not forced through the back of the kidney inadvertently by injudicious handling, which is not at all difficult to do!

Our dilatations are carried out in a single stage under neurolept or general anaesthesia with gentamicin cover. A typical exchange would involve J wire, Lunderguist wire, 8F, 12F, 16F, 20F, and 26F dilators passed one after another. If a two-stage procedure is contemplated (Miller 1983) once 26F dilatation has been attained an 8F pigtail can be passed into the collecting system. A 26F Whistle Tip Porges nephrostomy tube is then passed over the pigtail catheter into the kidney. We usually freeze these tubes to aid insertion. The tube is then sewn to the skin (two stitches) and carefully stuck down and connected to a drainage bag.

For one-stage procedures we use the Amplatz sheath (Rusnak et al. 1983, Fig. 2.9). This creates ideal conditions for endoscopy. It can also be used to allow nephrostomy tube placement.

Experimental Methods of Access

In the future, for selected cases, retrograde transureteric puncture of the collecting system and subsequent retrieval of the puncture wire through the loin may be used to facilitate stone removal. I first described this in 1983 (Miller 1983b) and the method has been successfully adopted by other American authors (Lawson et al. 1984, Hunter et al. 1984). The ideal will be the retrograde placement of the puncture wire under direct vision (ureteroscope) and retrieving it with the laparoscope from the loin. The wire then acts as a guide for antegrade dilatation in the manner described above.

Another method of potential benefit involves the use of a hydrophilic plastic tube which has the unique property of being able to expand in internal diam-

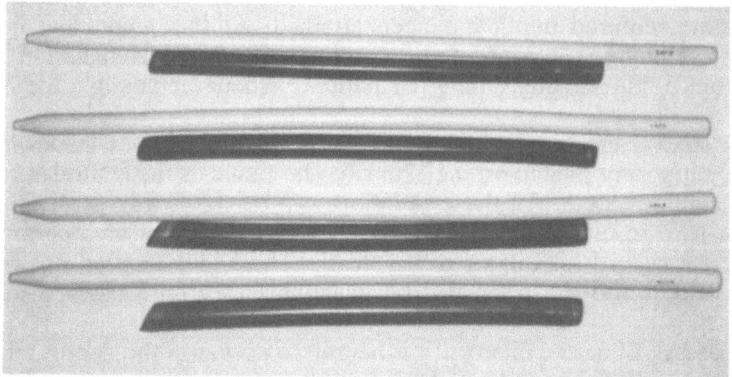

Fig. 2.9. Amplatz dilators. (Courtesy of Vance Products.)

eter when wetted without increasing its wall thickness. At the same time the
tube becomes extremely slippery. I have been working jointly with Mr. Peter
Fyderol and Mrs. Barbara Ringrose at the Royal Military College of Science to
develop this tube and it has been used successfully now in four patients. The
tube is wetted and dried onto a perforated taped plastic fascial bougie which is
then gamma sterilised. A 22F bougie with its imperceptible closely adherent
plastic sheath is then passed into the wound as described above. Normal saline
is introduced through the centre of the bougie alongside the guidewire. This
will leak through the perforations in the wall of the bougie and cause the
plastic to expand. The end result is a slippery 28F track. The bougie can then
be withdrawn from the centre of the dilator leaving a clear path into the
kidney. The expansion time is about 2 minutes. Further work is being carried
out into this method which shows enormous potential both for nephrostomy
dilatation and for ureteric access during ureteroscopy.

There are many other therapeutic and diagnostic manoeuvres which can be
performed by access through a percutaneous nephrostomy track. These include
split-function studies, pressure-flow measurements, ureteric embolisation,
pyelolysis, chemotherapy, stenting, stone dissolution and finally tumour resection. These techniques are beyond the scope of this chapter and are adequately
discussed elsewhere in the literature. Temporary drainage may easily be con-
verted to permanent drainage with a large-bore tube or even with a ring
nephrostomy tube.

Complications

The complications of percutaneous nephrostomy depend on the experience of
the operator and the size of the track required. Bleeding is the main problem but is usually self-limiting and rarely requires transfusion (Stables 1982;
Fernstrom 1983). Abnormalities of coagulation are an absolute contraindica-
tion to this method. Rarely, an AV fistula may be formed, but on the whole
these are self-limiting (Fernström 1983).

Infection is another recognised complication and is the reason we like to cover all our patients with antibiotics. High-pressure injection of contrast material into infected systems must be avoided.

Nausea, vomiting and ileus are frequently seen immediately post-puncture and are probably related to stimulation of the autonomic nerve plexus, anaesthetic agents, bleeding and perhaps rarely puncture of the large bowel lying anterior to the kidney with the preliminary needle puncture. On the whole these symptoms resolve spontaneously and soon.

Pulmonary complications including pneumothorax, hydrothorax, basal consolidation and lung perforation have all been described. They are rare with infra 12 puncture but commoner with supra 12 puncture especially if the surface markings of the pleural recess are not properly appreciated. Extravasation is also sometimes seen. This can be problematical during puncture of a grossly dilated system as it can cause the kidney to rotate and thus the track for large-calibre dilatation is lost. When dilating such a track it is advisable first to empty the collecting system prior to actual dilatation.

Transcolonic dilatation has occurred in a number of centres but has resolved on conservative management. It is a particular problem if the lateral approach is used in the supine patient. Professor Fernstrom recommends the injection of a small amount of contrast during needle passage to identify the peritoneal cavity should this lie in the way of the proposed needle track. This is a fairly elegant way of avoiding colonic perforation.

Clearly the spleen and liver are also at risk. Dr. Clayman tells me he has seen a late haemorrhage from a wide-bore nephrostomy track which was inadvertently dilated into a spleen. Although reports of isolated complications of percutaneous tube placement are scattered throughout the literature, it is quite clear that there can be no comparison with the complications which occur during open nephrostomy. Significant complications in experienced hands are thus minimal.

Conclusion

The ease with which percutaneous tubes are being placed has resulted in a veritable explosion of new radiological and endoscopic surgical techniques. Percutaneous nephrolithotomy has virtually replaced open renal surgery in some centres already. However, considerable care must be taken with the technique as serious complications may occur. Both urologists and radiologists must become familiar with this procedure. Finally it should again be stressed that antegrade drainage for terminal malignant disease can under certain circumstances be the greatest possible disservice a clinician can do for a patient.

Acknowledgements. I should like to thank Dr. Michael Kellett, not only for his great expertise in this field but also for teaching me many of his "tricks" during the $2\frac{1}{2}$ years we have worked so closely as a team. I should also like to thank Mr. John Wickham, my senior colleague, for his guidance and Mr. Larry Watkins for the hours of experimental work we have done together in the laboratory. I am endebted to Messrs William Cook, Europe and Vance products UK for the splendid illustrations in this chapter.

References

Alken P (1981) Teleskopbougierset zur perkutanen Nephrostomie. Aktuelle Urologie 12:216–219

Almgard LE, Fernström I (1974) Percutaneous pyelostomy. Acta Radiol 15:288–294

Barbaric Z, Wood BP (1977) Emergency percutaneous nephropylostomy: Experience with 34 patients and review of the literature. Am J Radiol 128:453–458

Bartley O, Chidekel N, Radberg C (1965) Percutaneous drainage of renal pelvis for uraemia due to obstructed urinary flow. Acta Chir Scand 129:443–446

Baron RL, Lee JKT, McLennan BL, Melson GL (1981) Percutaneous nephrostomy using real time sonographic guidance. Am J Radiol 136:1018–1019

Clayman RV (1983) Percutaneous removal of renal calculi: Use of the back loaded balloon catheter for rapid dilatation and instrumentation of the percutaneous track. Br J Urol (Supplement): 19–22

Fernstrom I (1983) Complications of percutaneous nephrostomy. Br J Urol (Supplement):23–24

Goodwin WE, Casey WC, Woolf W (1955) Percutaneous trocar (needle) in hydronephrosis. JAMA 157:891–894

Graves FT (1954) The anatomy of the intra-renal arteries and its application to segmental resection of the kidney. Br J Surg 42:132–139

Grunzig A, Vetter W, Meir B (1978) Treatment of renovascular hypertension with percutaneous transluminal dilatation of renal artery stenosis. Lancet 1:801–802

Günther R, Alken P, Altwein JE (1979) Percutaneous needle nephrostomy using a fine needle puncture set. Radiol 132:228–230

Haga JR, Zelch MG, Alfidi RJ, Stewart BH, Doherty JD (1977) C-T guided antegrade pyelography and percutaneous nephrostomy. Am J Radiol 128:621–624

Hunter PT, Hawkins IF, Finlayson B, Nanni G, Senior D (1984) Hunter Hawkins retrograde transcutaneous nephrostomy: A new technique. Urology 22:583–587

Kellett MJ, Miller RA, Wickham JEA (1983) The role of the Radiologist in percutaneous renal surgery. Br J Urol (Supplement):27–30

Lawson RK, Murphy JB, Taylor AJ, Jacobs SC (1984) Retrograde methods of percutaneous access to the kidney. Urology 22:581–582

Levy JM, Potter WM, Stegman CJ (1979) A new catheter system for permanent percutaneous nephrostomy. J Urol 122:442–443

Miller RA (1983a) Applied anatomy. In: Percutaneous renal surgery. Churchill Livingstone, Edinburgh, pp 1–16

Miller RA (1983b) Percutaneous nephrolithotomy and lithotresis. In: Percutaneous renal surgery. Churchill Livingstone, Edinburgh, pp 108–147

Miller RA, Wickham JEA, Kellett MJ (1983) Trans uretero pyelostomy. A new technique for percutaneous renal access. Br J Urol (Supplement):60–63

Pederson JF, Cowan DF, Kristensen JK, Holm HH, Homcke S, Jensen F (1976) Ultrasonically guided percutaneous nephrostomy. Radiology 119:429–431

Pfister RC, Yoder IC, Newhouse JH (1983) A new trocar cannula unit for percutaneous procedures. Br J Urol (Supplement):64–68

Raz S (1981) A simple method for pyonephrosis drainage. Lancet 2:529–530

Rusnak B, Castaneda-Zwiga W, Kotula F, Herrera M, Amplatz K (1982) An improved dilator system for percutaneous nephrostomies. Radiology 144:174

Saitoh M, Wantanabe H, Ohe H, Tanaka S, Hakura Y, Date S (1979) Ultrasonic real time guidance for percutaneous puncture. J Clin Ultrasound 7:269–272

Saxton H, Ogg CS, Cameron JS (1969) Percutaneous needle nephrostomy. Br Med J 4:657–660

Seldinger SI (1953) Catheter replacement of the needle in percutaneous angiography, a new technique. Acta Radiol 39:368–376

Stables DP (1982) Percutaneous nephrostomy: Techniques, indications and results: in Urol Clin North Am. 9:15–29

Chapter 3

Ureteric Stents

R.P. Finney and S.C. Hopkins

Introduction

Nearly twenty years ago, Willard Goodwin, originator of many commonly accepted urological procedures including the percutaneous nephrostomy, wrote a short essay entitled "Splint, Stent, Stint", in which he addressed the question of which word would be most appropriate. Prior to this article, the term "splint" denoted a catheter which was "left within the ureter and provided external drainage usually following surgery". In his essay Goodwin suggested that "stent" would be the most appropriate term (Goodwin 1972).

Some ten years later, Turner et al. (1982) published the results of a 1975 questionnaire completed by 1453 American urologists. Of this large number, 70% preferred the term "splint", whereas 30% believed the term "stent" to be more correct. In spite of this resistance to change, in the years since Goodwin's essay, "splint" has been used with increasing rarity and "stent" has become accepted. The vast majority of English-language medical publications now use the term "stent" as do most of the manufacturers of these devices. It is not within the scope of this chapter to decide whether or not the other terms are also correct, but as terminology evolves by common use it seems likely that "stint" and "splint" will gradually disappear.

Various words have also been used to describe a ureteric catheter which is positioned "completely inside the body" as opposed to one which "reaches the external environment". In this sense, the terms "indwelling", "inlying", and "internal" have been used interchangeably. "Indwelling", however, can refer to a drain or catheter which reaches the outside such as "an indwelling Foley catheter", and, although "inlying" is defined as "placed or situated inside or in the interior", for purposes of clarity, "internal" ureteric stent will be used specifically in this chapter.

During the nineteenth century, when production of gum elastic and rubber catheters became widespread, some method of standardisation was necessary. Joseph Charriere, a French instrument maker, devised a scale which is still the one most widely used today. This scale was based upon units of one-third of a millimetre such that a catheter one millimetre in diameter has come to be a "3 Charriere" in France, a "3 Ch." in Great Britain and a 3F (French) in the USA. In this section F will be used (Lytton 1975).

Anatomy of the Renal Collecting System and Ureter

The intrarenal collecting system, renal pelvis, and ureter form a hydro-dynamically integrated system to transport urine. The renal pelvis which lies within the renal sinus may occupy an intrarenal or extrarenal position relative to the parenchyma. Pelvic capacity, however, is frequently similar (4–8 ml), and in the patient requiring an internal stent, this anatomical variation is usually of no clinical significance.

Ureteral length in the adult varies between 25 cm and 34 cm and is dependent upon height, age and sex. The abdominal ureter, which is 14–16 cm long, descends to the brim of the bony pelvis. As it leaves the renal pelvis at the transverse process of the first lumbar vertebra and comes to lie on the psoas muscle, the ureter forms a lazy-S shaped curve. Although retroperitoneal, this portion of the ureter is closely adherent to the posterior parietal peritoneum (Davis et al. 1981).

As the ureter enters the true pelvis, it crosses anterior to the iliac vessels and comes to lie above each sacro-iliac joint. The pelvic ureter, which is also approximately 14–16 cm in length, courses along the side wall of the true pelvis to the level of the ischial spine where it turns medially to terminate at the ureteral orifice in the bladder. In the male, the pelvic ureter is crossed by the vas deferens. In the female, the ureter descends through the broad ligament and passes below the uterine artery, from where it courses medially and downward in front of the vagina to its entrance into the urinary bladder. The close relationship between the uterine artery and the pelvic ureter results in the relatively high incidence of surgical injury to the distal ureter in females (Davis et al. 1981).

In general, the calyces, renal pelvis, and ureter have a similar histological appearance (Velardo 1981). The lining of the upper collecting system is composed of transitional cell epithelium and is nearly identical to that of the bladder. Typically, however, no glandular elements are noted in the mucosa. The smooth musculature of the calyces, renal pelvis and ureter is also similar to that found in the bladder, but is less prominent. At the junction of each calyx and at the pyelo-ureteric junction, the muscle may be prominent and has been postulated to provide some sphincteric action (Kiil 1978; Davis et al. 1981).

The nerve supply to the intrarenal collecting system and ureter is abundant and is diffusely distributed throughout their entire length (Davis et al. 1981). Autonomic nerve fibres arise from the coeliac, aorticorenal, and mesenteric ganglia. The ureter may also receive innervation from the superior hypogastric and/or inferior hypogastric plexuses.

The exact role of the various autonomic nerves to the human ureter have not been clearly demonstrated. Excision or denervation of the ureter does not inhibit ureteral contraction; however, stimulation of nerve fibres in the renal hilum may double or even triple the peristaltic activity of the upper collecting system (Davis et al. 1981).

Although most texts adequately describe ureteral anatomy and its anatomical relationships, the functional internal ureteric diameter is not so well described. On histological section, the papillary infoldings of the mucosa may make this a moot point, but in the patient requiring internal urinary diversion, knowledge of the normal variation in ureteral calibre may be important.

Physiology of the Renal Collecting System and Ureter

Urine transport is accomplished by a coordinated and sequential contraction of smooth muscle bundles which propel the urine downwards in individual boluses. Muscle function is dependent upon many inter-related factors (Kiil 1978). The observation that electrical impulses and mechanical contraction begin above the pyelo-ureteric junction came from observations in animal models that contraction of the upper collecting system preceded every action potential and mechanical contraction in the ureter below, but that the converse was usually not true. Although peristalsis begins in the upper tracts, there is no evidence for one specific pacemaker site since any calyx or part of the renal pelvis can be removed without disturbing this electromechanical activity (Hanna 1981).

Infusion studies combined with pyelography and fluoroscopy have demonstrated that the renal calyces have the shortest refractory period and contract independently of the renal pelvis. Each calyceal contraction does not, however, result in measurable pressure fluctuations in the renal pelvis or ureter. This sequence of calyceal, renal pelvic, and ureteric electromechanical activity has been studied in the surgically isolated kidney (Hanna 1981). As the contractile wave is propagated from a calyx towards the pyelo-ureteric junction, it may be either recruited in the renal pelvis and propagated into the proximal ureter or fade out. As will be seen, an important property for any stent is that this activity should not be significantly impaired.

Once electrical recruitment and mechanical contraction of the renal pelvis occurs, there is a considerable change in the shape of the pelvis, but little change in volume and, as a result, pressure change is also small (Hanna 1981). This is important since urine must flow easily into and down a stent at relatively low pressures.

The mathematical equation for the relationship between volume and pressure in a tube is explained by Laplace's Law.

$$\text{Pressure} = \frac{\text{Tension} \times \text{Wall thickness}}{\text{Radius}}$$

Saline perfusion studies at physiological flow rates (0.5–2.0 ml/min) demonstrate that the normal intrapelvic pressure is $\leqslant 10$ cm H_2O and remains relatively unchanged as flow increases. Only when flow reaches supraphysiological rates (10–18 ml/min), or there is significant obstruction below, does the system decompensate – which results in changes in pressure and volume (Whitaker 1973; Pfister et al. 1982). Under these conditions, all modern stents preserve renal function, and, if anatomical changes have occurred, allow reversible factors to return to normal.

It is currently accepted that the pyelo-ureteric junction is functionally open during the resting or "diastolic" phase such that the pelvis and a short segment of the upper ureter fill with urine simultaneously. This upper segment of ureter forms the ureteric "cone or bulb" (Kiil 1978). When a propagated contraction reaches the ureteropelvic junction, this sphincter is occluded and a "trapped" urine bolus is transported down the ureter towards the bladder (Kiil 1978). This hypothesis has significant impact upon stent function. As will be seen, early ureteric "splints" (while attempting to preserve urine flow by means of a large lumen) did not take into account the effects of this sphincteric action upon urine bolus propagation. However, the development of "stents" with side-ports to allow flow into and out of the stent lumen was a major advance and reflected the increased attention paid to making stents work in harmony with normal upper tract physiology.

Urine transport down the ureter is also achieved by propagated electro-mechanical activity. During "diastole", the ureteral pressure is low (10 cm H_2O), and (according to Laplace's Law) reflects the low intrinsic tension of the resting ureteral wall. Ureteral "systole" induced by prior muscle distension results in pressure rises up to 20–40 cm H_2O, and at physiological flow rates (0.5–2 ml/min) peristaltic contractions occur at a frequency of 4–8/min, each lasting 2–5 s (Hanna 1981). Hence, the development of materials which are pliable but have sufficient resistance to physiological compression was a significant advance in stent design.

The frequency and force of ureteral peristalsis is thus determined by three main factors. These include (1) renal excretory volume, (2) urine flow rate, and (3) out-flow resistance. An adequate ureteric stent must take these factors into account in order to function effectively and in harmony with this complex hydrodynamic system.

In the 1940s and 1950s, many of the problems associated with the placement of "splints" were thought in part to result from rigid, non-biocompatible catheters which were proportionately too large for the ureteral lumen (Smart 1979). This frequently resulted in ischaemia, pressure necrosis and eventual stricture formation. Although most ureteric stents have a uniform outer diameter, the internal diameter of the human ureter varies within the same person, and from individual to individual. The distal intramural segment has the smallest potential lumen, but if dilated may tolerate flexible catheters of 7–10F without ischaemic sequelae. In the abdominal portion, catheters of 10–12F are often easily tolerated, although areas of physiological "narrowing" (requiring a smaller diameter catheter) are well recognised (Östling 1942).

As a result of these ischaemic complications with early rigid catheters, the largest outside diameter of modern stents does not exceed 11F, and for most models is 8.5, 9 or 9.5F (Gibbons 1982; Mardis et al. 1982; Finney 1982; Smith 1982a,c). The smaller outside diameter of these more pliable and bio-compatible stents has significantly decreased the incidence of stricture disease; however, to maintain adequate urine flow at physiological pressures, most stents have a minimum diameter of not less than 5F.

Flow Characteristics of Internal Ureteric Stents

The drainage efficiency of three commercial ureteric stents (Gibbons, Double Pigtail, and Double J) were recently evaluated under various obstructing conditions (Mardis et al. 1980). For each design, maximum flow at a mean pressure of 5 cm H_2O was directly proportional to the diameter of the stent used; however, adequate flow was maintained with 5F stents. The importance of side holes was demonstrated by the fact that each unported stent drained 40%–50% less efficiently than the identical catheter with side-ports (Fig. 3.1a).

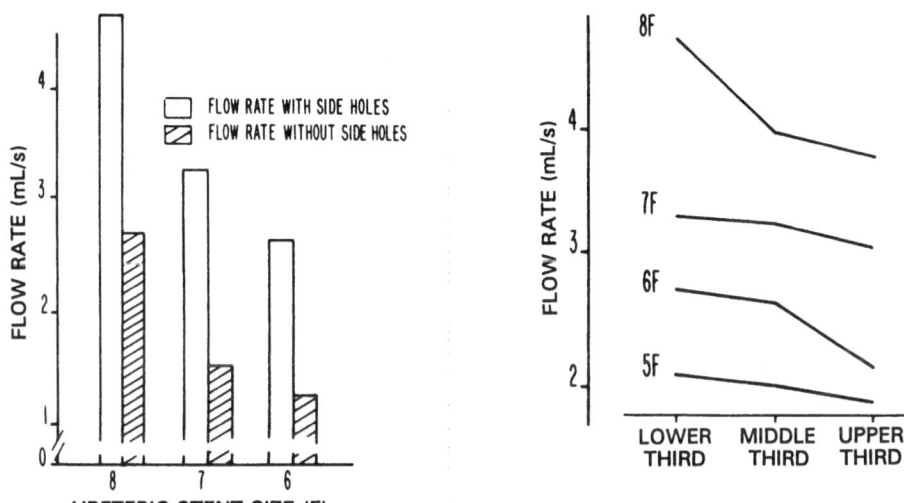

Fig. 3.1. **a** Flow through ureteric stents with and without side-ports. **b** Flow through pigtail stents in the presence of simulated lower, middle and upper ureteric obstruction. (From Mardis HK et al. (1982) Polyethylene double-pigtail ureteral stents. Urol Clin North Am 9:95–101, with permission.)

Interestingly, all stents demonstrated maximum efficiency when the blockage was placed at the lower end of the simulated ureter and, in each case, there was a reduction in flow of up to 20% as the blockage was serially advanced to the proximal segment (Fig. 3.1b). The length of the simulated blockage also correlated with a serial decrease in flow.

Although it was suggested that the Double Pigtail stent had the greatest overall drainage capacity, all three designs allowed physiological flow, regardless of site, length and relative degree of obstruction.

Stent Composition

During the past one hundred years many different materials have been used to fashion ureteric catheters and more recently, internal ureteric stents. After the 1950s it was recognised that the ideal stent would (1) allow adequate urine flow (0.5–2 ml/min) at physiological pressures (2–10 cm H_2O) and (2) interfere minimally with effective ureteral peristalsis. In addition, this stent would be composed of a substance which should be (3) non-wetting, (4) non-toxic, (5) non-absorbable, (6) easily fabricated, (7) compression-resistant, (8) capable of maintaining its position and shape over a long period of time, (9) capable of being heat sterilised, (10) resistant to encrustation by urinary salts, (11) radio-opaque, and (12) not too costly (Hepperlen et al. 1978; Finney 1978; Kearney et al. 1979).

Although many of the criteria for the ideal internal stent have to some degree been satisfied by modern stenting devices, an historic review of stent materials is of interest, and may be particularly helpful to the practising urologist who does not have a suitable commercial stent readily available, and must fashion his own (Mangelson et al. 1968; Kearney et al. 1979).

Latex Rubber

Since gum elastic became available in the last century, latex rubber has been used extensively for the manufacture of urethral catheters. Little attention was paid by the early manufacturers to the toxicity of their products, however, and through the years chemicals were added to the latex to produce desired mechanical properties with little consideration of the deleterious effects they had on body tissues (Lytton 1975). Despite the use of these hardening agents, rubber ureteric catheters required an internal stiffening wire as the rubber was too pliable. Latex rubber does not have a non-wetting surface and resists encrustation poorly. Hence, it was recognised early that this would not be a suitable material for the manufacture of a longterm ureteric stent (Blum et al. 1963).

Woven Fabric

Until relatively recently, standard non-disposable ureteric catheters were fashioned by weaving a fine fabric to cover a mandrel and then dipping this repeatedly in various varnish compounds to produce the desired rigidity and water tightness (Brown and Harrison 1951). Although catheter placement was easy, and generally in the short-term situation worked reasonably well, the exposed lumenal crevices in the fabric resulted in rapid encrustation by blood and urine salts, causing catheter plugging. This undoubtedly accounted for the limited popularity of surgical stenting for many years (Smart 1979).

Polyvinyl Chloride (PVC)

Polyvinyl chloride (PVC) became available in the 1940s and over the next decade was used to fashion open-ended "indwelling ureteric splints" (Ferris and Grindley 1948; Davis 1951). This plastic, which is available in the form of disposable infant feeding tubes, is inexpensive, but when used as a ureteric stent has several serious disadvantages. Plasticisers (chemicals added to the vinyl in order to make it soft and pliable) are leached out of the plastic after prolonged contact with urine, and in time can result in a hard, brittle catheter. This caused marked mucosal irritation and severe ureteric scarring (Brown and Harrison 1951). In addition, PVC tended to encrust relatively rapidly (Blum et al. 1963). For these reasons no commercial stent at present is made of vinyl.

Polytetrafluorethylene (PTFE, Teflon)

PTFE has several properties which make it a good material for the construction of a ureteric stent. It is non-wetting and non-toxic to body tissue, and may be autoclaved at high temperatures without deteriorating. Its major drawback is that, like PVC, it is relatively hard and brittle. PTFE also does not resist encrustation as well as many other materials (Blum et al. 1963).

Acrylic and Nylon

These synthetic materials, which also became available in the 1940s, were noted to cause little body-tissue reaction. They are currently used to make biocompatible bone cement and suture material. But, as with untreated vinyl, and PTFE, the rigidity of these compounds precluded their use in fabricating ureteric stents (Brown and Harrison 1951).

Polyethylene and Other Plastics

Polyethylene is, as the name implies, a polymer of ethylene with each molecule containing 200–1000 ethylene units. This plastic has many properties which make it a good material for the manufacture of disposable urethral catheters. It is flexible, odourless, translucent, and non-reactive in the body (Brown and Harrison 1951). For these reasons, early hand-made ureteric stents were fashioned from commercial polyethylene tubing (Ferris and Grindley 1948). These catheters proved to be superior to those of latex rubber or woven fabric, and for a time many disposable ureteric stents were composed of polyethylene.

Although polyethylene resists encrustation well (albeit somewhat less than silicone) and is easily moulded, it has a low melting point and cannot be autoclaved. Therefore, it must be gased with ethylene oxide to ensure sterilisation. In addition, this plastic is not particularly pliable, and as a result stents tend to be rather stiff (Mardis et al. 1982). Flexion while in the ureter has led to spontaneous depolymerisation and frequent stent breakage, which make endoscopic removal difficult (Mardis et al. 1982). Because of this, most manufacturers no longer use this material.

More recently, newer plastic polymers have become available and are represented by such names as polyurethane, C-Flex, Bio-flex and Siltex. These materials are said to be more pliable than polyethylene and may resist encrustation and breakage better (Mardis 1984 personal communication). Whether they will stiffen after prolonged exposure to urine, and how well they actually resist encrustation, have not been determined.

Siloxan (Silicone)

The family of silicone rubber polymers was developed during the 1940s for use in military aircraft. Silicone molecules, when substituted for carbon-based methyl groups, produce various greases, synthetic rubbers and other materials which are more resistant to high temperatures than their organic precursors (Blum et al. 1963). Tubing made of this rubber can be moulded or extruded and the softness or stiffness of the tubing can be partly controlled by the degree to which it is polymerised. Repeated flexion does not make this polymer brittle, and it may be repeatedly sterilised by autoclaving. A specific advantage of silicone rubber is that it is extremely biocompatible (Mangelson et al. 1968) and as a result medical-grade silicone is widely used to produce implantable prostheses including cardiac pacemakers, penile implants and urinary incontinence devices.

Although silicone resists encrustation well, unequivocal evidence of its superiority is lacking and is even disputed (Mardis 1984 personal communication). However, the other properties of this elastomer satisfy many of the criteria for the ideal internal stent, and many commercial designs incorporate it.

Historical Stents

The function of any ureteric stent is to facilitate low-pressure urine drainage from the kidney to the bladder in cases of ureteric obstruction or to prevent leakage of urine from the kidney or ureter following surgery. A stent can also serve to keep the ureteric lumen patent during healing thereby preventing stricture formation, and surgically placed stents may prevent a mobilised ureter from becoming sharply angulated during the healing process (Persky and Krause 1981).

Early catheters of woven fabric coated with varnish were helpful as temporary surgical stents, but were not satisfactory when prolonged ureteric drainage was necessary. These rigid catheters usually required either direct drainage to the outside or were brought out through the urethra. In addition, although they could be coiled up in the bladder, their intrinsic rigidity caused significant irritation to the bladder mucosa, and as a result they were debilitatingly uncomfortable to the patient (Brown and Harrison 1951).

The internal diameter of these woven catheters was small, and flow through the lumen was limited unless very large catheters were used. Hence, because of their composition, fabrication and small, rough internal surface they not only encrusted and obstructed rapidly (Brown and Harrison 1951), but frequently injured the ureter (Persky and Krause 1981).

A significant problem recognised early was the fact that there were no side-ports along the length of these ureteric catheters. A bolus of urine enters the abdominal ureter by the coordinated peristaltic relaxation of the pyelo-ureteric junction and upper ureteral segment which then contracts to propel the urine bolus further downward. When a ureteric catheter with no side-ports is used as a stent proximal to the ureteropelvic junction, much of the urine bolus passes around the outside of the catheter beyond the proximal drainage holes, and this bolus must then find its way towards the bladder. This urine is very likely to be forced through the site of injury or surgery into the surrounding tissues if the ureter has been previously injured or if surgery has been performed, which often resulted in inflammation, scarring and stricture formation. Because of the prevalence of these not insignificant problems, some earlier authors did not see much benefit to stenting (Smart 1979).

Other early attempts were made to stent the ureter with small, latex rubber urethral catheters or commercial polyethylene tubing. These were brought out through the urethra or a flank incision and emptied into an external drainage system. The latex, however, was too soft, reacted poorly with the body tissues and also facilitated rapid encrustation. In addition, both types of "indwelling" catheters served as pathways for the entrance of infection (Brown and Harrison 1951).

In the 1960s medical-grade silicone rubber tubing became available for longterm implantation in the body (Dow Corning). In 1963 Blum and associates noted that silicone rubber left in the bladder became less encrusted than patches of other synthetic materials. They also noted that surgically implanted silicone was biocompatible as a ureteric prosthesis in animals for up to 57 months with no evidence of inflammation.

Four years later, Zimskind reported on the first use of open-ended silicone tubing as a completely internal ureteric stent in order to palliate patients having malignant ureteric obstruction or to bypass uretero-vaginal fistulae (Zimskind et al. 1967). This tubing consisted of commercial silicone (Dow Corning) which was 7.3 or 9.6F in outside diameter. A 4F or 5F well-lubricated whistle-tip ureteral catheter was inserted inside the stent lumen to provide temporary rigidity and serve as an obdurator. The tubing was precut to length (30–34 cm), such that after placement in the ureter a few centimetres protruded into the bladder.

These tubes (without side holes) were implanted through a panendoscope in retrograde fashion. The silicone tubing was passed to the renal pelvis, the tube grasped near its point of exit from the ureteric vesical orifice with foreign-body forceps and the whistle-tip ureteric catheter withdrawn. Zimskind and associates described 16 patients who had successful implantation of these silicone catheters over 6 weeks to 19 months. The advantage of this stent was that in contrast to individuals having conventional "indwelling" catheters, these patients did not require an external collection device, were freely ambulatory, and remained uninfected.

Although these authors, as others before them, depended upon tube calibre to resist expulsion by providing a snug fit at the site of obstruction, this does not detract from the fact that they were among the first to demonstrate that longterm, entirely internal stenting was feasible, and that if made relatively compression-resistant, silicone rubber was superior to other then-available materials.

Three years later, Marmar modified Zimskind's stent, by closing the proximal end with silicone adhesive (Dow Corning) to facilitate its retrograde passage. In addition, three holes were cut near the sealed end to promote intralumenal urine flow from the proximal ureter. A 4F ureteric catheter with a wire stylet was again used to stiffen the stent, and after retrograde passage through a cystoscope, a catheter deflector positioned on the distal end of the stent allowed withdrawal of the ureteric catheter and stylet. Marmar was able to use this technique successfully on four of five patients with ureteric obstruction secondary to malignancy (Marmar 1970).

Orikasa and associates (1973) suggested another modification to Zimskind's technique. These authors first inserted a 5F ureteric catheter containing a stiffening wire stylet through the ureter into the renal pelvis. They then threaded an appropriate length of 9F silicone tubing over the catheter to the kidney. Instead of grasping forceps to hold the silicone in place during removal of the ureteric catheter, a rigid plastic positioning tube threaded behind the stent held the silicone tubing in place, allowing removal of the ureteric catheter and stylet. This modification of the "Seldinger" technique (Seldinger 1953) was successful in 17 patients and the silicone catheters remained in place from 2 weeks to 8 months.

These early stents, while providing satisfactory drainage without undue pressure and ischaemia, were still nothing more than compressible straight tubes with no means of preventing distal or proximal migration. Some were expelled into the bladder while others migrated above the ureterovesical junction making retrieval difficult especially since they were not radiopaque.

In 1974, Gibbons and associates published their results on 12 patients who were successfully treated with a compression-resistant internal silicone stent. This stent was a major modification from the open-ended straight tubes used by previous authors. The catheters were precut to 24 cm in length and were bevelled and sealed at the proximal end as suggested by Marmar. In addition, the distal end of the stent was also modified by placing an acorn-shaped collar of silicone rubber cement 2 cm from the distal end. Holes of 1 mm in diameter were placed every centimetre distal to the proximal end and every 5 mm distal to the acorn-shaped collar. These stents were again fashioned from straight commercial silicone tubing and had outside diameters of 6, 7.3, or 9.6F. Stent placement was accomplished by the retrograde technique of Zimskind (1967).

The distal acorn-shaped collar was designed to pass just above the intramural ureter and wedge at this site to reduce the chance of downward migration and expulsion. Of the first 12 patients, however, upward migration occurred in 2 and the stent was expelled in 4 others. Because of these problems, Gibbons et al. modified their design resulting in the first of the commercially available "modern" internal ureteric stents (Gibbons 1976).

Modern Internal Stents

Gibbons Stent

In 1975, Gibbons designed a stent made of compression-resistant silicone tubing with winged or "dentate" protrusions at fixed intervals in its middle third in order to wedge the stent above an obstructing lesion. A distal flange was also incorporated into the design to prevent upward migration, but since this flange had to be small enough to pass through the cystoscope it was not invariably successful. The Gibbons stent which is currently available (Heyer-Shulte/Mentor) has been gradually improved over the past years by various other modifications (Gibbons et al. 1976; Gibbons 1982) including a distal radiopaque collar that has a retrieval tail to facilitate stent removal in case of upward migration (Fig. 3.2a).

This stent which comes in two diameters (8.0 and 9.5F) and three lengths (15, 23 and 29 cm) is especially useful when the lower ureter is obstructed by malignancy (Fig. 3.2b). Since the stent depends upon an obstruction in the mid or lower one-third of the ureter to prevent expulsion, the tip need not extend up to the ureteropelvic junction, but should extend at least 3 cm above the obstruction in order to be functionally effective. Occasionally, however, the ureter above may kink (Schneider et al. 1976) and, as has been suggested by Gibbons, there are the additional disadvantages of the retaining wings: (1) the wings must be passed above the site of obstruction in order to prevent stent expulsion, thereby making the stent ineffective if the obstruction is at the pyelo-ureteric junction or the upper one-third of the ureter, (2) the wings increase the stent diameter, hence an 8.0F stent wedged into the ureter may in fact have a functional diameter of 11F and (3) in the situations of ureteral

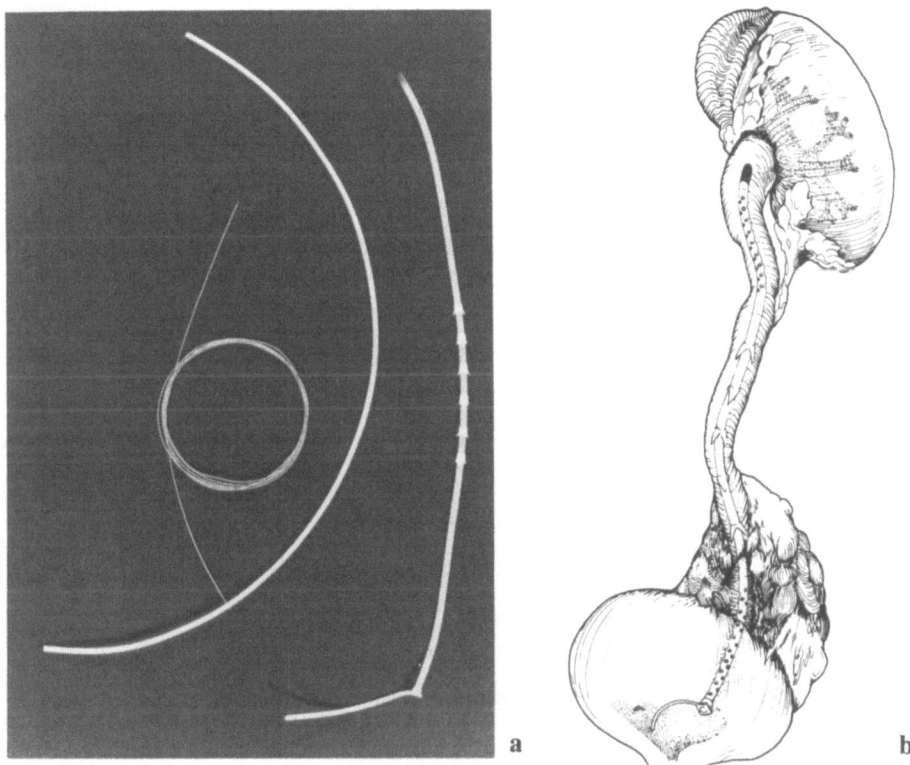

Fig. 3.2. a Gibbons stent kit includes a stent, stent positioner, and guidewire. **b** This stent is most effective for distal ureteric obstruction secondary to malignancy, and, when the proximal ureter is severely kinked. (From Gibbons R (1982) Gibbons ureteral stents. Urol Clin North Am 9:85–88, with permission.)

fistula or surgical anastomosis, the wings could keep the fistula open or protrude through the suture line. Nonetheless this stent is particularly useful in select situations of lower ureteric malignant obstruction.

Single Pigtail Stent

In 1978, Hepperlen, Mardis and Kammandel reported the use of a polyethylene "Suspension-type" stent (similar to the "Shepherds-crook" design by McCullough 1974) with a preformed single pigtail which, when placed above the pyelo-ureteric junction, would spontaneously coil and prevent downward migration. In the distal end of the stent there was a flange to prevent upward migration. This stent was inserted with a guidewire and a plastic stent positioner using the Seldinger technique as suggested by Orikasa et al. The suspension modification was a significant improvement over previous designs since the pigtail did not functionally increase the diameter of the stent but, by coiling within the renal pelvis, provided excellent protection against downward migration. The distal flange, however, was not adequate to prevent proximal migra-

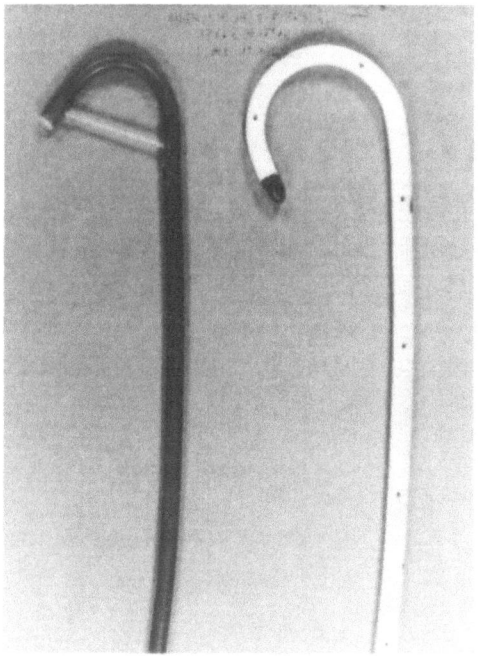

Fig. 3.3. Prototype of the Double J stent with a hand-made silicone bowstring (left) compared with the commercial Double J with molded hooks on both ends. (From Finney R (1982) Urol Clin North Am 9:89–94, with permission.)

tion and as a result problems with stent retrieval were not uncommon (Collier et al. 1979; Camacho et al. 1979).

Double J Stent

Finney (1978) reported his experience with the Double J design (Surgitek). The prototype for this stent had been a hand-made prosthesis of radiopaque silicone tubing which formed a J-shape at each end by means of a fine strand of silicone rubber which bent the tip back on itself like a bow-string (Fig. 3.3). The J hooks on either end could be straightened with a wire stylet while the stent was being passed into the ureter. When the stylet wire was removed the Js reformed and the stent became self-retaining. In addition, these prototype stents had the proximal end sealed and were also provided with 1-mm side-port holes each centimetre along the entire length.

The commercial Double J Silicone Stent (Surgitek) became available with the two Js moulded into the elastomer and formed in opposite directions to facilitate coiling in the renal pelvis and bladder (Fig. 3.4B). The second J in the bladder resolved the previous problems of stent migration and bladder irritation (Camacho et al. 1979; Mardis et al. 1982). In distinction to other stents the commercial Double J was provided with both ends sealed. This allowed the stent to be used intraoperatively such that the catheter may be passed both

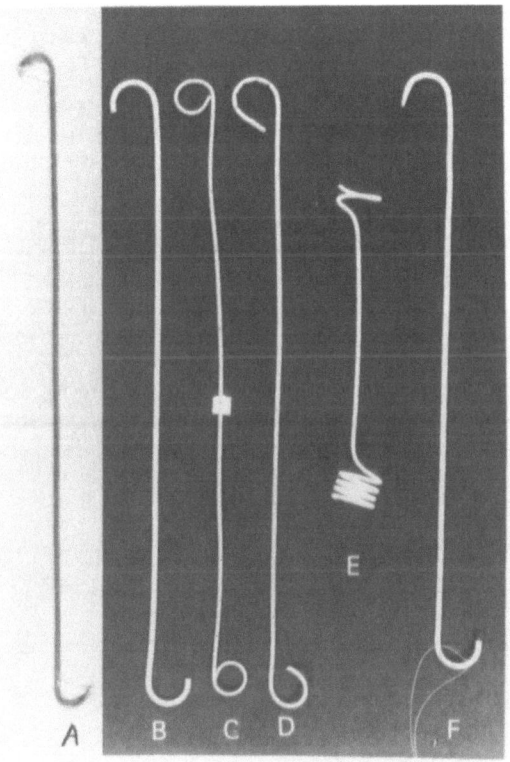

Fig. 3.4. Prototype and modern ureteric stents. A, prototype silicone ureteric stent; B, double J ureteric stent; C, double pigtail/Mardis stent; D, uropass stent; E, coil stent; F, percutaneous antegrade double J stent.

antegrade and retrograde through any standard ureterotomy or pyelotomy incision without first passing a guide wire (Fig. 3.5). For endoscopic passage the distal tip was trimmed, exposing the lumen. The Double J Ureteral Stent kit is available in three diameters (6, 7 and 8.5F) and four lengths (16, 26, 28 and 30 cm). The kit includes a stylet wire and a stent positioner, and the catheters are marked at 5-cm intervals to facilitate proper endoscopic or surgical placement.

The Percutaneous Antegrade Double J Stent kit (Surgitek) allows the antegrade passage of this stent through a percutaneous nephrostomy when retrograde endoscopic placement is not possible (Fig. 3.4F).

Double Pigtail Stent

In 1979, Mardis and associates reported their results using the Double Pigtail ureteric stent (Cook) (Fig. 3.4C). Because of spontaneous depolymerisation

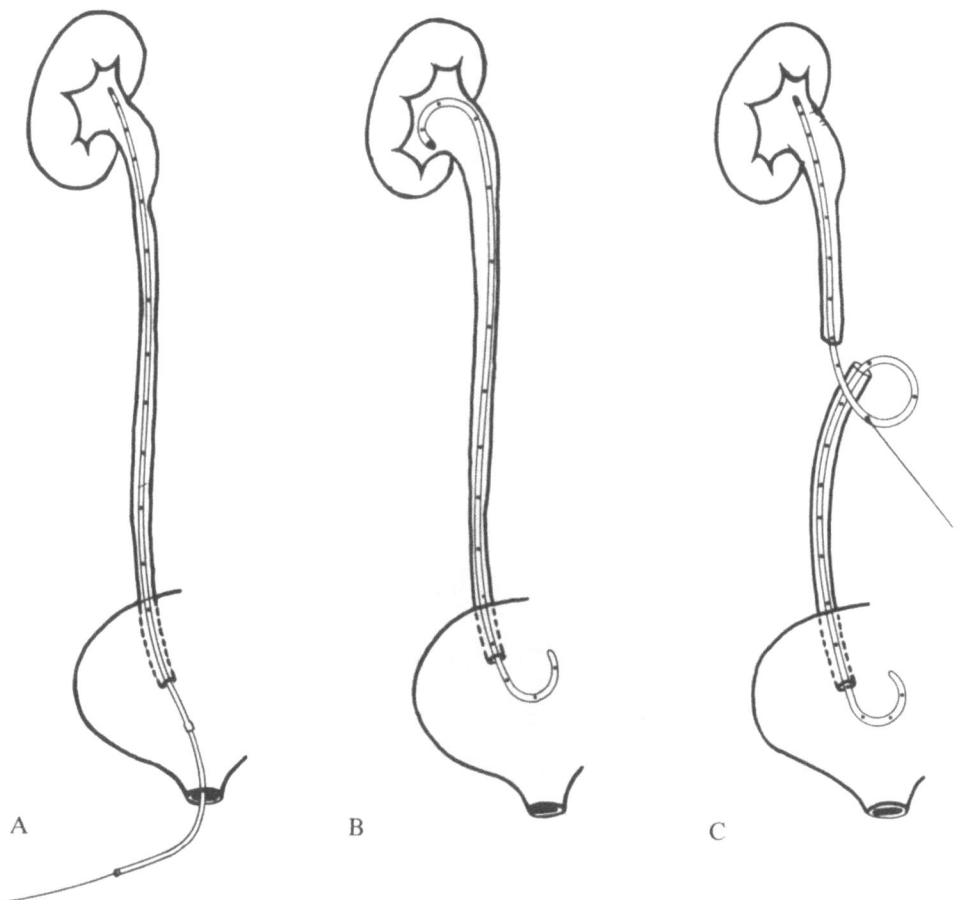

Fig. 3.5. Retrograde and intraoperative insertion of the double J stent. A, the guidewire straightens the stent; B, the stent positioner prevents stent dislodgement as the guidewire is withdrawn. The distal J coils spontaneously in the bladder once the guidewire is removed; C, intraoperatively, threading the guidewire through side-ports straightens the stent and permits passage down into the bladder and up into the kidney. (From Finney R (1978) Experience with new-double-J ureteral catheter stent. J Urol 120:678–681, with permission.)

and breakage this polyethylene-based design is now made of polyurethane (Cook) or C-Flex (Van-tec). Four diameters (5, 6, 7 and 8F) and varying lengths are available (8–30 cm). As previously mentioned, although these two new plastics have a non-wetting smooth surface, they are more rigid and firmer than silicone. In addition, their longterm resistance to breakage and encrustation is unknown.

The Double Pigtail Stent kit includes a flexible tip guidewire, a graduated ureteral catheter and a stent positioner. Although the Double Pigtail and the Double J stents are similar in design, the Double Pigtail stent is closed at one end only, to allow retrograde passage: by trimming this end, passage may be achieved using the Seldinger technique (Fig. 3.6).

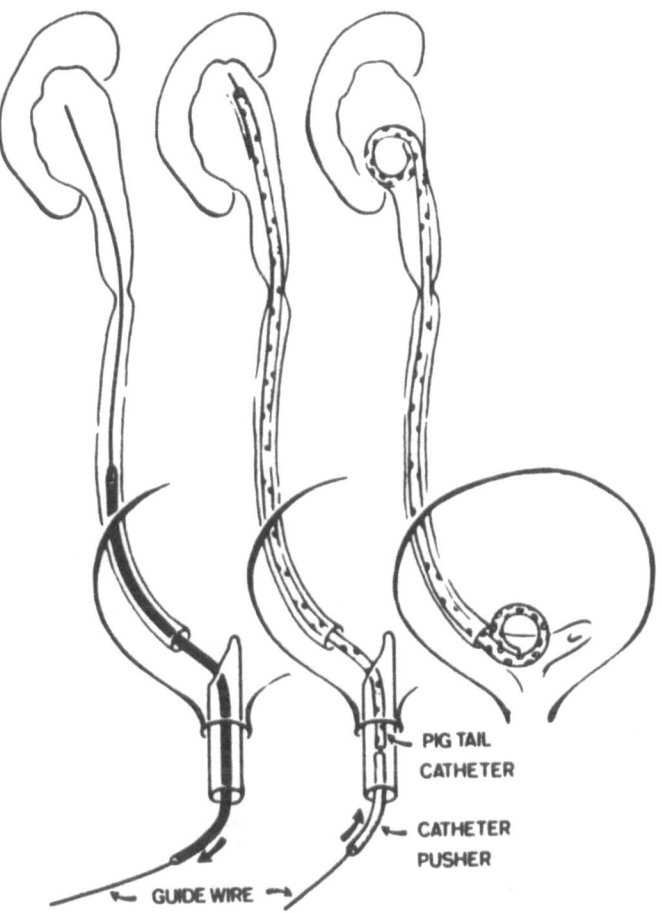

PIG TAIL
CATHETER

CATHETER
PUSHER

GUIDE WIRE

Fig. 3.6. Seldinger technique for endoscopic insertion of the Double Pigtail, Mardis, or the Uropass stent. The guidewire is passed up the ureter followed by a ureteric catheter. The "dilating" catheter is then withdrawn and the stent manipulated over the guidewire by a push catheter. Severe ureteric tortuosity may be overcome by insertion of the guidewire and ureteric catheter simultaneously. (Courtesy of HK Mardis.)

Coil Stent

In 1983, the "Coil Stent" (Bard) was introduced (Fig. 3.4E). This stent is a further modification of the Double J and Double Pigtail designs. The salient feature of this stent relates to the distal end which is coiled into four turns. At the proximal or renal end there is one retention coil, designed to prevent downward migration. Following insertion into the ureter, the excess coils in the bladder end can be removed endoscopically or, if stent length can be determined accurately before insertion, the excess coils can be removed then. As with the Double J and Double Pigtail stents the Coil Stent is made in various diameters (5, 6, 7 and 8F), but there is only one length, which is adjustable from 12 cm to 30 cm.

Uropass Stent

In 1984 the Uropass Stent (Surgitek, Racine, Wisconsin, USA) was introduced (Fig. 3.4D). This Silitek plastic stent (by the use of a novel proximal tip design) may be passed either over a guidewire (Seldinger technique) or in standard retrograde fashion, and may be particularly useful for percutaneous stent placement. The Silitek plastic is softer and more elastic than other plastic stents and should produce less tissue reaction.

Nephrostomy Stents

Universal Stent

Although most commercial stents to date are of the internal variety and are supplied in various materials, diameters, and lengths, Smith has suggested that it may cause logistics problems for a hospital to stock them all, for reasons of space and money. In addition, for patients with inoperable ureteral obstruction who live some distance away from a hospital, occlusion may result in terminal uraemia or sepsis before stent replacement or other surgical intervention is possible (Smith 1982a,c).

This has lead to the development of a "Universal" silicone stent (Heyer-Schulte) which requires placement through a percutaneous nephrostomy (Fig. 3.7a). The Universal stent provides internal drainage similar to the other designs but the proximal end is brought out as a nephrostomy, thus allowing a "safety" mechanism for decompression of the kidney (by the patient) if the internal part of the stent should become occluded. This stent is available in one diameter (8F) and one length (79 cm).

The Universal stent, because of its external nephrostomy component, may be more prone to infection and encrustation than other forms of purely internal drainage. An advantage of this design is that it may be possible to clear the blockage (if not firmly plugged) by percutaneous irrigation if the stent becomes occluded, or if stent replacement is required, a guidewire may be passed through the stent into the bladder allowing the old stent to be removed and a new one to be threaded over the guidewire in antegrade fashion (Smith 1982c).

Nephrostent

The most recent stent to become available, the Nephrostent, is somewhat similar in configuration to the Universal stent except that it is designed to be passed intra-operatively (Fig. 3.7b). Basically, it is a Double J Stent with an attached nephrostomy tube. A trocar is supplied to pass the stent through the renal parenchyma and flank musculature. This stent has a proximal and distal J to help prevent migration and it can also be passed over a wire by the percutaneous route. Both Cook and Van-Tec also produce stents combined with a nephrostomy which are designed to be placed by percutaneous techniques.

Caution is advisable when using percutaneous nephrostomy stents in patients too ill to tolerate open surgery. Each percutaneous manipulation carries some risk of possible haemorrhage and urine extravasation which may then require open surgical intervention. The potential risks must be weighed against possible advantages.

The various types, sizes, and manufacturers (USA) of stents are listed in Table 3.1.

Indications for Ureteral Stents

Management of the patient with pain or uraemia secondary to ureteric obstruction has been a challenge to the urological surgeon for decades. These individuals can be extremely ill and, as a result may be poor candidates for surgery. Supravesical diversion either as a temporary or permanent measure has often resulted in significant morbidity and mortality. In 1973, Grabstald and McPhee reported a 3% operative mortality in 170 patients who underwent surgical nephrostomy for diversion of malignant ureteral obstruction. Of these patients, 43% died before leaving the hospital as a result of complications of the procedure or superimposed progression of the disease. Brin and associates (1975) also were discouraged by the finding that 41% of their patients who required surgical nephrostomy died of complications. This has led some authors to suggest limiting indications for palliative urinary diversion (Holden et al. 1979).

The introduction of ureteric stents has made invasive surgical management of the patient with malignant urinary obstruction less urgent, and in selected patients, has allowed adequate palliation in the face of limited survival (Singh et al. 1979; Hepperlen et al. 1979). In addition, for those individuals with acute ureteral obstruction secondary to a benign process, the ureteric stent has improved not only quality and quantity of life, but has also allowed earlier discharge from hospital (Finney 1982; Andriole et al. 1984).

In patients who have sustained injury to the ureter either as a direct result of surgery, or as a consequence of external trauma, the stent has been proclaimed as the "safety valve" which prevents undue urine extravasation of the site of injury or repair. This reduces the potential for secondary infection, ischaemia, and scarring, and again allows earlier patient ambulation and discharge. The indications for ureteral stents therefore, include:

Ureteral obstruction
  Neoplasm
  Stone disease
  Retroperitoneal fibrosis
  Uretero-vesical obstruction
  UPJ obstruction
  Ureteric stricture
  Pregnancy
  Miscellaneous conditions

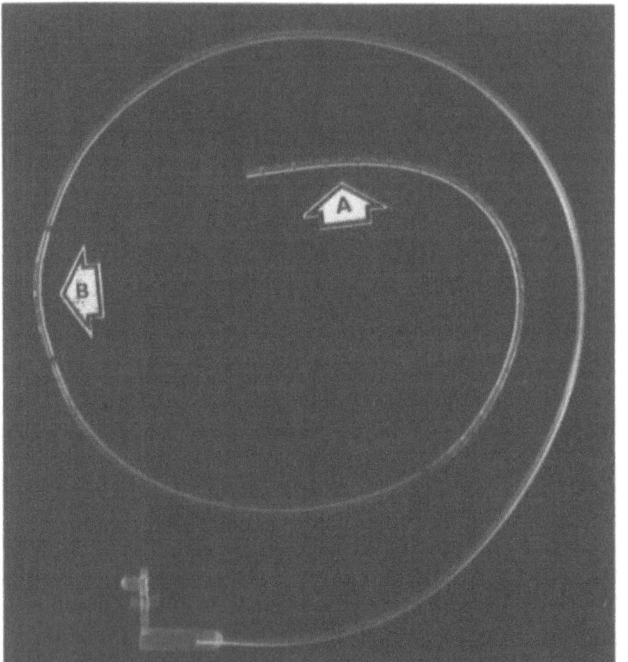

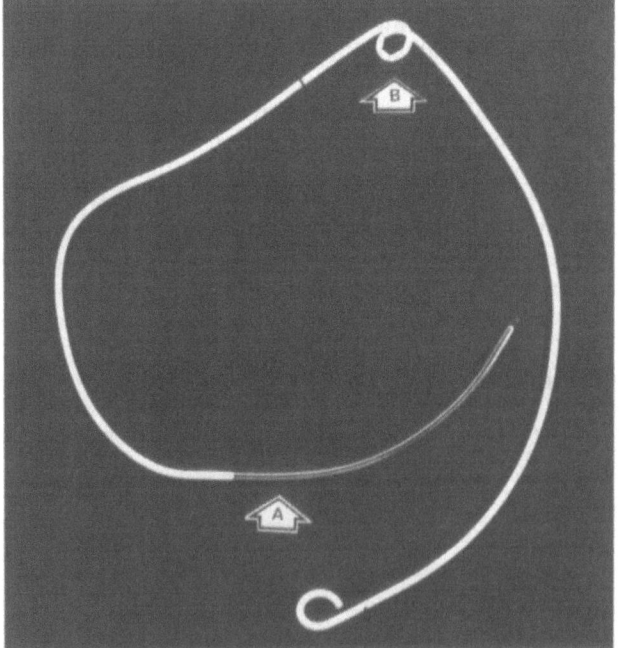

Fig. 3.7. **a** The Universal stent is designed to be passed through a percutaneous nephrostomy and down the ureter into the bladder. The bladder end (A) may be trimmed to the proper length while mid stent holes (B) are positioned within the renal pelvis. **b** The nephrostent is designed for placement in the operating room. A trocar (A) allows passage of the stent out through the renal cortex and the flank muscles. A mid stent "loop" (B) which is perforated with holes is positioned within the renal pelvis while the ureteric portion is passed in to the bladder over a guidewire.

Caution is advisable when using percutaneous nephrostomy stents in patients too ill to tolerate open surgery. Each percutaneous manipulation carries some risk of possible haemorrhage and urine extravasation which may then require open surgical intervention. The potential risks must be weighed against possible advantages.

The various types, sizes, and manufacturers (USA) of stents are listed in Table 3.1.

Indications for Ureteral Stents

Management of the patient with pain or uraemia secondary to ureteric obstruction has been a challenge to the urological surgeon for decades. These individuals can be extremely ill and, as a result may be poor candidates for surgery. Supravesical diversion either as a temporary or permanent measure has often resulted in significant morbidity and mortality. In 1973, Grabstald and McPhee reported a 3% operative mortality in 170 patients who underwent surgical nephrostomy for diversion of malignant ureteral obstruction. Of these patients, 43% died before leaving the hospital as a result of complications of the procedure or superimposed progression of the disease. Brin and associates (1975) also were discouraged by the finding that 41% of their patients who required surgical nephrostomy died of complications. This has led some authors to suggest limiting indications for palliative urinary diversion (Holden et al. 1979).

The introduction of ureteric stents has made invasive surgical management of the patient with malignant urinary obstruction less urgent, and in selected patients, has allowed adequate palliation in the face of limited survival (Singh et al. 1979; Hepperlen et al. 1979). In addition, for those individuals with acute ureteral obstruction secondary to a benign process, the ureteric stent has improved not only quality and quantity of life, but has also allowed earlier discharge from hospital (Finney 1982; Andriole et al. 1984).

In patients who have sustained injury to the ureter either as a direct result of surgery, or as a consequence of external trauma, the stent has been proclaimed as the "safety valve" which prevents undue urine extravasation of the site of injury or repair. This reduces the potential for secondary infection, ischaemia, and scarring, and again allows earlier patient ambulation and discharge. The indications for ureteral stents therefore, include:

Ureteral obstruction
  Neoplasm
  Stone disease
  Retroperitoneal fibrosis
  Uretero-vesical obstruction
  UPJ obstruction
  Ureteric stricture
  Pregnancy
  Miscellaneous conditions

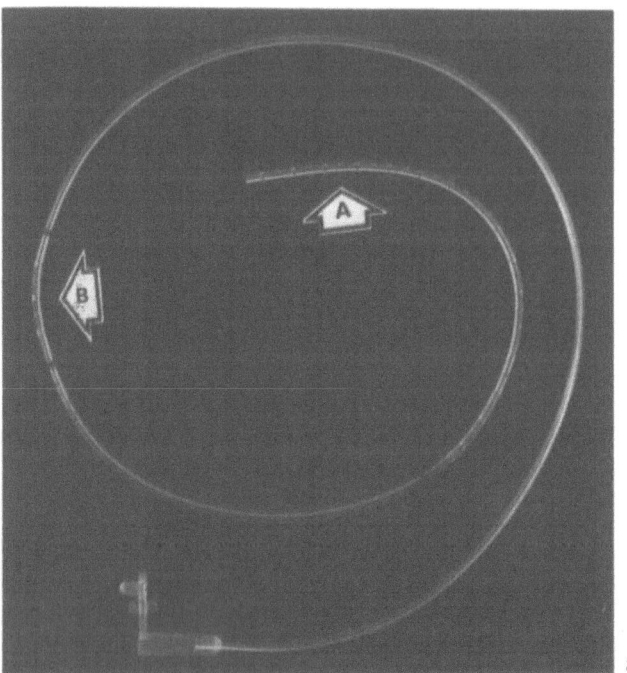

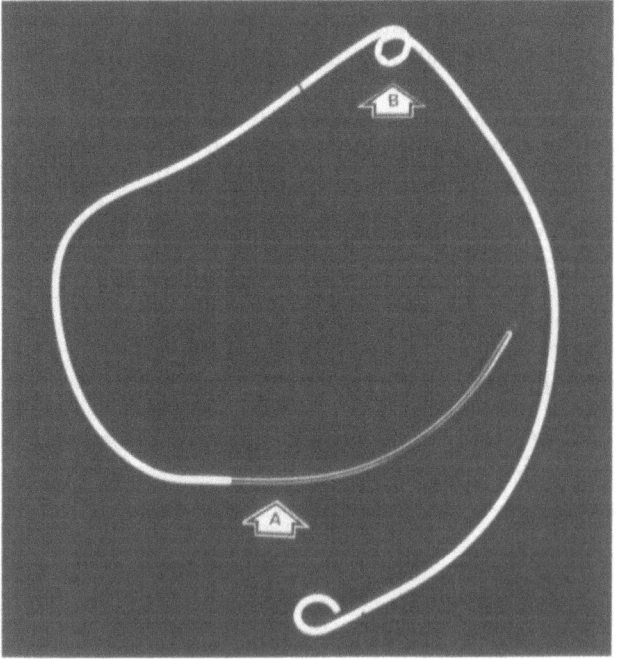

Fig. 3.7. **a** The Universal stent is designed to be passed through a percutaneous nephrostomy and down the ureter into the bladder. The bladder end (A) may be trimmed to the proper length while mid stent holes (B) are positioned within the renal pelvis. **b** The nephrostent is designed for placement in the operating room. A trocar (A) allows passage of the stent out through the renal cortex and the flank muscles. A mid stent "loop" (B) which is perforated with holes is positioned within the renal pelvis while the ureteric portion is passed in to the bladder over a guidewire.

Table 3.1. Commercial Stents Available in the United States of America

Manufacturer	Name	Sizes (F)	Lengths (cm)	Composition	Radiopaque	Kit	Placement[a]
Surgitek Inc. 3037 Mt. Pleasant Street Racine, WI 53404, USA	Double J stent	6, 7, 8.5	12, 16, 20, 24, 26, 28, 30	Silicone	Yes	Wire guide stent positioner	E, I
	Percutaneous Double J stent	8.5	26, 28	Silicone	Yes	Mineral oil stent positioner	P
	Uropass obstruction stent	7, 8.5	22, 24, 26, 28	Silitek (Plastic)	Yes	Double diameter wire guide	E, I
	Nephro-Stent (Nephrostomy stent)	8.5	27 (Stent) 30 (Percutaneous portion)	Silicone	Yes	Trocar wire guide stopcock skin disc and tie	I
Heyer-Schulte (Mentor) 600 Pine Avenue Goleta Ave, CA 93017	Gibbons stent	8, 9.5	15, 23, 29	Silicone	Markers	Wire guide stent positioner nipple	E
	Universal stent	8	79 (Trimmable)	Silicone	Markers		P
Cook Urological (V.P.I.) 1100 West Morgan Street P.O. Box 227 Spencer, IN 47460	Double Pigtail	5	8 to 30 Even	Polyurethane (Plastic)	Yes	Wire guide stent positioner	E, I
	Double Pigtail	6, 7, 8	18 to 30 (Even)				
Van-Tec P.O. Box 26 Spencer, IN 47460	Mardis stent	5	8–30 (Even)	C-Flex	Yes	Wire guide stent positioner	E, I
	Mardis stent	6, 7, 8	18–30 (Even)	C-Flex	Yes		
	Combination Nephrostomy stent	7, 8	30 (Stent) 27 (Percutaneous portion)	C-Flex	Yes		P
Bard Urological C.R. Bard Inc. Murry Hill, NJ 07974	Coil stent	5, 6, 7, 8	30 (Adjustable)	Silicone	Yes	Wire guide stent positioner	E, I
Dow Corning Medical Products Division Midland, Michigan 48640	Medical grade tubing	Numerous diameters	Up to 15 meters	Silicone	No		

[a] E, Endoscopic (Retrograde); I, Intra-operative; P, Percutaneous (Antegrade).

Post-operative drainage
  Complicated pyelolithotomy
  Complicated ureterolithotomy
  Surgery on a solitary kidney
  Pyeloplasty
  Uretero ureterostomy
  Complicated uretero-neocystostomy
  Uretero-intestinal anastomosis
Upper urinary tract injury
  Penetrating
  Blunt
Ureteral fistulae
  Uretero-cutaneous
  Uretero-vaginal

Malignant Obstruction

As previously discussed, the first hand-made internal stents were fashioned in order to provide palliative drainage of ureters obstructed by malignant tumours primarily from the bladder, prostate, uterus, ovaries and intestinal tract (Brown and Harrison 1951; Zimskind et al. 1967; Marmar 1970; Orikasa et al. 1973). While stenting can be beneficial to some, careful thought must be given as to the quality of life that each individual will lead following placement of the stent. Prolongation of life in association with severe disabling pain is *not* advisable. In addition, once the stent is in place, it is invariably difficult later in the progression of disease to suggest stent removal with either the patient or family.

Ureteric obstruction from malignancy should be anticipated whenever possible, and confirmed by early intravenous urography (Fig. 3.8). Early stent placement preserves renal function, and can be accomplished once partial obstruction is first detected. Delay on the part of the physician or rapid tumour progression may make subsequent retrograde stent placement difficult or impossible, thereby requiring percutaneous placement at a later date when the patient may be acutely ill. Purely prophylactic stent placement is, however, also inadvisable.

An internal stent may also benefit the patient with partial ureteric obstruction who is receiving therapeutic external beam irradiation and/or chemotherapy. Swelling and degeneration of the malignant cells may produce rapid marked obstruction, and when this is anticipated stents can be implanted prior to treatment and then removed when the ureters appear to be open. If no tumour regression is noted, the stents can be left inlying and changed as required.

Obstetric Obstruction

By the second trimester of pregnancy, bilateral ureterohydronephrosis is seen radiographically with the dilatation occurring above the pelvic brim. This dilatation is accompanied by progressively poorer peristaltic activity until the eighth month when ureteric function stabilises (Williams 1982).

During this period, the occasional patient may develop a superimposed acute mechanical obstruction as a result of a renal calculous or external compression requiring narcotic analgesia and/or hospitalisation. The endoscopic placement of a ureteric stent under topical anaesthesia can frequently alleviate the pain and temporise until term delivery. Serial urines must be obtained to preclude infection (Fisher et al. 1982). Ureteric stents have also been recommended for treating obstruction occuring during pregnancy (Lowes et al. 1987).

Stone Disease

Acute obstruction of the ureter by a stone (urate or cystine) or a sloughed papilla may at times be managed non-surgically (Smith 1982c; Finney 1982;

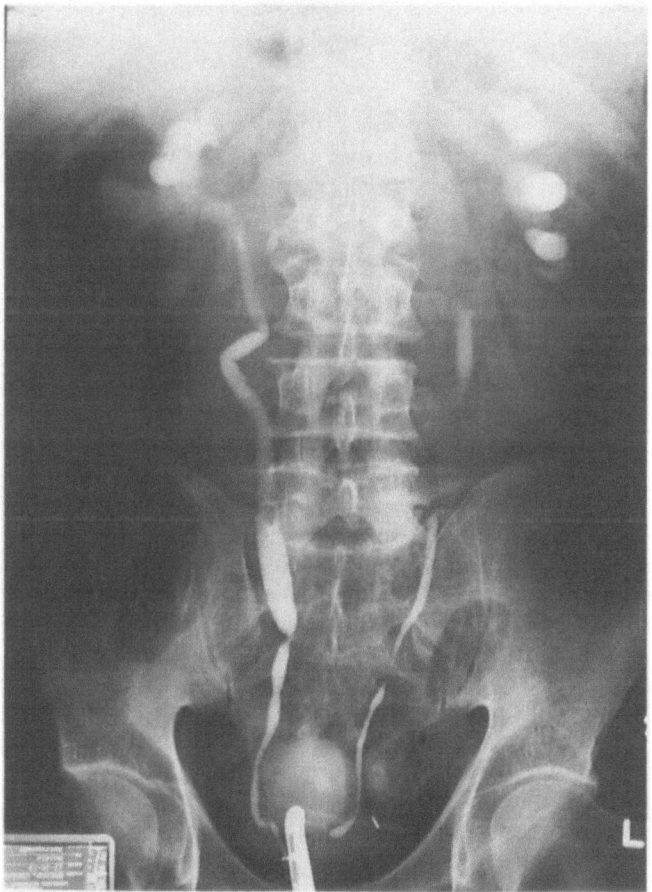

Fig. 3.8. a Radiograph of a patient having ureteric obstruction secondary to adenocarcinoma of the rectosigmoid colon. **b** (*page 54*) After endoscopic insertion of bilateral Mardis Ureteric Stents drainage was restored and renal function normalised. The patient had no further genitourinary problem until death. (From Mardis HK et al. (1979) Double pigtail ureteral stent. Urology 14:23–26, with permission.)

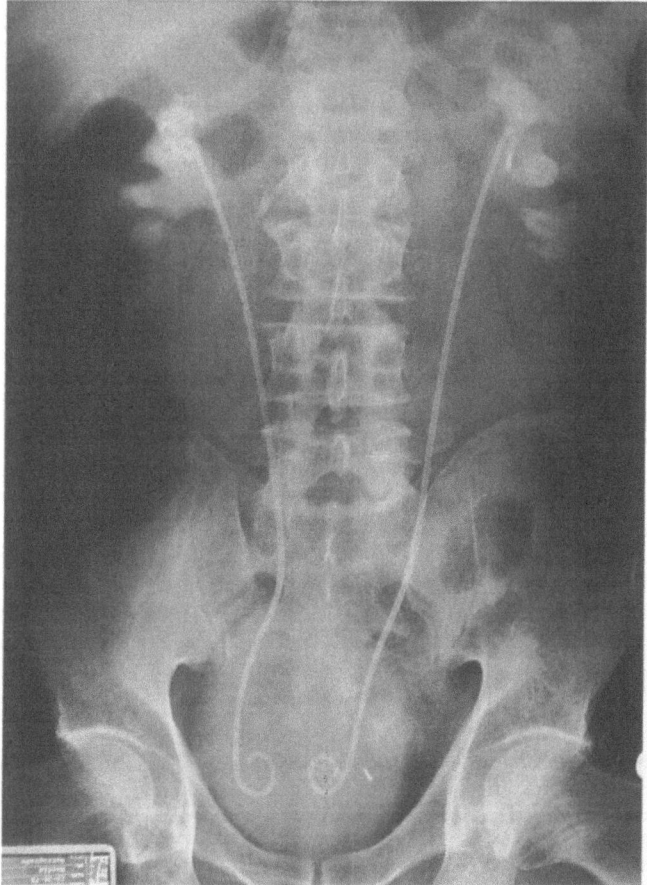

Fig. 3.8. b

Andriole et al. 1984). If a stent can be passed beyond the site of obstruction a urate or cystine stone can often be dissolved by chemolysis, including alkalinisation of the urine by diet and sodium bicarbonate. If this is not sufficient, pharmacological manipulation with carbonic anhydrase inhibitors or acetyl cysteine may also be used.

Patients with pyonephrosis secondary to stone obstruction and infection can present with acute sepsis, and occasionally in shock. If a stent can be passed endoscopically, this frequently provides sufficient time to treat the shock and infection and permits definitive surgery when the patient can better tolerate it (Brown and Harrison 1951; Finney 1978; Kearney et al. 1979). The use of stents in association with lithotripsy has introduced a new field of stent usage.

Ureteric Strictures

Strictures of the ureter have at times been treated by internal ureteric dilatation and/or internal stents (Orikasa et al. 1973; Barbaric et al. 1977; Smith et al. 1979; Bigongiari et al. 1979; Banner et al. 1983). A decade ago, Orikasa and associates described good (80%) short-term results in 13 patients. Eight patients had ureteric strictures secondary to surgery or radiation, and five had strictures secondary to tuberculosis.

More recently, Banner and associates reported their experience with dilating and stenting ureteric strictures which had formed as a result of earlier surgery. Twenty-three strictures were dilated and stented in conjunction with, or subsequent to, percutaneous nephrostomy, while four strictures were dilated and stented in retrograde fashion. Dilatation was accomplished by either a balloon catheter or flexible dilators (Cook, Van-Tec), and the strictures were then stented over a period ranging from 1 day to 6 months. Their overall success however, was only 48%. Three strictures which developed following ureterolithotomy were successfully treated, while only seven of eleven (64%) strictures which occurred following prior uretero-intestinal anastomoses were also corrected. Their results were less impressive when the strictures resulted from devascularization as a result of pelvic radiation and surgery (Banner et al. 1983).

These findings are not surprising when an analogy is made between the ureter and urethra, i.e., soft dilatation and longterm stenting of a urethral stricture with a urethric catheter does not necessarily preclude stricture recurrence. As uretero-renoscopy becomes widely used, direct vision internal ureterotomy followed by ureteric stenting may improve results, and in select cases eliminate the need for open surgical repair (Wickham and Miller 1983).

Ureteral Surgery

An internal stent following a ureteric anastomosis, or surgery associated with a solitary kidney can at times eliminate the need for a diverting nephrostomy (Dorr et al. 1974; Sieben et al. 1978; Pitts and Peterson 1981). A water-tight closure using closely spaced absorbable suture frequently permits the patient to be ambulant soon after surgery, without drainage paraphernalia. Although extraperitoneal tissue drains should always be used, reduced or absent leakage permits early drain removal and more repaid patient discharge. Usually the stent is removed in 6–8 weeks, or, when complete healing has occurred. It should be remembered that most absorbable sutures require at least 4 weeks to dissolve and complete healing cannot occur until this has taken place.

Correction of a complicated obstruction of the uretero-pelvic junction, where a significant leak of urine may be likely, is an ideal procedure for ureteric stent, although, for routine procedures this is not recommended (Smart 1979). Again, the largest calibre catheter which the ureter can accept should be used to provide adequate drainage without ischaemia (8–9F in the adult). In these cases, the stent may be passed from the renal pelvis to the bladder just prior to completion of the closure. The use of a small nephrostomy tube may also have some merit. The nephrostomy may then be clamped after several days and removed if no urine extravasation occurs. The stent can then be left in place for 1–3 months to assure proper healing once the periureteral inflammation has subsided. It may then be removed endoscopically under topical anesthesia. Longterm stent placement to dilate a previously failed pyeloplasty has not been uniformly successful (Banner et al. 1983), nor is it of uniform benefit in the surgical correction of reflux (Fort et al. 1983).

Although some transplant surgeons have recommended routine use of an internal ureteric stent at the time of renal transplant, the fact that most resorbable sutures require at least 4 weeks to dissolve should be recalled.

Correction of a complicated ureteropelvic-junction obstruction where a significant urine leak may be likely is an ideal procedure for a ureteric stent, although, for routine procedures this is not recommended (Smart 1979). Again, the largest calibre catheter which the ureter can accept should be used to provide adequate drainage without ischaemia (8–9F in the adult). In these cases, the stent may be passed from the renal pelvis to the bladder just prior to completion of the closure. The use of a small nephrostomy tube may also have some merit. The nephrostomy may then be clamped after several days and removed if no urine extravasation occurs. The stent can then be left in place for 1–3 months to assure proper healing once the periureteral inflammation has subsided. It may then be removed endoscopically under topical anaesthesia. Longterm placement of the stent to dilate a previously failed pyeloplasty has not been uniformly successful (Banner et al. 1983), nor is it of uniform benefit in the surgical correction of reflux (Fort et al. 1983).

Although some transplant surgeons have recommended routine use of an internal ureteric stent at the time of renal transplant, the majority reserve stent placement for those cases in which a secondary uretero-neocystostomy becomes necessary because of a urine leak (Berger et al. 1980; Tremann and Marchioro 1977). Shorter stents for this purpose are available (Finney 1982).

Retroperitoneal Fibrosis

The surgical management of retroperitoneal fibrosis is often unsatisfactory. These ureters are frequently encased and compressed by dense fibrous tissue which not only results in obstruction (patients not infrequently present after renal function has already been significantly impaired), but also compromises the ureteric blood supply. Mobilisation of the ureters from this fibrous plaque is difficult, and often they do not function properly following lateralisation or intraperitonealisation (Ormond 1981).

In retroperitoneal fibrosis, the early placement of bilateral internal ureteric stents can usually be accomplished easily and provides free drainage of the kidneys. This allows time to stabilise the patient, make the proper diagnosis, evaluate renal function, and decide on further therapy. Occasionally, it may be advisable to leave the stents inlying for a prolonged period following surgical exploration and biopsy to allow the inflammatory process time to resolve spontaneously.

Urinary Intestinal Diversion

Special Single J stents (Surgitek) are specifically available for use during urinary diversion into an isolated segment of bowel or the intact sigmoid colon (Fig. 3.9a). These stents have a retaining J in the proximal end only, and are 95 cm long such that the distal protruding end may be trimmed to proper length. Drainage holes are supplied only in the proximal end of the stent to allow easy flushing as well as retrograde pyelography in the event of significant urine leakage (Fig. 3.9b).

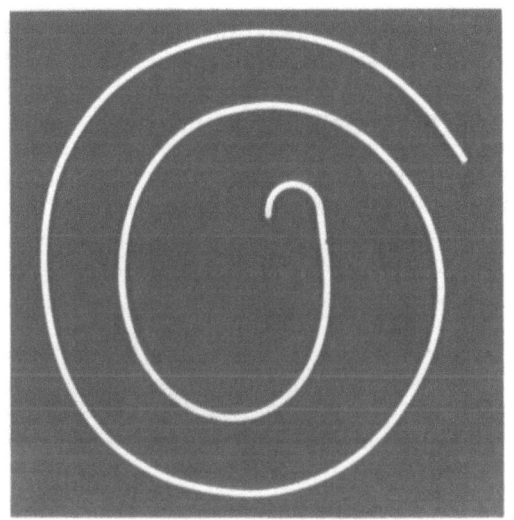

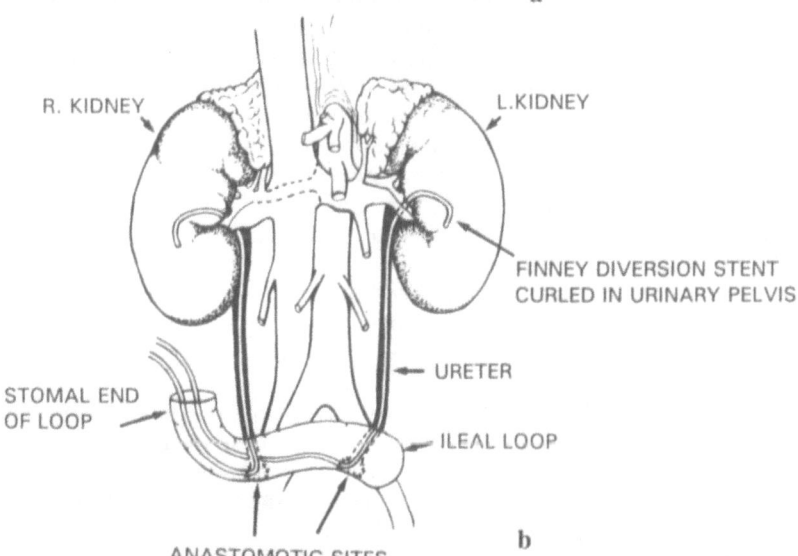

Fig. 3.9. a The diversion stent has side-ports in the proximal J end only. Additional holes have been omitted since these may become plugged with bowel mucus which can lead to stent obstruction and sepsis. **b** Diversion stents significantly reduce leakage at the anastomosis of the ureter to the bowel which can be a very serious complication for any intestinal urinary diversion. (From Jarowenko MV et al. (1983) Use of single J diversion stents in intestinal urinary diversion. Urology 22:369–370, with permission.)

Prior to completion of the uretero-intestinal anastomoses, the Single J stents are passed to the kidney and then through the lumen of the bowel to the outside. The protruding ends are then sutured to the skin at the stoma site to prevent accidental dislodgement, but remain inside the urine collection bag. The Nephrostent and the Universal stent can also be used for this purpose (Smith 1982c).

Single J Diversion stents have significantly decreased the incidence of leakage at the uretero-intestinal anastomosis which can be a grave complication. In the postoperative period, bilateral urine cultures can be obtained as well as bilateral creatinine clearance studies if so desired. Usually, the stents are removed prior to discharge (Finney 1982).

The use of standard stents having holes along their entire length is *not* advisable as that portion which traverses the bowel may become rapidly plugged with mucus, promoting rather than decreasing leakage at the anastamosis.

Stent Placement

Endoscopic Stent Placement

Internal ureteric stents have become an established therapeutic procedure in the acute or longterm management of many patients with ureteral obstruction or injury (Andriole et al. 1984). Although early models had major problems with placement, stent migration, encrustation, and compression, at the time these were acceptable complications in the management of the acutely ill or terminal patient in whom external urinary diversion would be the only other alternative (Zimskind et al. 1967; Marmar 1970; Orikasa et al. 1973).

Each of the currently manufactured internal stents have significantly decreased the aforementioned problems and their use has become rapidly accepted by the urological community.

All internal designs are specifically devised for endoscopic placement which, although conventionally is best done under spinal or general anaesthesia, can also be performed under topical anaesthesia. This may be advantageous for the acutely ill, poor-risk patient.

The two primary techniques for catheter placement (Retrograde and Seldinger) have been well described (Figs. 3.5, 3.6). These techniques arose as a natural outgrowth of much trial and error in order to insert open or close-ended straight polyethylene or silicone tubing past the site of obstruction or injury (Zimskind et al. 1967; Orikasa et al. 1973).

In all cases the largest calibre stent that will bypass the obstruction should be used. In order to maximise flow, Gibbons suggested that prior to placement of his stent, ureteral dilatation should be performed with successively larger bore catheters or dilators to allow the permanent catheter easily to bypass the obstruction (Gibbons 1982). This is not usually necessary for most of the other designs, however the practice is useful prior to the passage of any ureteric stent (Becker and Schellhammer 1982; Finney 1982).

All stents can be inserted through a number 24F panendoscope or cystoscope. Most kits come equipped with a wire stylet which is either inserted into the distal end of the stent and passed up its entire length (Gibbons, Double J, Coil Stent, Uropass) or is passed up the ureter first, allowing the stent to be threaded over it (Double Pigtail, Mardis, Uropass) (Gibbons et al. 1976; Finney 1978; Mardis et al. 1979). The stylet offers two advantages: (1) it straightens the coiled ends of the stent to allow placement in the ureter, and

(2) it acts as a rigid guide to facilitate stent placement through the obstruction. Prior to insertion of the stylet in the lumen of a silicone stent, sterile mineral oil should be injected to facilitate its removal. The mineral oil decreases the inherent friction between the silicone elastomer and the metal, especially when they are wet. Lubrication of the outside of the stent is also helpful to facilitate stent insertion.

Most kits also supply a push catheter or "stent positioner" which is threaded over the stylet wire behind the stent. This is used to push the stent up into the ureter and allows stylet removal without dislodging the stent itself.

Because internal stents create a freely refluxing system from the bladder into the upper collecting system, stent patency and position may be checked by a static cystogram. In some cases a higher than normal intravesical pressure may be required to produce reflux and occasionally as much as 100 cm of water pressure is necessary in order to visualise contrast reflux into the upper collecting system. An alternative method of determining stent patency is to watch the efflux of previously administered intravenous methylene blue or indigo carmine from the stent orifice. In the presence of a solitary kidney, adequate drainage through the stent may be monitored by periodic determination of the serum creatinine clearance (Finney 1982).

Operative Stent Placement

Four of the modern internal ureteral stents, including the Double J, Uropass and Double Pigtail and Mardis variations are particularly useful during open procedures in the upper urinary tract. In addition to bypassing obstruction resulting from malignancy, stone disease, retroperitoneal fibrosis or trauma, intra-operative placement of these suspension stents can be employed in conjunction with plastic repair of the (proximal or distal) ureter and renal pelvis (Maar et al. 1976; Sieben et al. 1978; Fort et al. 1983). In the case of the Double J stent, each end of the wire stylet is passed into an appropriate side hole and is abutted against each of the closed ends (Fig. 3.5C). The appropriate length stent is next threaded in the ureter, first in one direction and then in the other. Double J stent placement can be easily performed through incisions in the renal pelvis or ureter or during procedures in the urinary bladder (Finney 1978). In the case of the Double Pigtail stent, the stylet is passed first above and then below and the stent is then threaded over it (Fig. 3.10) (Mardis et al. 1979). Because of its tapered but open ends, the Uropass (Fig. 3.4C) stent can be inserted by either method.

During any intra-operative procedure, precaution is advised to make sure that the entire "J" or "Pigtail" of the stent has reached the bladder below and the renal pelvis above. This can be ensured by choosing a stent that is several centimetres longer than the ureter to be traversed. Prior to stent insertion, ureteral length from the ureterotomy site to the bladder can be accurately determined by threading a graduated ureteral catheter (4–5F) into the ureter while aspirating with a syringe. When urine appears, the bladder has just been entered and the appropriate length, usually 4–5 cm longer than the ureter, can be inserted to allow adequate coiling within the bladder (Finney 1982). If only the stent tip reaches the bladder the J or Pigtail cannot form and upward migration often occurs.

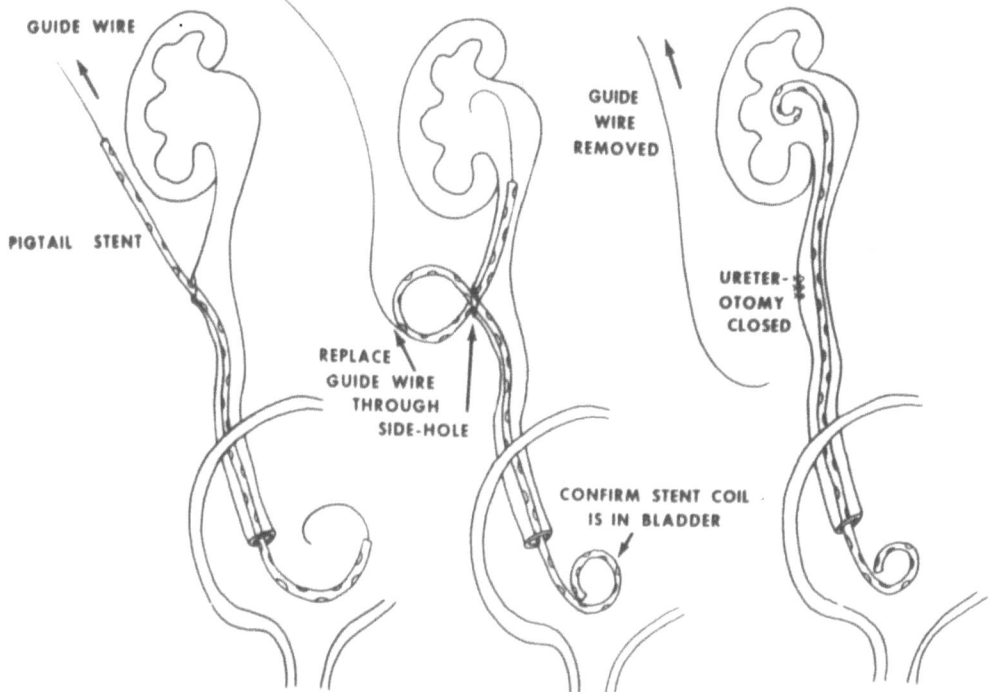

Fig. 3.10. Intra-operatively, the Double Pigtail, Mardis, and Uropass stents are inserted using a modified Seldinger technique. A guidewire is first passed down to the bladder and a portion of the stent is threaded over this. Removal of the wire allows the distal loop to reform. The same technique positions the proximal loop within the renal pelvis. (From Mardis HK et al. (1982) Polyethylene double-pigtail ureteral stents. Urol Clin North Am 9:95–101, with permission.)

Surgically placed stents can usually be left in place for 6–12 weeks to allow for complete tissue healing. At the proper time endoscopic stent removal can usually be accomplished on an out-patient basis (Finney 1982).

Percutaneous Stent Placement

Although retrograde stent insertion is the initial technique of choice, not infrequently (in up to one-third of cases) the procedure is unsuccessful. Causes of failure may include (1) inability to see the ureteral orifice (2) significant lateral displacement of the ureter (3) severe ureteric stenosis or obstruction and (4) an impassable ureteral fistula. Antegrade stent placement through a percutaneous nephrostomy will frequently overcome most of these difficulties (Stables 1982).

A "blind" technique for percutaneous insertion of a nephrostomy tube had been described as early as 1955 by Goodwin and associates, but it required sophisticated imaging equipment and techniques to allow consistently successful placement of angiographic needles and larger bore catheters through the renal parenchyma into the collecting system (Bartley et al. 1965; Jonson et al. 1972). These techniques have not only advanced both the diagnosis and therapy of upper tract obstruction but have also allowed the development of even more sophisticated techniques to thread catheters and stents down the ureter past the obstructing lesion. As a result, in many instances the internal stent has precluded use of the nephrostomy itself (Mardis 1965; Bigongiari et al. 1980a,b; Fritzsche et al. 1981; Levine et al. 1982; Elyanderani et al. 1982b).

In general, nephrostomy and stent insertion can be performed under topical anaesthesia which may be of particular advantage to the poor-risk patient. The first stage of the procedure, the percutaneous nephrostomy, may be performed under fluoroscopic, ultrasound or computed tomography scan control (Lang et al. 1979; Smith et al. 1978, 1979a,b; Mazer et al. 1979; Elyanderani et al. 1982a,b). Prior to insertion of the nephrostomy tube, each patient is screened for bleeding tendencies. In addition, if there is any suspicion of infection antibotics are prescribed pre-operatively (Smith et al. 1979).

Although percutaneous stent placement had been successfully reported in anecdotal cases and animal models previously (Barbaric et al. 1977; Stables 1982), two of the clinical innovators in stent techniques, Smith and Bigongiari, independently and about the same time used the Seldinger method to thread flexible, or floppy, tipped rigid guidewires down the ureter past the site of obstruction and into the bladder. In a second stage a stent was then either threaded or pulled up the ureter in retrograde fashion (Fig. 3.11) (Smith et al. 1978, 1979a,b; Bigongiari et al. 1978, 1979, 1980a,b). In Smith's description, PTFE dilators (up to 8F) followed by a 7F angiographic catheter were first advanced over the guidewire in order to dilate both the tract and the site of obstruction. After 24 h, the guidewire and catheter were retrieved cystoscopically per urethrum; a 5F filiform and a 10F follower followed by a Gibbons stent were then attached to the distal end of the angiographic catheter

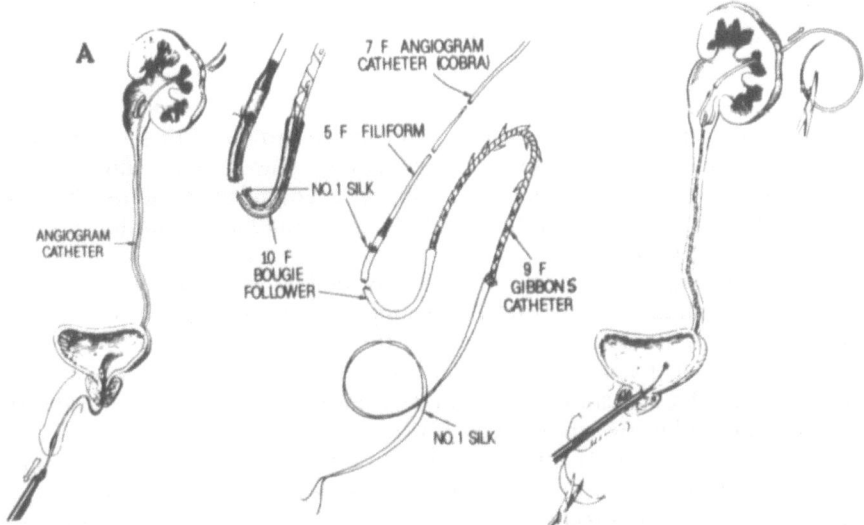

Fig. 3.11. The two-stage percutaneous and retrograde technique for placement of the Gibbons Stent. (From Smith AD et al. (1978) Introduction of the Gibbons ureteral stent facilitated by antecedent percutaneous Nephrostomy. J Urol 120:543–44, with permission.)

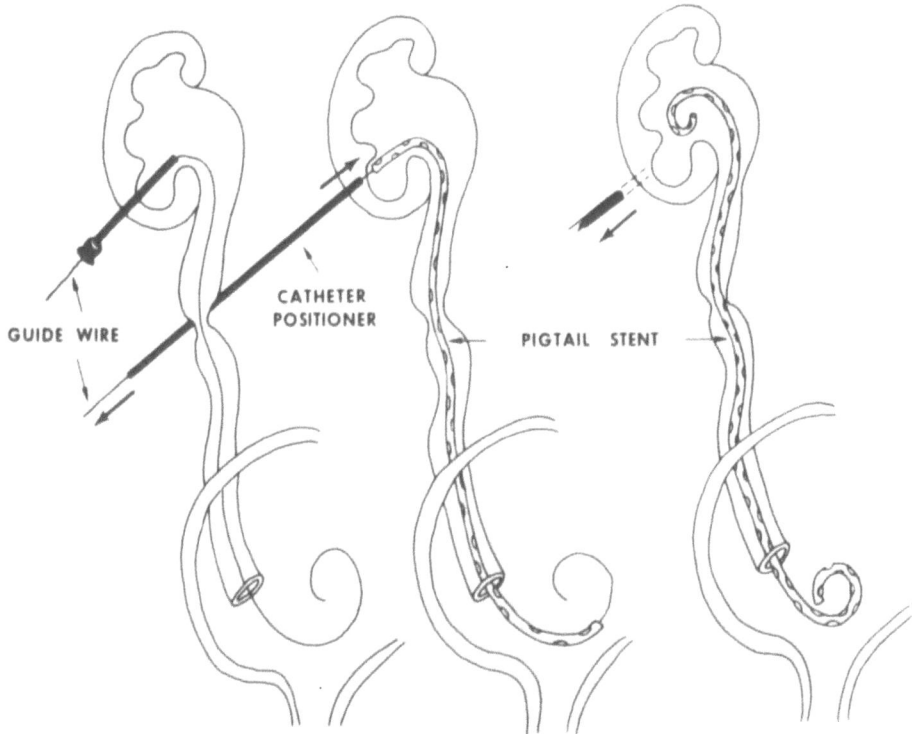

Fig. 3.12. Percutaneous one-stage stent insertion (double pigtail/Mardis uropass, double J percutaneous) is accomplished by positioning a guidewire down the ureter and into the bladder. The stent is then threaded over this wire until its distal segment is also within the bladder. The guidewire is then removed. (From Mardis HK et al. (1982) Polyethylene double-pigtail ureteral stents. Urol Clin North Am 9:95–101, with permission.)

which was pulled back into the bladder and up the ureter until the stent was wedged above the site of obstruction. The angiographic catheter, filiform and follower were subsequently detached. This is a complicated multistep procedure and should not be attempted without careful reading of Smith's description (Smith et al. 1979b).

In the intervening years, this cumbersome and occasionally difficult technique has been simplified such that the second stage of retrograde stent placement is frequently no longer required for the newer suspension-type stents. After percutaneous passage of the guidewire to the bladder, the catheter positioner is used to position the stent (Uropass, Double J PC, Mardis or Double Pigtail) within the ureter (Fig. 3.12).

Percutaneous insertion of internal ureteric stents is now a widely accepted procedure. Recent literature suggests that when using either the Double J or Double Pigtail stents, the technique can be successfully employed in more than 90% of failed endoscopic cases (Mazer et al. 1979; Smith et al. 1979a; Fowler et al. 1980; Elyanderani et al. 1982a; Banner et al. 1983). These techniques are also currently used to insert the new nephrostomy stents as well, although the softer silicone may make one-stage insertion more difficult (Lang et al. 1979; Smith 1982a,c).

Complications

Stent Insertion

Endoscopic stent placement is usually no more difficult than passing a standard ureteric catheter, but in the face of obstruction, infection, and haematuria adequate preparation and considerable patience may be required. Silicone stents (Double J, Gibbons, Coil stent) have a high coefficient of friction with metal and, as already mentioned, it is advisable to lubricate the stent and the guidewire with sterile mineral oil prior to insertion. Plastic stents (Uropass, Double Pigtail) may not require additional lubrication. The smallest endoscope (21 or 24F) which can contain the stent should be used to reduce the possibility of traumatic haematuria and to prevent the stent from buckling inside the endoscope sheath during retrograde passage. The rubber endoscope nipple should be large enough to allow the stent easily into the endoscope but not so large as to permit significant leakage.

In the patient having an invasive cancer of the bladder trigone or severe trabeculation and diverticulae, locating the ureteric orifices can be most difficult and considerable patience and prolonged observation may be necessary. Often the renal function of an obstructed system is decreased to the point where intravenous methylene blue is not concentrated by the kidney to a sufficient degree to allow visualisation, and very careful observation for a weak jet of urine may be necessary to identify the ureteric orifice.

If the ureteric orifices cannot be located by observation then gentle probing may be successful. In the presence of prostatic carcinoma the ureters are often more lateral than normal. If only one ureter is to be stented but is obscured, its orifice is usually in the mirror image position, or, somewhat more lateral than the unobstructed orifice.

Once the orifice has been visualised it is often prudent to first pass a 5 or 6F standard ureteric catheter and then successively dilate with larger catheters until the stent size has been reached (Gibbons 1982; Finney 1982; Becker and Schellhammer 1982). Tapered dilators or a balloon catheter are also quite satisfactory for this purpose. If the stent itself cannot be passed even with dilation then the largest size standard ureteric catheter which can be threaded up the ureter may be left in place for 1 to 2 days, after which the stent may be more readily passed. Again, patience is the key. Too vigorous an attempt to pass a stent through the intramural ureter or through an obstruction is likely to produce a false passage or even frank ureteric perforation (Kidd et al. 1980). A severely kinked or tortuous ureter above an inferior ureteric obstruction may best be managed with the Gibbons stent; however, a flexible tipped guidewire may successfully traverse a tortuous ureter after which a suspension-type stent may be passed over the wire by using the Seldinger technique (Mardis et al. 1982).

When the obstruction has been bypassed, the endoscopist may not be able to tell by tactile means when the stent has reached the renal pelvis; and in all cases of stent placement radiographic control must be used (Oswalt et al. 1979). Forceful stent advancement can perforate the renal pelvis and parenchyma or even enter the hilar vessels necessitating open surgery (Kidd et al. 1980).

If endoscopic insertion is not feasible or is unsuccessful, the percutaneous route should be attempted (Elyaderani et al. 1982a,b).

In-situ Complications

Bacteriuria

Prophylactic antibiotics are not required in the absence of infection, but the urine should be monitored frequently (Mardis et al. 1982). If bacteriuria is present, every effort should be made to sterilise the urine prior to passing the stent (Gibbons 1976; Finney 1982). Infection, especially that caused by urea-splitting organisms such as *Proteus* or *Pseudomonas* can cause rapid encrustation. In addition to antimicrobial agents and a high fluid intake, aceto-hydraxamic acid (AHA) can be most helpful. This drug, which is available in the USA under the trade name of Lithostat has the ability to inhibit urease formation, which in turn prevents ammonia formation and alkalinisation of the urine. While not without undesirable side effects this new drug can be most useful (Griffin et al. 1979).

Sterile Pyuria

Sterile pyuria is not infrequent and reflects foreign body reaction to the stent. In the absence of infection, proved by culture, pyuria is generally inconsequential (Mardis et al. 1982).

Reflux

Reflux can be anticipated for any properly placed ureteric stent, but in the absence of bacteriuria only rare sequelae have been noted (Kearney et al. 1979; Mardis et al. 1982). This had not been the case in renal transplant recipients, however, and stents are not routinely indicated (Tremann and Marchioro 1977). The occasional patient who notes flank pain while voiding can usually be treated symptomatically.

Bladder Irritation and Trigonal Erosion

Minor bladder irritation is not uncommon with the more rigid internal stents and can usually be controlled by antispasmodics (Mardis et al. 1982; Kearney et al. 1979). A stent which is too long and thus pressing on the trigone or kidney is a frequent cause of this irritation, and exchange for a shorter stent may resolve the problem. Trigonal erosion is exceedingly rare and usually occurred with the early rigid straight stents (Zimskind et al. 1967).

Haematuria

Microscopic haematuria is not uncommon with all ureteric stents, but there may be less irritation from the softer, more flexible silicone stents than from those made of plastic (Gibbons et al. 1976). Gross haematuria is rare and may indicate that the proximal or distal stent tip is eroding into the surrounding tissues (Zimskind et al. 1967). The fact that haematuria can also be caused by the primary disease or other concomitant conditions should also not be over-looked. Gross haematuria following upper-tract surgery can completely obstruct any stent with clots, and if this is anticipated it is advisable to place a temporary nephrostomy. The nephrostomy may be removed as soon as the urine clears.

Spontaneous Breakage

Although silicone ureteric stents have not been reported to fracture sponta-neously, a number of polyethylene stents have broken in-situ (Fig. 3.13), and this material is no longer used (Mardis 1984). Other plastic stents made from materials such as Silitex, Bio-Flex, C-Flex and polyurethane are more flexible than polyethylene and may prove to be more resistant to breakage.

Stent Migration

It is not difficult to position the distal stent loop within the bladder endo-scopically since this is accomplished under direct vision. Migration of properly placed suspension-type stents is exceedingly rare and the greatest chance for error occurs during open surgery when the distal stent segment is to be passed through a ureterotomy into the bladder (Finney 1978; Hepperlen et al. 1978). As mentioned, not only must the distal tip of the stent reach the bladder but an additional length (4–5 cm) must be passed to allow formation of the distal retaining loop. If this loop does not form, then upward migration is not prevented. Proximal stent passage can be facilitated by its palpation within the renal pelvis (Finney 1982).

Encrustation and Obstruction

Although a thin film of urinary salts or mucoid eventually deposits over any known foreign body in the urinary system, internal stents may drain for months or years without obstructing provided that the urine is kept dilute (high fluid intake), acidic (diet and occasionally acidifying drugs) and infection-free (Blum et al. 1963; Gibbons 1976; Mardis et al. 1982). An alkaline, low volume, infected urine can rapidly encrust and obstruct any stent (Fig. 3.14) (Schneider et al. 1976; Finney 1982). Once blocked, the stent must be changed, although the Double Pigtail and Uropasss stents which have both ends open may at times be temporarily unblocked by the passage of a wire stylet through their lumen. However, the distal end of the stent which is curled within the bladder

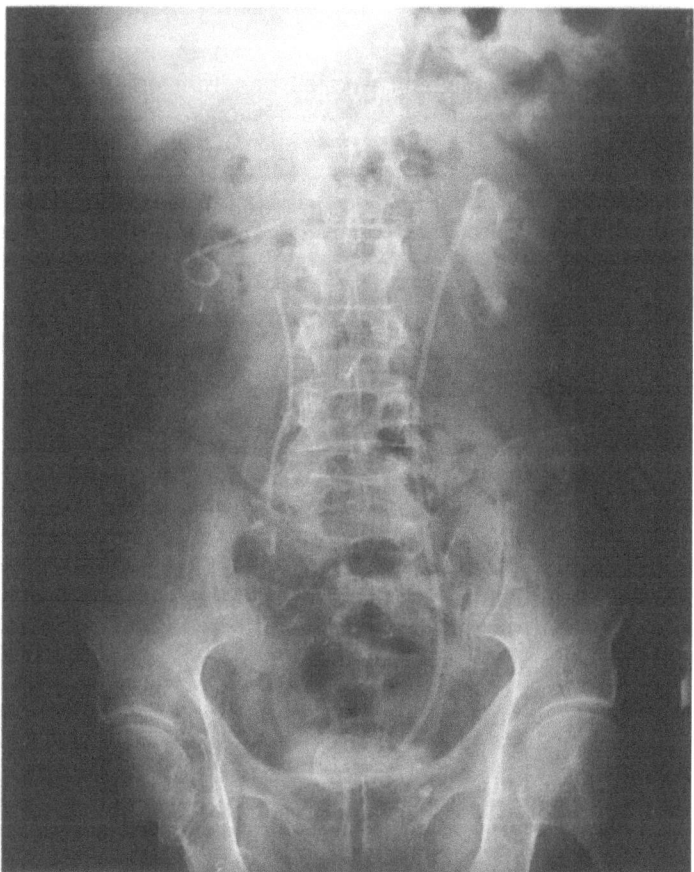

Fig. 3.13. Multiple spontaneous breaks of a polyethylene pigtail stent with retained segments in the ureter. This patient had previously failed three attempts at surgical ureterolysis for retro-peritoneal fibrosis. Endoscopic removal of such stent fragments can be exceedingly difficult although the newer percutaneous and endoscopic equipment may make this more feasible. (Courtesy of HK Mardis.)

must be positioned to allow wire passage and usually it is simpler to perform a stent change.

A stent may also become encrusted and obstructed in the patient having abnormally high levels of excretion of uric acid. Stent obstruction by urate has been seen in patients with chronic ureteric obstruction and high levels of uric acid in the serum. With stent placement the urate is excreted in quite high concentrations and may rapidly precipitate within the stent. In these cases, one stent change is usually required, after which the urate concentration is insufficient to produce recurrent obstruction (Finney 1978).

The Siphon Effect

Under certain circumstances a patient having an open nephrostomy and stent or a newer nephrostent draining one obstructed urinary system may not void

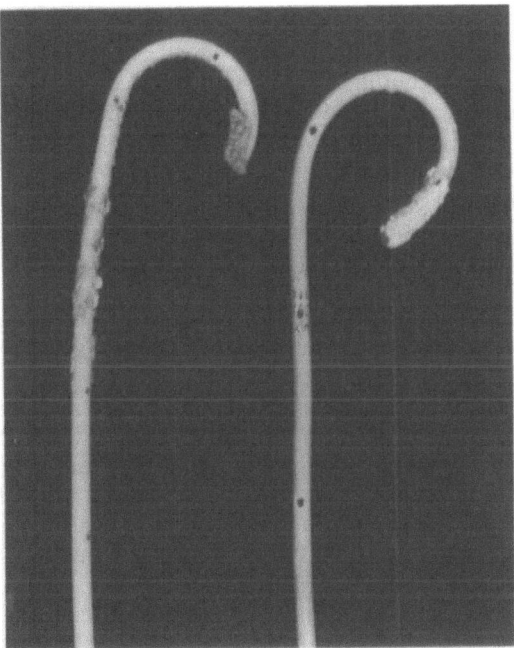

Fig. 3.14. Encrustation of the proximal ends of two stents removed from chronic stone-formers. Much of the external encrustation broke off during handling. The portions within the renal pelvis and bladder were heavily encrusted while the middle segment had been wiped clean by ureteral peristalsis. This phenomenon has been noted on numerous occasions and stents have been designed with external grooves to permit improved drainage in the face of encrustation. (From Finney R (1982) Double-J and diversion stents. Urol Clin North Am 9:89–94, with permission.)

even though his contralateral kidney is functioning well. If the nephrostomy is connected to an external drainage bag, this is usually kept below the level of the bladder, particularly when the patient is recumbent. The column of urine within the drainage tubing can then exert a negative pressure within the kidney, which is transmitted down the stent into the bladder such that urine produced by the contralateral kidney is also drawn or "siphoned" out of the bladder, through the nephrostomy into the collection bag. If this siphon effect is not understood, the surgeon may bacome alarmed that the contralateral kidney is no longer functioning when in truth all urine from both kidneys is passing out of the nephrostomy (Finney 1978).

Problems with Stent Removal

Removal of a properly placed internal ureteric stent can be accomplished on an out-patient basis under topical anaesthesia. The distal loop is usually easily visualised in the bladder and may be grasped with foreign-body forceps or a small wire hook protruding from the tip of a standard ureteric catheter. Once the end has been engaged, the stent should be removed by withdrawing the endoscope and stent together (Smith 1982b).

A major problem arises when the stent has been improperly positioned or has migrated above the ureteric orifice such that it may not be directly visualised. Many ingenious devices and techniques have been devised to engage these malpositioned stents (Firlit and Brown 1972; Hinman and Palubinskas 1980).

The Gibbons stent is provided with a tail which may remain within the bladder and can be grasped to effect removal (Fig. 3.3b). If the stent has migrated further, an angiographic balloon or embolectomy catheter can be passed inside its lumen, the balloon inflated and removal accomplished (Niendorf and Kamhi 1975).

The distal loops of the Double J, Pigtail, and Uropass stents when positioned in the ureter are usually directed somewhat to the side, and these have been successfully removed by retractable stone baskets. The stone basket is passed into the ureteric orifice and the basket opened slightly below the stent. Continued retrograde passage of the basket by using a rotary motion may be successful in looping one or more of the wires around the end of the stent. When it is thought that the stent has been engaged, the stone basket is tightly closed and withdrawn. Multiple attempts may be necessary to effect stent removal; these manoeuvres can usually be facilitated by a radiographic image intensifier but this is not essential.

A migrated stent can also be removed by using foreign-body forceps or a wire loop under image intensification (Fig. 3.15). The standard endoscopic forceps designed for use in the bladder are often too rigid and short for any but the most minimally displaced stents. However, longer, smaller, and more flexible foreign-body forceps made for use in gastrointestinal endoscopic instruments or special ureteric forceps (Fig. 3.15) can be adapted to this purpose.

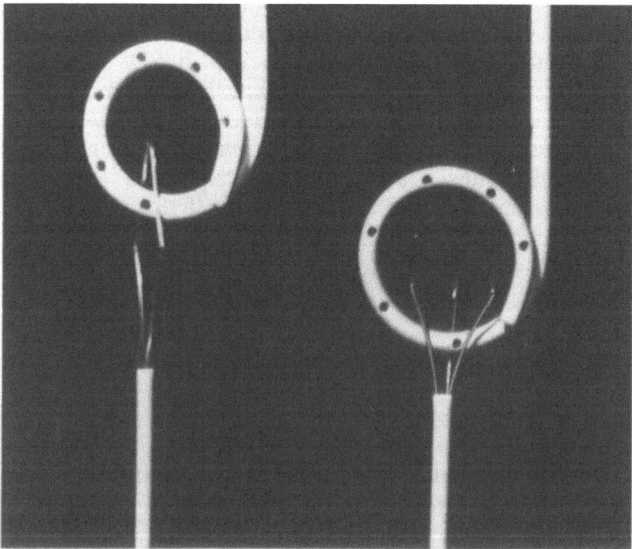

Fig. 3.15. Instruments used to engage and extract displaced stents. The wire loop (left) and grasping forceps (right) are manipulated with the aid of image intensification or under direct vision. (Courtesy of Cook Urological.)

Under image-intensification control these forceps can be threaded up the ureter to the distal end of the migrated stent, the jaws opened and rotated to the proper direction and the stent grasped and removed (Finney 1982). An assistant should open and close the forceps allowing the endoscopist to use two hands for proper positioning of the instruments.

While many hospitals do not possess urological tables equipped with image intensification, most will have a portable "C-Arm" image intensification unit used for placement of cardiac pacemakers, etc. These C-Arm units may be used on standard urological endoscopy tables if the surface is radiolucent and if the carriage designed to hold the film can be removed or positioned to the head of the table. If this is not possible, endoscopy and stent removal may be performed in the radiological suite.

The newer ureteric-renoscopes permit direct visualisation of a migrated ureteric stent and facilitate engagement and removal with a loop or flexible forceps. If endoscopic methods fail and if the proximal end of the stent is lying within the kidney, removal can be accomplished through a percutaneous nephrostomy.

Ureteric obstruction from mucosal oedema can arise following stent removal. This is secondary to ischaemia caused by the use of too large a stent. This transient obstruction, frequently associated with a superimposed infection, is usually distal but can occur anywhere. In severe cases, proximal nephrostomy drainage may be required for 5–7 days (Levine et al. 1982) or a smaller stent can be reinserted.

Summary

The development of internal ureteric stents and indwelling nephrostomy stents which are capable of providing excellent drainage from the kidney to the bladder for long periods of time have produced profound changes in the management of many urological conditions. A significant cost saving has been effected since many patients previously requiring open surgical intervention may now be managed endoscopically. In addition, patients who were previously required to remain in the hospital for prolonged periods because of external drainage tubes and excessive urine leakage may now be sent home with an internal stent at a much earlier date. One less day in hospital can more than make up the cost of the stent.

Future research should be directed primarily toward finding a material (possibly one of the hydrophylic polymers), that will not encrust even when immersed in infected and salt-saturated urine. A great deal has been accomplished recently and we may have great expectations for the future.

References

Altwein, JE, Alken P (1980) Internal urinary diversion by a percutaneous ureteric splint. Br J Urol 51:165

Andriole GL, Bettmann MA, Garnick MB, Richie JP (1984) Indwelling double-J ureteral stents for temporary and permanent urinary drainage: experience with 87 patients. J Urol 131:239–241

Banner MP, Pollack HM, Ring EJ, Wein AJ (1983) Catheter dilatation of benign ureteral strictures. Radiology 147:427–433

Barbaric ZL, Gothlin JH, Davies RS (1977) Transluminal dilation and stent placement in obstructed ureters in dogs through the use of percutaneous nephro-pyelostomy. Invest Radiol 12:534–536

Bartley O, Chidekel N, Radberg C (1965) Percutaneous drainage of the renal pelvis for uremia due to obstructed urinary ourflow. Acta Chir Scand 129:433–446

Becker W, Schellhammer P (1982) Placement of double-pigtail ureteral stent via cystoscope. Urology 20:310–311

Berger RE, Ansell JS, Tremann JA, Herz JH, Rattazzi LC, Marchioro TL (1980) The use of self-retained ureteral stents in the management of urologic complications in renal transplant recipients. J Urol 124:781–782

Bigongiari LR, Lee KR, Mebust WK, Foret J, Weigel J (1978) Transurethral conversion of a percutaneous ureteral stent to an indwelling stent. AJR 131:1089–1099

Bigongiari LR, Lee KR, Moffat RE, Mebust WK, Foret J, Weigel J (1979) Percutaneous ureteral stent placement for stricture management and internal urinary diversion. AJR 133:865–868

Bigongiari LR, Lee KR, Moffat RE, Mebust WK, Foret J, Weigel J (1980a) Subcutaneous implantation of percutaneous ureteral stents. Clin Radiol 31:707–709

Bigongiari L, Lee KR, Moffat RE, Mebust WK, Foret J, Weigel J (1980b) Conversion of percutaneous ureteral stent to indwelling pigtail stent over guidewire. Urology 15:461–465

Blum J, Skemp C, Reiser M (1963) Silicone rubber ureteral prosthesis. J Urol 90:276-280

Boyarsky S, Labay P (1981) Principles of ureteral physiology. In: Bergman H (ed) The ureter. Springer-Verlag, Berlin, Heidelberg, New York pp 71–104

Brin EN, Schiff M Jr, Weiss RM (1975) Palliative urinary diversion for pelvic malignancy. J Urol 113:619–622

Brown HP, Harrison JH (1951) The efficacy of plastic ureteral and urethral catheters for constant drainage. J Urol 66:85–93

Camacho MF, Carrion H, Lockhart J, Bondhus M, Politano VA (1981) Easier way to introduce pigtail ureteral stents. Urology 18:402

Camacho MF, Pereiras R, Carrion H, Bondhus M, Politano V (1979) Double-ended pigtail ureteral stent: useful modification to single-end ureteral stent. Urology 13:516–520

Chodak G, Huffman J, Schoenberg H, Lyon ES (1982) Technique for replacing indwelling double-J ureteral stents. Urology 19:544–545

Collier MD, Jerkins GR, Noe HN, Soloway MS (1979) Proximal stent displacement as complication of pigtail ureteral stent. Urology 13:372–375

Cordonnier JJ, Roane JS (1950) Ureteral splinting: an experimental evaluation of prolonged ureteral splinting. Surg Clin North Am 30:1523–1527

Danoff DS (1977) The Gibbons indwelling silicone ureteral stent catheter. J Urol 117:33

Davis DM (1951) Intubated ureterotomy. J Urol 66:77–84

Davis JE, Hagedoorn JP, Bergman LL (1981) Anatomy and ultrastructure of the ureter. In: Bergman H (ed) The ureter. Springer, Berlin, Heidelberg New York pp 55–70

Dorr RP, Ratliff RK, Hyndman CW (1974) Technique of ureteral repair using an indwelling ureteral stent. J Urol 111:481–482

Elyaderani MK, Belis JA, Kandzari SJ, Gabriele OF (1982a) Facilitation of difficult percutaneous ureteral stent insertion. J Urol 128:1173–1176

Elyaderani MK, Gabriele OF, Kandzari SJ, Belis JA (1982b) Percutanous nephrostomy and antegrade ureteral stent insertion. Urology 20:650–656

Ferris DD, Grindley JH (1948) Use of the polyethylene and polyvinyl tubing in ureterostomy, nephrostomy and cystostomy. Mayo Clin Proc 23:385

Finney RP (1978) Experience with new double J ureteral catheter stent. J Urol 120:678–681

Finney RP (1982) Double-J and diversion stents. Urol Clin North Am 9:89–94

Firlit CF, Brown JL (1972) Ureteral stents: a device for removal. J Urol 108:954

Fisher HAG, Bennet AH, Rivard, DJ, Caputo T, Goldman M (1982) Non-operative supravesical urinary diversion in obstetrics and gynecology. Gynecol Oncol 14:365–372

Fort KF, Selman SH, Kropp KA (1983) A retrospective analysis of the use of ureteral stents in children undergoing ureteroneocystotomy. J Urol 129:545–548

Fowler JE Jr, Raife MJ, Sennott R (1980) A method for placement of a ureteral stent following supravesical intestinal diversion. J Urol 124:547–549

Fritzsche P, Moorhead D, Axford PD, Torrey RR (1981) Urologic applications of angiographic guide wire and catheter techniques. J Urol 125:774–780

Gerber WL, Narayana AS (1982) Failure of the double-curved ureteral stent. J Urol 127:317–319

Gibbons RP (1976) New ureteral stent for long-term drainage. Mod Med 44:15, 111

Gibbons RP (1982) Gibbons ureteral stents. Urol Clin North Am 9:85–88

Gibbons RP, Correa RJ Jr, Cummings KB, Mason JT (1976) Experience with indwelling ureteral stent catheters. J Urol 115:22–26

Gibbons RP, Mason JT, Correa RJ Jr (1974) Experience with indwelling silicone rubber ureteral catheters. J Urol 111:594–599

Goldin AR (1977) Percutaneous splinting. Urology 10:165–168

Goodwin WE (1972) Splint, stent, stint. Urol Digest 11:13

Goodwin WE, Casey WC, Woolf W (1955) Percutaneous trochar (needle) nephrostomy in hydronephrosis. JAMA 157:891–894

Grabstald H, McPhee M (1973) Nephrostomy and the cancer patient. South Med J 66:217–220

Griffith DP, Moskowitz PA, Carlton CE Jr (1979) Adjunctive chemotherapy of infection-induced staghorn calculi. J Urol 121:711–715

Hanna Moneer K (1981) Clinical application of hydrodynamics of the ureter and renal pelvis. In: Bergman H (ed) The ureter. Springer, Berlin, Heidelberg New York pp 163–178

Hepperlen TW, Mardis HK, Kammandel H (1978) Self-retained internal ureteral stents: a new approach. J Urol 119:731–734

Hepperlen TW, Mardis HK, Kammandel H (1979) The pigtail ureteral stent in the cancer patient. J Urol 121:17–18

Hinman F, Palubinskas AJ (1980) Catheter retriever. J Urol 123:527

Holden S, McPhee M, Grabstald H (1979) The rationale of urinary diversion in cancer patients. J Urol 121:19–21

Jonson M, Lindberg B, Risholm L (1972) Percutaneous nephro-pyelostomy in cases of ureteric obstruction. Scand J Urol Nephrol 6:51–53

Kearney GP, Mahoney EM, Brown HP (1979) Useful technique for long-term urinary drainage by inlying ureteral stent. Urology 14:126–134

Kidd RV III, Confer DJ, Ball RP Jr (1980) Ureteral and renal vein perforation with placement into the renal vein as a complication of the pigtail ureteral stent. J Urol 124:424–426

Kiil F (1978) Physiology of the renal pelvis and ureter. In: Harrison JH, Gittes RF, Perlmutter AD, Stamey TA, Walsh PC (eds) Campbell's urology. WB Saunders Company, Philadelphia London Toronto, pp 55–86

Kramer SA, Anderson EE (1980) Fixation of temporary ureteral stents. Urology 15:408

Lang EK, Lanasa JA, Garrett J, Stripling J, Palomar J (1979) The management of urinary fistulas and strictures with percutaneous ureteral stent catheters. J Urol 122:736–740

Levine RS, Pollack HM, Banner MP (1982) Transient ureteral obstruction after ureteral stenting. AJR 138:323–327

Lowes IJ Mackenzie JC, Abrahams PH, Gingell JC (1987) Acute renal failure and acute hydronephrosis in pregnancy: use of the double J stent. JR Soc Med 80:524–525

Lytton B (1975) Catheters and sounds. In: Perspectives in urology. AUA Monograph. Roche Laboratories, Nutley, New Jersey

Maar K, Meridies R, Dettmar H (1976) Indwelling and transrenal splint techniques for pyeloplasty. Urology 8:19–21

Mangelson NL, Kado RT, Cockett ATK (1968) Silicone rubber uses in the lower urinary tract. J Urol 100:573–577

Mardis HK (1965) Technical considerations in renal arteriography: some modifications in retrograde femoral catheterization technique. J Urol 93:627–630

Mardis HK (1983) A new self-retained internal ureteral stent (Abst. 287) Proc. 78th Ann Meeting Am Urol Assoc, p 163

Mardis HK, Hepperlen TW, Kammandel H (1979) Double pigtail ureteral stent. Urology 14:23–26

Mardis HK, Kammandel H, Hepperlen TW (1980) Drainage efficiency of self-retained internal ureteral stent catheters. (Abst. 590) Proc. 75th Ann Meeting Am Urol Assoc, p 270

Mardis HK, Kroeger RM, Hepperlen TW, Mazer MJ, Kammandel H (1982) Polyethylene double-pigtail ureteral stents. Urol Clin North Am. 9:95–101

Marmar JL (1970) The management of ureteral obstruction with silicone rubber splint catheters. J Urol 104:386–389

Mazer MJ, LeVeen RF, Call JE, Wolf G, Baltaxe HA (1979) Permanent percutaneous antegrade ureteral stent placement without transurethral assistance. Urology 14:413–419

McCullough DL (1974) "Shepherds-crook" self-retaining ureteral catheter. Urologists' Letter Club:32:54

Niendorf DC, Kamhi B (1975) Retrieval of indwelling ureteral stent utilizing Fogarty catheter. Urology 6:622–623

Orikasa S, Tsuji I, Siba T, Ohashi N (1973) A new technique for transurethral insertion of a silicone rubber tube into an obstructed ureter. J Urol 100:184–187

Ormond JK (1981) Idiopathic retroperitoneal fibrosis. In: Bergman H (ed) The ureter. Springer, Berlin, Heidelberg New York pp 225–245

Östling K (1942) The genesis of hydronephrosis. Acta Chir Scand (Suppl) 72:86

Oswalt GC Jr, Bueschen AJ, Lloyd LK (1979) Upward migration of indwelling ureteral stents. J Urol 122:249–250

Pais VM, Spellman RM, Stiles RE, Mahoney SA (1975) Internal ureteral splints. Urology 5:32–36

Parker M, Riehle RA Jr (1982) Operative placement of indwelling ureteral stent. Urology 20:540–541

Persky L, Krause J (1981) Splinting versus nonsplinting in ureteral surgery. In: Bergman H (ed) The ureter. Springer, Verlag, Berlin, Heidelberg New York pp 187–192

Pfister RC, Newhouse JH, Hendren WH (1982) Percutaneous urodynamics. Urol Clin North Am 9:41–49

Pingoud EG, Bagley DH, Zeman RK, Glancy KE, Pais OS (1980) Percutaneous antegrade bilateral ureteral dilatation and stent placement for internal drainage. Radiology 134:780

Pitts JC III, Peterson ME (1981) Penetrating injuries of the ureter. J Trauma 21:978–982

Raghavaiah NV (1981) New self-retaining ureteral catheter. J Urol 126:29–30

Schneider RE, DePauw AP, Montie JE, Thompson IM (1976) Problems associated with Gibbons ureteral catheter. Urology 8:243–246

Seldinger SI (1953) Catheter replacement of the needle in percutaneous arteriography: a new technique. Acta Radiol 39:368–376

Sieben DM, Howerton L, Amin M, Holt H, Lich R Jr (1978) The role of ureteral stenting in the management of surgical injury to the ureter. J Urol 119:330–331

Singh B, Kim H, Wax SH (1979) Stents versus nephrostomy: is there a choice? J Urol 121:268–270

Smart WR (1979) Surgical correction of hydronephrosis. In: Harrison JH, Gittes RF, Perlmutter AD, Stamey TA, Walsh PC (eds) Campbells' urology. WB Saunders Company, Philadelphia London Toronto, pp 2047–2116

Smith AD (1982a) The universal ureteral stent. J Urol 127:892–893

Smith AD (1982b) Retrieval of ureteral stents. Urol Clin North Am 9:109–112

Simth AD (1982c) The universal ureteral stent. Urol Clin North Am 9:103–107

Smith AD, Lange PH, Miller RP, Reinke DB (1978) Introduction of the Gibbons ureteral stent facilitated by antecedent percutaneous nephrostomy. J Urol 120:543–544

Smith AD, Lange PH, Miller RP, Reinke DB (1979a) Percutaneous dilatation of uretero-ileal strictures and insertion of Gibbons ureteral stents. Urology 13:24–26

Smith AD, Miller RP, Reinke DB, Lange PH, Fraley EE (1979b) Insertion of Gibbons ureteral stents using endourologic techniques. Urology 14:330–336

Stables DP (1982) Percutaneous nephrostomy: techniques, indications and results. Urol Clin North Am 9:15–29

Trachenberg J, Winfield H, Stein L (1983) Alternative to nephrostomy by internal urinary diversion (Abst. 288). 78th Ann Meeting Am Urol Assoc, p 163

Tremann JA, Marchioro TL (1977) Gibbons ureteral stent in renal transplant recipients. Urology 9:390–393

Turner MD, Witherington R, Carswell JJ (1982) Ureteral splints: results of a survey. J Urol 127:654–656

Velardo JT (1981) Histology of the ureter. In: Bergman H (ed) The ureter. Springer, Berlin, Heidelberg New York pp 13–54

Vermeulen CW, Grove WJ, Goetz HD, Ragins HD, Correll NO (1950) Experimental urolithiasis. I. Development of calculi upon foreign bodies surgically introduced into the bladder of rats. J Urol 64:541–548

Whitaker RH (1973) Methods of assessing obstruction in dilated ureters. Br J Urol 45:15–22

Williams TJ (1982) The ureter in obstetrics and gynecology. In: Bergman H (ed) The ureter. Springer, Berlin, Heidelberg New York pp 583–624

Zimskind PD, Fetter TD, Wilkerson JL (1967) Clinical use of long-term indwelling silicone rubber ureteral splints inserted cystoscopically. J Urol 97:840–844

Chapter 4

Urethral and Suprapubic Catheters

M.C. Bishop and R.J. Lemberger

History (Herman 1973; Murphy 1972) (Fig. 4.1)

The need and ability to drain retained urine from the bladder has been recognised from prehistoric times. Man's ingenuity was nowhere better exemplified than in the variety of materials and objects used to catheterise the urethra. Reeds and straws were commonly used. The Chinese accomplished the task with the dried, rolled up, outer leaves of a species of onion. In the eastern Mediterranean the Sumerians, Babylonians and Egyptians used gold and silver to manufacture catheters. Metal catheters were also recovered in the excavations at Pompeii. Galen devised an "S"-shaped catheter which indicated his clear understanding of the natural curves of the male urethra.

There were no significant developments in catheter design until the early nineteenth century when, under the auspices of the French school of urological surgery, the use of new materials was explored. Woven silk impregnated with linseed oil or varnished was particularly popular. Flexibility was introduced with the development of manufacturing processes in the rubber industry and in particular the Goodyear process, introduced in 1844, which facilitated the moulding of rubber whilst retaining its malleable properties after heating.

Several early attempts were made to incorporate a self-retaining function. Reybard designed a catheter terminating in a bag made of sausage skin and inflated through a separate lumen. Ultimately the prototype Foley catheter developed in 1930, a direct descendant, consisted simply of a balloon with an inflating tube attached to a longitudinally grooved catheter. Shortly afterwards the drainage and evacuating channels became integrated into the form which is now familiar. Other forms of self-retaining catheters than those dependant on the inflatable balloon were also developed pari passu. In general they were held in place by some form of rubber moulding. In practice their only application was for suprapubic vesical drainage. They have mainly been replaced by plastic catheters in which the detachable introducing trocar is integrated.

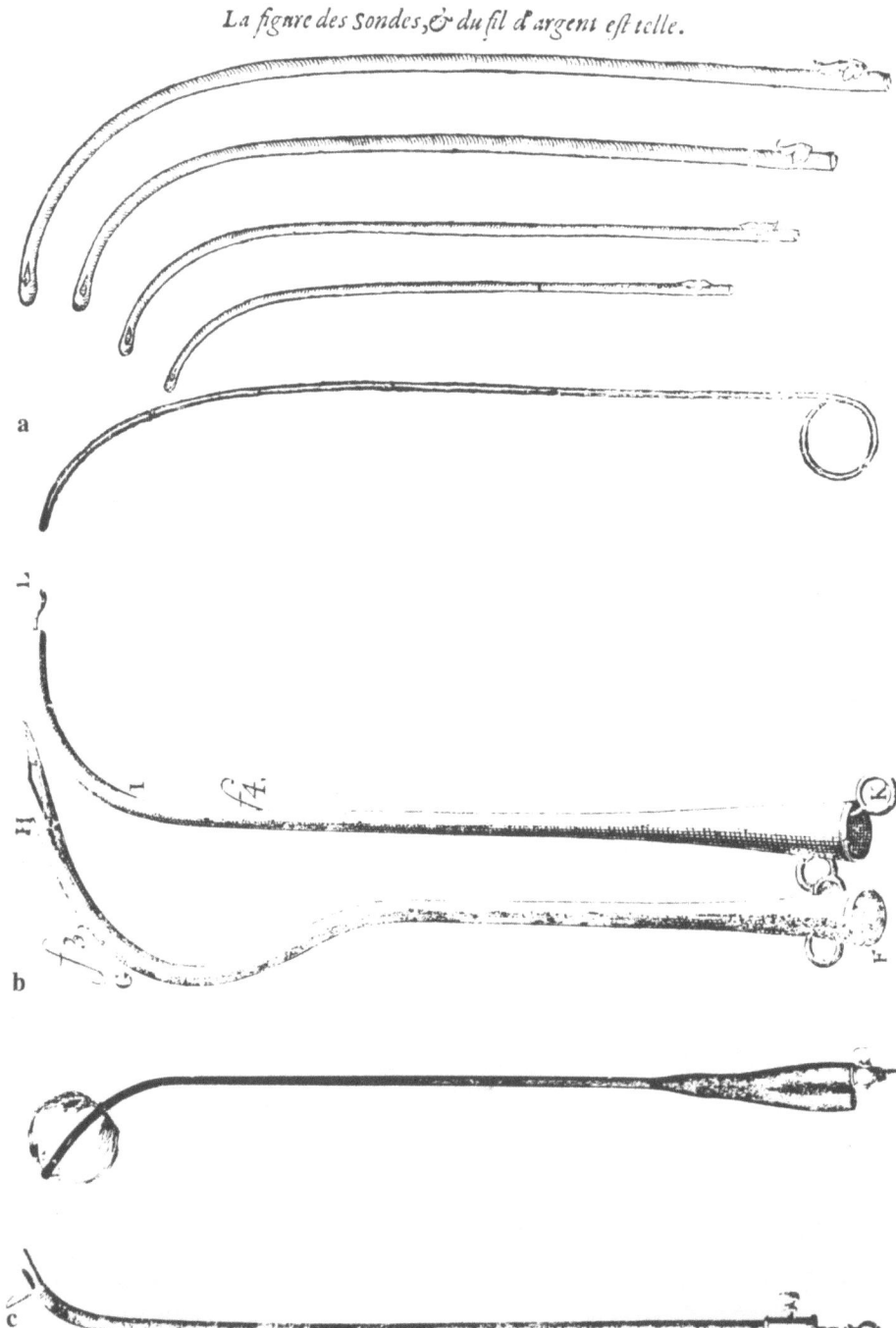

Fig. 4.1a–c. Historical aspects. **a** Selection of silver catheters and stylet, 1564. Paré. The side drainage aperture was a comparatively recent innovation. **b** Two silver catheters in common use in the seventeenth century. f3, double curved instrument with oblique side apertures; f4, catheter traversed by a metal wire ending in a small button occluding its orifice during introduction. **c** Two self-retaining catheters designed by Reybard (1853). One is held in place with a movable flange. The other, a double lumen gum elastic catheter, fitted with an inflatable balloon is the prototype of the modern Foley catheter. (From Murphy 1972.)

Variety of Catheters and Accessories

Types of Catheters

Catheters vary in dimension, shape of terminal portion and site and number of drainage ports. It must be emphasised that the external diameter may not necessary reflect lumen size. Clearly the irrigation channel of a 3-way catheter will limit the space available for drainage. However, the principal factor limiting flow is the dimension of the outlet port at the tip. It is, of course, pointless for this to exceed the cross-sectional area of the lumen.

The coudé and Tiemann catheters are so designed to negotiate the natural bends in the bulbar membranous urethra. However, the shape of a straight catheter can be fixed more certainly with an introducer (see below).

Catheters may vary in the number and site of drainage perforations. The second hole behind the self-retaining balloon of the Roberts' catheter can be helpful in situations where the tip eye is occluded, e.g., by the balloon itself (*see* Complications). Further drainage holes along the shaft of a self-retaining catheter may have some advantage in allowing evacuation of urethral secretions and blood after urethral surgery (Smith and Ball 1984; Turner-Warwick 1973).

The Gibbon catheter consists of a narrow gauge plastic intra-urethral part and a very long section between the meatus and collection device and was originally designed for longterm drainage of the neuropathic bladder. The retaining straps obviate the need for a balloon which can be an extra cause of bladder irritation and hence instability and infection (Gibbon 1976). The narrow gauge itself minimises irritation to the urethra and facilitates drainage of secretions collecting between the urothelium and catheter. Nowadays this catheter may have more application to paediatric practice and short-term use, e.g., after hypospadias surgery. The variation in catheter design is considerable and in many cases has been "personalised" according to a particular urologist's whims. There is little point in itemising every variation.

Materials

The choice of catheter is often based on the tendency of one or other material to induce urethral inflammation or encrustation in relation to cost and sometimes availability (Nacey et al. 1985; Engel et al. 1972; Painter et al. 1971; Binder et al. 1969; Keitzer et al. 1968). Recent comparative studies show significant differences between the different materials (Talja et al. 1990; Ohkawa et al. 1990).

Latex Rubber

The cheapest catheters are made from uncoated latex. It has a relatively rough surface which is all too apparent on high power scanning electron micrographs. Possibly for this reason it is prone to cause urethral irritation and should only be used in the short term.

Coated Latex

Coating with silicone elastomer or Teflon provides a smooth surface which is less prone to encrustation than uncoated latex. Such catheters can be used for several weeks but are perhaps slightly more irritant than those constructed from pure silicone rubber.

Silicone

Arguably, this material causes least irritation to epithelial tissues. Most manufacturers recommend that such catheters can be left in situ for 3 months or more. However, the majority of patients will react by producing a certain amount of debris and a small proportion, considerable catheter encrustation if it is left for much beyond 6 weeks. Silicone rubber is also not as pliable as latex and another disadvantage is that it will not re-seal after needle puncture if urine aspiration from the closed drainage system is attempted.

Polyvinylchloride (PVC)

Polyvinylchloride provides a rigid catheter which is most effective for irrigation of clot or debris. However, its lack of flexibility can lead to bladder perforation and to discomfort although the material is said to soften at body temperature.

Lofric Catheters

See Carroll, Chap. 6.

Other Materials

Red rubber is still used by some manufacturers. It is very prone to encrustation and is much more likely to irritate the urothelium than modern materials but it is cheap and has considerable resilience. It may still be suitable for short-term use, particularly single catheterisation and perhaps after prostatectomy since its ability to withstand negative pressure may have particular application during aspiration of clot which would otherwise collapse the lumen. However, for this purpose a PVC plastic catheter or a latex catheter reinforced with an internal wire spiral is nowadays more often used.

Catheters are also available manufactured from gum elastic, a traditional material popular in Europe and particularly in France. It has the disadvantage that a self-retaining balloon cannot be incorporated. However, the material is relatively non-reactive and of great resilience so that it compares with the more recently developed PVC. Gum elastic is also used in the manufacture of graded, flexible bougies for urethral dilatation. These can be constructed in a system of filiforms and followers with a lumen for urinary drainage.

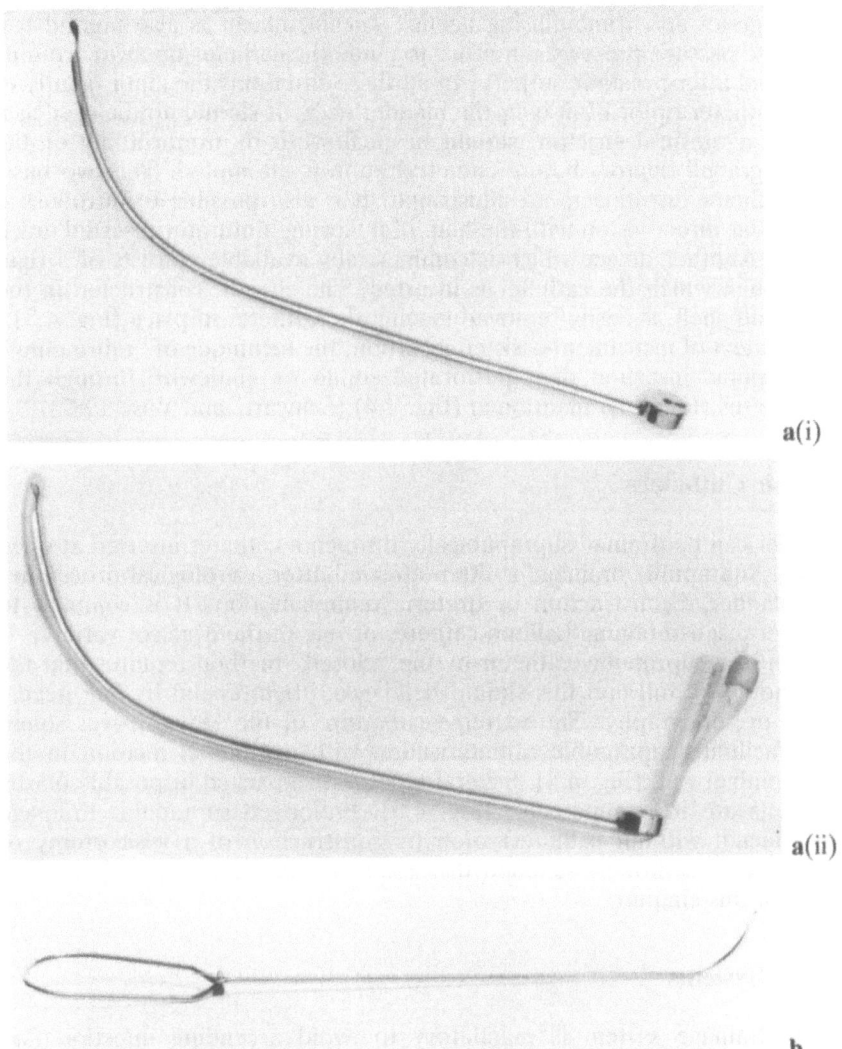

a(i)

a(ii)

b

Fig. 4.2a,b. Catheter introducers. **a** Maryfield type: (i) introducer; (ii) catheter applied over groove on introducer. **b** Metal bougie-shaped rod inserted through catheter lumen. The importance of rigid construction is emphasised.

Catheter Introducers (Fig. 4.2)

An introducer may be required in situations where despite the use of adequate lubricant the urethra is too rigid though not necessarily too narrow for easy passage. Further manipulations lead only to the catheter being concertinaed, generally at the level of the prostate. This is particularly prone to occur with a very much enlarged, benign prostate (and hence a high bladder neck) or perhaps in prostatic malignancy. Occasionally intense spasm at the bladder neck will prevent the passage of the catheter despite reassurance and even the use of analgesics and tranquillising agents. An introducer is also helpful if a urethral false passage pre-exists in order to guide the catheter tip away from its entrance, and after prostatic surgery. In all these situations the aim is gently to guide the catheter tip or lift it over the bladder neck. It should not be used as a dilator and a urethral stricture should be dealt with by urethrotomy or the passage of graded dilators before catheterisation is attempted. The two basic types of catheter introducers are illustrated. It is also possible to introduce a catheter under direct vision with the help of a viewing obturator inserted down the lumen. Another device which is commercially available consists of a rigid sheath through which the catheter is inserted. The sheath, constructed in the form of a half shell, is easily removed leaving the catheter in place (Fig. 4.3).

In the context of instrument-assisted insertion, the technique of "railroading" after suprapubic insertion of a perforated sound or guidewire through the internal meatus should be mentioned (Fig. 4.4) (Schwartz and Wise 1982).

Suprapubic Catheters

The bladder can be drained suprapubically through a catheter inserted at open cystotomy. Suprapubic drainage is often effected after a urological procedure, such as bladder reconstruction or ureteric reimplantation. It is common to insert either a self-retaining balloon catheter or one of the Malecot variety.

Insertion of a suprapubic catheter by the "closed" method requires that the bladder should be full and this should be checked beforehand by fine needle aspiration or sonography. The extreme curvature of the Hey–Groves sound can also facilitate suprapubic catheterisation with a minimal incision in the lower abdominal wall (Fig. 4.4). Several types of pre-packed disposable plastic catheter sets are in common use (Fig. 4.5). Prolonged suprapubic drainage can be effected without catheterisation by construction of a vesicostomy or suprapubic neo-urethra. A detailed discussion of these techniques is beyond the scope of this chapter.

Collection Systems

A closed drainage system is mandatory to avoid ascending infection (*see* Complications). The use of a simple spigot with intermittent release is to be

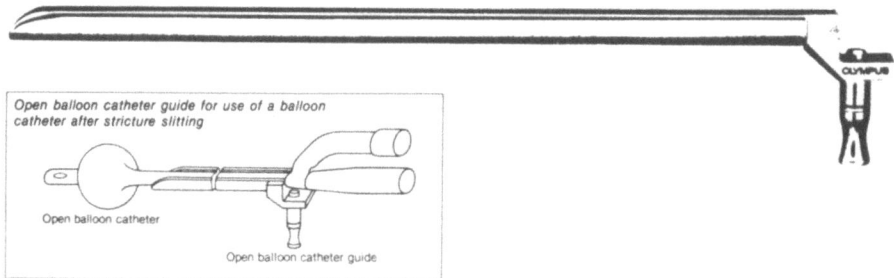

Fig. 4.3. Sheath to facilitate catheterisation, e.g., after transurethral resection, internal urethrotomy.

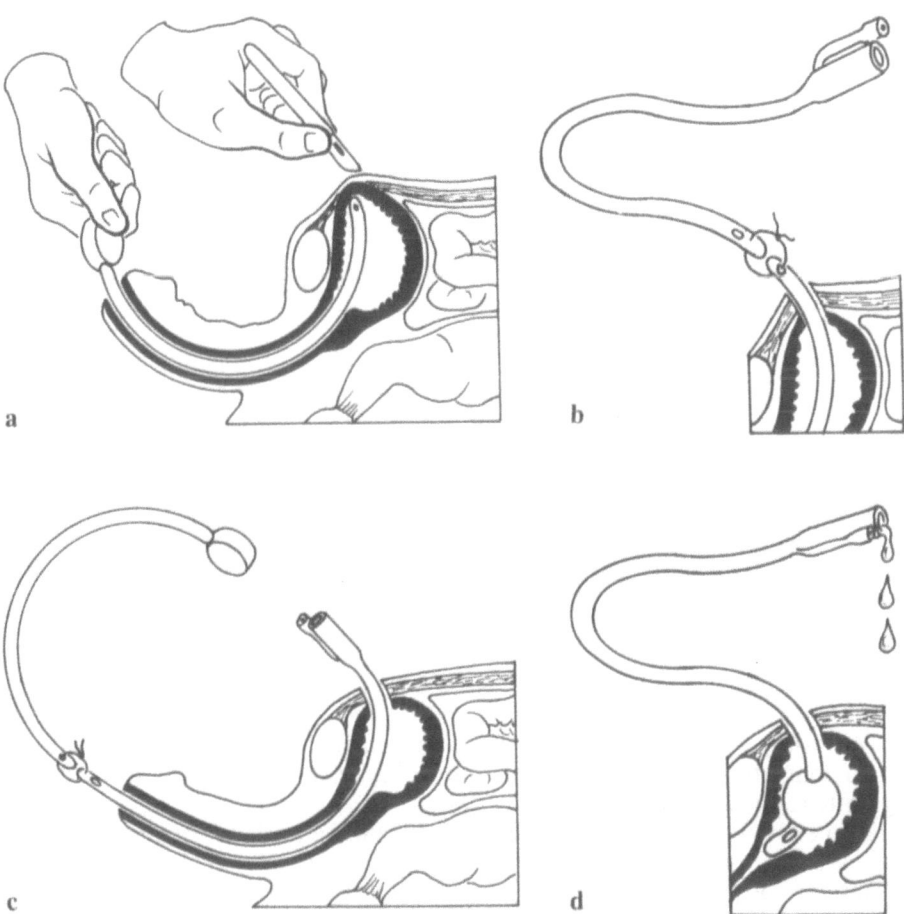

Fig. 4.4a–d. Suprapubic catheterisation using the Hey-Groves sound and minimal abdominal incision. **a** The semicircular sound is passed into the bladder which should contain at least 100 ml of fluid. The abdominal wall is tented in the midline. Care is taken to ensure that the bladder is extraperitoneal at this point. A stab incision is made on to the sound whose tip is pushed out through the skin. **b** A thick suture fixes a catheter to the eye of the sound. **c** The sound is withdrawn so that the catheter emerges from the penis and the suture is removed. **d** The catheter is withdrawn until urine just begins to drain (i.e., when the catheter enters the bladder and the balloon is inflated). The same procedure can be used antegradely through a cystotomy to introduce a urethral catheter.

deprecated. A flap valve or drip chamber in the plastic drainage bag ensures one-way drainage provided precautions are taken to prevent blockage by clot or debris at this junction. Modifications of the basic design provide integral devices for accurate volume measurement and for aspiration of urine specimens without breach of the closed system. For patients undergoing prostatic or bladder surgery a disposable device incorporating a suction balloon between catheter and bag can facilitate irrigation of clot without disconnection of catheter and drainage tube. There may be limited indications for these but too often their wholesale use adds needlessly to the expense of bladder drainage.

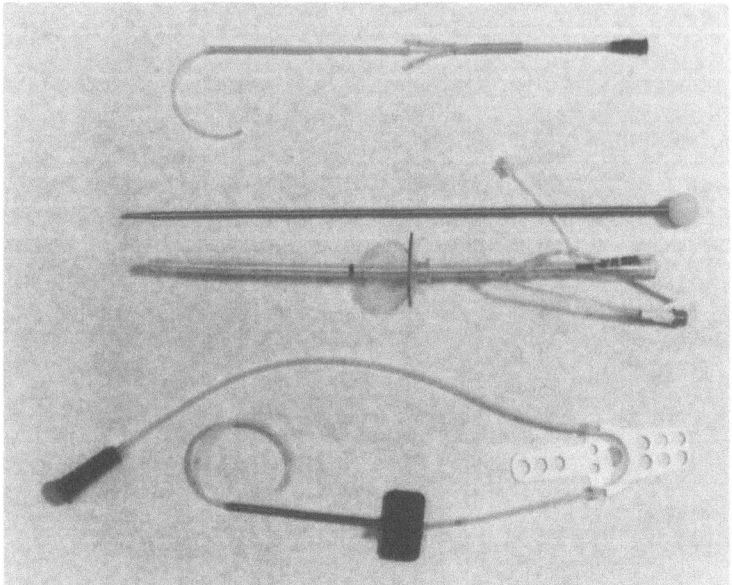

Fig. 4.5. Varieties of suprapubic catheters. From the top: Bonanno type; Ingram type; "Cystofix" catheter, the most suitable for paediatric use.

A variety of drainage bags exist for attachment to the leg to allow patients with longterm indwelling catheters to be fully ambulant. These contribute greatly to their full rehabilitation.

Some text-books of surgery and nursing continue to show complicated drainage systems, in particular to facilitate slow decompression in chronic retention. These are obsolete (see below).

Indications for Bladder Catheterisation

The indications for catheterisation are listed in Table 4.1.

Retention

Acute decompensation of detrusor function may be due to physical occlusion of the bladder outflow, acute detrusor failure or a combination of the two. Stable chronic obstruction, i.e., low flow, high voiding pressure, with or without increased residual urine volume, can decompensate with a sudden fluid load. Acute retention can occur as a culmination of deteriorating outflow obstruction with or without a previous history of urinary symptoms.

Chronic retention, or painless enlargement of the bladder, is not necessarily an indication for catheterisation or even treatment. However, prostatism, recurrent infection or obstructive nephropathy will necessitate surgery and

Table 4.1. Indications for catheterisation

Urethral
Retention of urine
  acute
  chronic: if symptomatic or in association with upper tract dilatation and nephropathy
Incontinence: particularly from the neuropathic bladder
For assessment of urine output
  in severe acute medical and surgical illness
  in oliguric renal failure
After genito-urinary or pelvic surgery where retention, haemorrhage into urine or urinary
extravasation are anticipated
In selected cases of urethral trauma: particularly disruption of membranous urethra, after
surgical realignment
Determination of residual urine volume (probably obsolete with development of calibrated
ultrasound)
To obtain clean specimen of urine if midstream specimen contaminated. Suprapubic aspiration
preferable
For contrast studies of lower urinary tract, e.g., micturating cystography
For lower and upper tract urodynamic studies, e.g., videocystomanometry; Whitaker test
For Helmstein bladder distension
To assist retention of ureteric catheters

Suprapubic
Acute/chronic retention + failure to pass urethral catheter
Acute retention + urethral trauma
After penile/urethral surgery
In conjunction with TUR prostate as a means of providing continuous low pressure irrigation

prior catheterisation is desirable. After chronic retention with upper-tract dilatation and, later on, with renal failure, a post-obstructive diuresis frequently
occurs, though is not invariable (Bishop 1985; Vaughan and Gillenwater 1973).
It is difficult to predict which patients will react thus but the likelihood is
greatest where the basal bladder pressure pre-decompression is elevated and
filling urodynamics demonstrate instability (Abrams et al. 1978). Although
some surgeons feel that definitive treatment should be offered without delay, it
seems desirable to wait for post-decompression diuresis to be concluded and
renal function stabilised. Diuresis is usually associated with a fall in plasma
creatinine but the converse does not necessarily apply. Management of the
considerable output of salt and water is surely best accomplished out of the
context of any post-operative problems.

Traditionally, chronic retention was treated by slow decompression with
the intermittent release of small volumes of urine. The aim was to prevent
severe haematuria and even to limit the diuresis which might otherwise occur
through rapid decompression. It is now clear that these manoeuvres are pointless as bladder pressure will fall very rapidly with the release of only very
small volumes. Moreover these complications are not related to the rate of
decompression.

Suprapubic versus Urethral Catheterisation in Retention

Urethral catheterisation undoubtedly causes damage to the urethral mucosa,
particularly if attempted in difficult circumstances. This may be avoided by

invariably relieving retention by suprapubic catheterisation. It has the added advantage that the catheter can be used for low pressure continuous irrigation during the subsequent transurethral resection (Reuter and Jones 1974).

Catheterisation and the Neuropathic Bladder

Interference with bladder innervation produces detrusor atony (lower motor neuron lesion) or spasticity which can include the outflow musculature (upper motor neuron lesion). Retention can result from either. The other common complication, incontinence, may be due to overflow or as a result of detrusor instability. Renal failure was formerly a common cause of morbidity and mortality due to ascending infection aided by neuropathic vesicoureteric reflux and hypertonicity (Gibbon 1976).

Catheterisation is central in the management of the neuropathic bladder. In an acute neuropathy or myelopathy, the functional disorder may change from atony to spasticity. Catheterisation may be required in the early stages until cord reflexes allow automatism. Complete bladder emptying must be achieved and this may require a longterm indwelling catheter. However, sphincterotomy even at the expense of creating incontinence may be desirable, particularly as improved devices for male incontinence become available.

One of the outstanding results of the rigid discipline imposed by Guttmann in the routine management of spinal injuries, was reduction in the incidence of early renal complications and introduction of a system of bladder training giving continence with minimal residual urine (Guttmann and Frankel 1966). In the early days of spinal units the advantages of frequent, regular, intermittent aseptic catheterisation as against longterm indwelling catheters with elaborate measures to prevent local infection, were fiercely contested. Nowadays there is much less emphasis on asepsis and asymptomatic bacteriuria is often disregarded.

The management of chronic stable neuropathic bladder is undergoing a revolution due to the development of reconstructive techniques and of artificial sphincter implants (Stephenson and Mundy 1985). However, longterm intermittent or continuous catheterisation are still of vital importance to the patients who cannot achieve spontaneous micturition (Barrett and Furlow 1984).

Clean Intermittent Catheterisation (CIC)

This has been established as a simple alternative to urinary diversion. Its feasibility was established in the treatment of spinal injuries but initially as an aseptic procedure. Since the first report by Lapides et al. (1972), a large number of publications have described similar satisfactory results (Rickwood et al. 1983; Crooks and Enrile 1983). These can be summarised: the bladder can be drained efficiently by three to four times daily catheterisation. Recurrent acute ascending infection can thus be prevented. Continence can also be achieved, even in the unstable patient, with the assistance of regular oral anticholinergic agents such as propantheline or oxybutynin (Mulcahy et al. 1977). In selected cases augmentation or substitution cystoplasty may also be necessary to relieve instability and hyperreflexia. A striking and permanent improvement can be obtained in upper tract dilatation and progressive renal

Table 4.2. Change in status of the upper urinary tracts of children with spina bifida after ileal conduit diversion and CIC

	Ileal conduit				
	Before conduit	After conduit (early)		After conduit (late)	
		Unchanged	Improved	Stable	Deteriorated
28	Normal	28	–	9	19
20	Hydronephrosis	1	19	2	18
	CIC				
		After CIC			
		Stable	Improved	Deteriorated	
64	Normal	64	–	–	
36	Hydronephrosis	19	11	6	

From Crooks and Enrile (1983).

functional impairment can be limited, though the presence of vesicoureteric reflux combined with detrusor sphincter dyssynergia make this goal more difficult to achieve (Borzyskowski et al. 1982). Intermittent catheterisation without full aseptic techniques will often lead to chronic bacteriuria but this is generally asymptomatic and seems to be of little account. It certainly does not warrant treatment with prophylactic antibiotics. CIC can be self-administered and even quite young children can be taught the technique, though it is more likely to be successful in females. Provided some sphincter function is present and a functional capacity of 200 ml or more can be achieved, a successful result from CIC can be anticipated whether the bladder is atonic or unstable. The technique can be used safely after renal transplantation. A variety of catheters can be used: a simple PVC catheter of appropriate length is generally suitable. Although disposable it can be used several times and kept in an antiseptic solution (e.g., sodium hypochlorite) after washing with soap and water. Others favour the use of a silver catheter.

Since ileal or colonic conduit diversion was until recently popular for the same patients who can now be managed by CIC, it is useful to summarise the complications of diversion and compare the results for one typical study (Table 4.2).

The Indwelling Catheter

Success with CIC is limited by a functional bladder capacity which might be insufficient to allow 3–4 hours of dryness. This is clearly not suitable for patients of limited intelligence or inco-ordinated limb movements. Since the disadvantages of diversion, particularly in the longterm, are now obvious an acceptable alternative in girls is still an indwelling catheter (Table 4.3). If boys with congenital neuropathic bladder and atony or outlet obstruction cannot be taught CIC, they can at least be managed with a penile urinal after sphincterotomy, but again indwelling catheterisation may still be acceptable.

An indwelling catheter can undoubtedly cause complications but it can certainly be effective in maintaining renal function which would otherwise be

Table 4.3. Factors predisposing to management by indwelling catheter in neuropathic bladder (i.e. failure of CIC)

Female
High lesion (above D12)
Wheelchair bound
High adduction deformity
Sphincter weakness incontinence

From Rickwood et al. (1983).

compromised by outflow obstruction, and keep the individual dry. It is still the most realistic form of management in children with severe disability. The same principles apply to adults with neuropathic bladder dysfunction. CIC is now appropriate where diversion used to be practised. An indwelling catheter is still a satisfactory compromise in the elderly, infirm and immobile patient. The choice of catheter for longterm use is important. Urethral irritation and discharge are reduced with a small diameter catheter (14–16F). A small balloon size (5–10 ml) generally lessens problems with leakage, infection and debris collection (*see* Complications).

Urine Measurement

Urine Output

Immediate assessment of urine output is of obvious importance in a wide variety of serious medical and surgical illnesses. The production of urine is a good sign of renal perfusion and hence satisfactory cardiac output. Intravenous fluid replacement can be vigorous provided venous return, weight and urine output can be monitored.

The assessment of oliguric renal failure requires the passage of a catheter, both to exclude a misdiagnosis of retention and to monitor output carefully if the patient is challenged with a large dose of diuretic or a fluid bolus when a pre-renal contribution to renal failure is in question. To have the information withheld on the grounds that catheterisation may cause infection is patently absurd. However, extreme care should be experienced in any patient suspected of a urethral injury perhaps associated with severe pelvic or abdominal trauma.

Residual Urine

An abnormal volume of residual urine must indicate either bladder outflow obstruction, detrusor failure or a combination of the two. Although the passage of a catheter will allow the volume to be measured accurately, in practice this is seldom necessary nor does it warrant the attendant risk of introducing infection. Other methods of measuring residual urine indirectly include an assessment of the post-micturition film of the bladder on the urogram and its comparison with the bladder outline on the control film, measurement of the "bladder phase" during isotope renography (Sherwood et al. 1980) and abdominal ultrasound (Poston et al. 1983; Ravichandran and Fellows 1983). For the latter it is possible to calibrate the instrument and an accurate measurement can be made.

Urodynamics

Catheters are also required in the study of lower tract urodynamics (Whiteside and Bates 1979). In general these are passed urethrally, two being inserted in tandem, the larger for bladder filling and a fine catheter attached to a transducer for the measurement of pressure. The catheters may also be passed suprapubically. The latter technique has the advantage that the structure and function of the bladder outflow can be studied unimpeded by the catheter. However, there is some possibility that introduction of a cannula through the bladder wall can give misleading results in terms of spurious instability. A catheter must also be inserted for measurement of bladder pressure in upper urinary tract urodynamic studies. The diagnosis of ureteric obstruction is made from the difference between intrarenal and bladder pressures during a simulated diuresis (Whitaker 1973).

Recovery of Urine Specimens for Microbiological Study

Culture of mid-stream urine specimens may be unsatisfactory in persistently showing contamination by commensal organisms, particularly in the diagnosis of infection by fastidious organisms. In these circumstances there may be some advantage in collecting catheter urine. Suprapubic aspiration is likely to yield the cleanest specimen (Savage et al. 1983) and has been used for many years, particularly in diagnosis of urine infection in the paediatric age group. However, potential contamination from single shot urethral catheterisation might be improved by using an open-ended catheter (Murphy et al. 1984).

Catheterisation in Association with Operative Urology

Drainage after Prostatectomy

After prostatectomy the catheter must provide efficient drainage so that blood is evacuated before clots can form, for irrigation and, if bleeding is severe, to effect haemostasis in the prostatic bed. A variety of catheters and techniques are used. Some favour the use of a PVC plastic catheter with its advantage of rigidity so that clot can be evacuated more easily. Others use the more expensive reinforced latex haematuria catheter. Most surgeons agree that if adequate haemostasis can be achieved at operation a coated latex catheter is adequate. The majority use a self-retaining catheter. However, if open prostatectomy is performed it is possible for a simple wide-bore catheter to be retained in the bladder by a stitch through the tip traversing the bladder wall and fixed over a gauze roll or metal bar on the surface of the abdomen. The advantage of a non-self-retaining catheter is of course that a wider channel for evacuation can be provided than for a balloon catheter of the same circumference. The use of a "two-way" catheter after prostatectomy requires that very careful haemostasis should be achieved and a good urine flow encouraged with diuretics and a high intravenous fluid load. For those who feel that there may be inherent dangers of fluid overload, particularly in the elderly patient, the bladder can be irrigated using a third line on the catheter (three-way). However, there is probably little advantage of one method over the other in terms of blood loss, infection and catheter patency in the post-operative period. Irrigation with the three-way catheter requires the use of saline rather than hypotonic fluid or an isotonic irrigant which is low in electrolyte since there is a risk of haemolysis with one and haemodilution with the other. It is possible to obtain clear effluent with the three-way catheter although the bladder is full of clot and the nursing staff should be especially vigilant of this possibility (*see* Complications).

If bleeding is heavy after prostatectomy haemostasis can be achieved with the catheter balloon. The technique involves withdrawing the catheter with a semi-inflated balloon back into the prostatic cavity. The balloon is then over-inflated (50 ml+) (Mauermayer 1983). Another technique is to apply traction of the catheter with the balloon over-inflated so that it impacts on the trigone. There seems very little logic in this though admittedly if the traction is applied by a meatal swab tied around the catheter, then the bleeding should be contained in a closed system and haemorrhage should be arrested by a tamponade, but compression of veins at the bladder neck may be involved. If the latter method is used the swab must not be forgotten and should in any case be removed after a maximum of 20 min lest pressure necrosis of the meatus ensues.

Urethral Surgery

After urethroplasty or hypospadias repair a catheter will be required to splint the anastomosis or reconstruction. The same catheter may be used for urinary drainage or a separate suprapubic catheter can be inserted. For boys undergoing such surgery the "Cystofix" suprapubic catheter is very convenient for this purpose. Alternatively, the Gibbon catheter is effective since the plastic "wings" can be included in the penile dressing. The use of a fenestrated catheter has also been advocated to allow the passage of blood and urethral secretion down the lumen away from the site of the anastomosis, thus lessening the danger of secondary infection (Smith and Ball 1984).

After complete membranous urethral rupture it is important to bridge the gap with a catheter to limit the length and complexity of the stricture which would otherwise subsequently develop (Blandy 1975). In general the catheter is railroaded back through the internal meatus through the opened bladder during suprapubic exploration after the pelvic fracture (Mundy 1984). It is probably important that separate sutures through the bladder and pelvic floor should be employed to hold the "free floating" bladder in place rather than to use traction on the catheter balloon for this purpose. If the latter is done there is a grave risk of pressure necrosis of the bladder neck and possibly of the already damaged external sphincter mechanism.

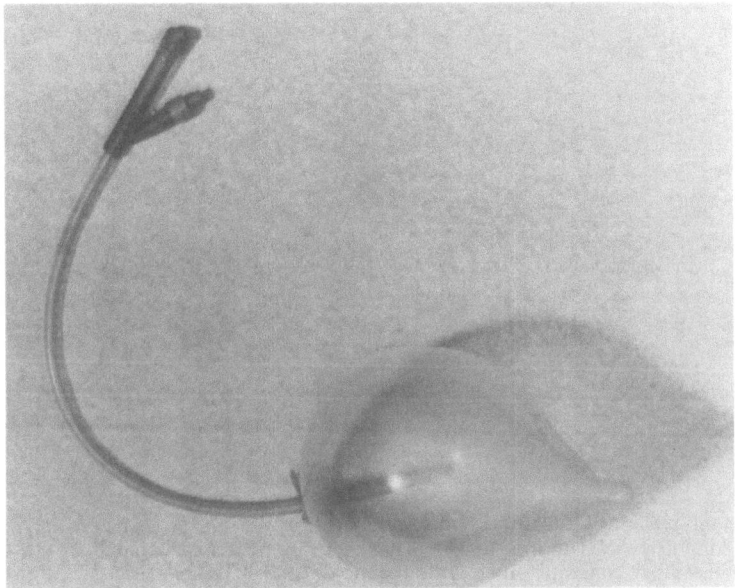

Fig. 4.6. Catheter used in prolonged hydrostatic dilatation of the bladder (Helmstein).

Bladder Surgery

Cystotomy for any purpose requires two-layer closure and continuous catheter drainage for a minimum period of 5 days. If there is a danger of clot retention through the single catheter it is wise to insert an additional suprapubic catheter to provide a second port of exit and also an entry point for continuous irrigation.

Prolonged Bladder Distension

Prolonged hydrostatic bladder dilatation by the Helmstein technique requires the use of a special catheter. Unfortunately, the quality of the distending balloon in manufactured catheters can vary such that the compliance is unpredictable. A better result may be achieved with a condom attached to a plastic catheter at the time of surgery (Fig. 4.6). This technique has been used with some success in the control of multiple superficial bladder tumours, of bleeding in haemorrhagic cystitis and in the treatment of urge and urge incontinence associated with detrusor instability (Wolk and Bishop 1981; Pengelly et al. 1978; Ramsden et al. 1976; Whitfield and Mayo 1975).

Fixation of Ureteric Catheters

A urethral catheter may be used to retain a ureteric catheter (Fig. 4.7). This method is particularly useful where longterm ureteric drainage is required.

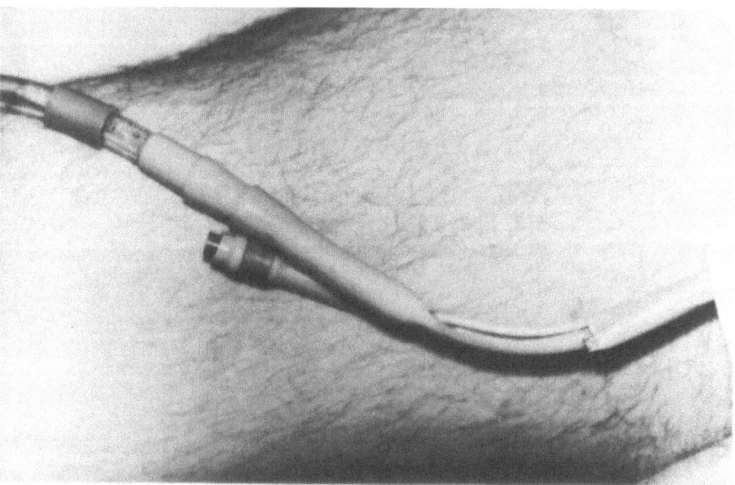

Fig. 4.7. Use of self-retaining bladder catheter to retain ureteric catheter. The end of the ureteric catheter is passed through a small incision in the Foley catheter outlet and allowed to drain into the lumen of the drainage bag connecting tube. The ureteric catheter is secured to the stem of the Foley catheter with "sleek".

Conventional fixation in a separate specimen bottle is very likely to lead to dislodgement.

Complications

During Insertion

Difficulty in Passing the Catheter (Fig. 4.8)

It should be obvious that a catheter of the smallest diameter to effect adequate drainage should be used after the injection of adequate quantities of lubricant. Sufficient delay should be allowed to elapse after infiltration of local anaesthetic gel to permit adequate local anaesthesia. If the procedure causes pain or anxiety (Fig. 4.8b), spasm at the external sphincter or bladder neck may impede the insertion. Unfortunately, it can be difficult to anaesthetise the urethra adequately beyond the point of a stricture, though this problem is usually obvious to the operator.

Unfamiliarity with the anatomy of the external genitalia, particularly of females, can cause problems in identifying the external urethral meatus. Difficulties can be encountered in the male whose external meatus is hypospadiac, particularly as a deep but blind pit is often seen at the tip of the meatus and some distance anterior to the true meatus which can be situated anywhere along the midline from the corona to the perineum. The presence of an incomplete prepuce ventrally should always raise the suspicion of hypospadias in the male. The condition can also occur in the female, in which case the meatus may be situated well inside the introitus.

Difficulty may be encountered due to the presence of a urethral stricture. In the male this may occur at the meatus, particularly where there is evidence of balanitis xerotica, or nappy rash, in a baby which can lead to meatal ulcer and stenosis; submeatally, at the posterior limit of the navicular fossa; at the peno-scrotal junction, particularly after a gonococcal infection or perhaps due to previous catheterisation; in the bulbar urethra, due to direct trauma and in the membranous urethra, as a result of a previous pelvic fracture and urethral disruption. Difficulty may also be encountered due to a high bladder neck with narrowing though not necessarily fixed stenosis of the urethra. In the un-circumcised male, phimosis may even prevent insertion of a catheter into the preputial sac. In the female, occasionally urethral stenosis may be present, as a result of atrophic vulvovaginitis, previous surgery or perhaps radiotherapy.

Perforation

Perforation can occur in the normal urethra if catheterisation is attempted by a heavyhanded, ignorant operator. It is particularly likely with the inexperienced use of an introducer in situations where difficulty is encountered. Provided the bladder is palpable the alternative solution is suprapubic catheterisation. If the patient is known to have a urethral stricture this should be treated by optical internal urethrotomy under general or regional local anaesthesia. The less acceptable alternative is bouginage. This is done under local anaesthetic with rigid sounds (Clutton's, Lister, Benique). However, flexible gum elastic bougies are probably safer, particularly if used as followers to threaded fili-forms. Perforation of the urethra with the formation of a false passage is extremely easy to accomplish through the delicate mucosal layer and the underlying areolar tissue and spongiosum. Occasionally the operator may be fortunate enough to force the catheter back into the urethral lumen. However, the catheter may also be passed across Denonvillier's fascia into the rectum or into a long, blind passage behind the bladder neck (Fig. 4.9). Further injury to the urethra is much more likely to occur after attempted catheterisation in patients with pre-existing urethral injury.

In acute trauma, either through direct injury to the perineum and hence bulbar urethra or indirectly with disruption of the membranous urethra after severe pelvic fracture, urinary retention is the rule. Many advocate that this should always be relieved by suprapubic catheterisation. If urethral injury is in doubt, acute urethrography seems safe and certain and if no perforation is seen, gentle catheterisation can be undertaken.

Perforation of the bladder itself by a catheter is possible particularly if there is some abnormality causing diminution in the thickness of the wall, such as a diverticulum, after radiotherapy, or with severe perivesical inflammation. It is perhaps a little more likely to occur with the use of indwelling PVC catheters although these are said to soften at body temperature. It is of course well described with the use of the Helmstein bladder distension catheter. Bladder perforation can occur intra or extraperitoneally. In either situation the bladder will usually heal with a period of catheter drainage though if intraperitoneal perforation has occurred with the passage of considerable volumes of urine into the peritoneal cavity, many surgeons would feel that the bladder should be repaired at open operation. Bladder rupture during Helmstein distension

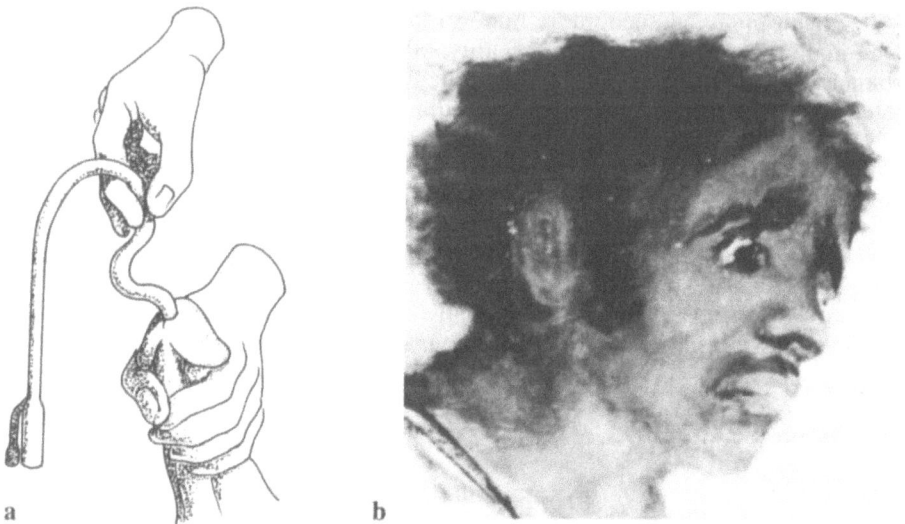

a   b

Fig. 4.8a–d. Difficulties/hazards in catheterisation. **a** Inadequate lubricant. **b** Pain and anxiety can cause muscle spasm in the proximal urethra (after F. Goya). **c** Hypospadias in male and female. **d** Organic obstruction. Examples of causative factors in parentheses.

usually has a remarkably benign course and it is said that such patients may even obtain a better result, particularly if the indication is bladder instability (Higson et al. 1978). Extraperitoneal bladder rupture is recognised from the development of a tender, suprapubic mass though without evidence of extravasation in the genitalia. The latter can only occur if urine tracks superficial to the deep fascia and beneath the deep layer of the superficial fascia (Scarpa's and/or Colles' fasciae). Intraperitoneal rupture is recognised by the presence of urinary peritonitis. At first the symptoms of this are usually mild unless the urine is infected. Perforation with a three-way catheter which is not recognised early on may lead to absorption of large quantities of irrigant giving symptoms and signs of circulatory overload, though without haemodilution found in the TUR syndrome and assuming that physiological saline is used as the irrigant.

Bacteraemia

Catheter insertion may be followed by the rapid onset of rigors and perhaps bacteraemic shock (Ferrie et al. 1979; Drach 1976; Feingold 1970). This is more likely if prolonged attempts are made at a difficult catheterisation, particularly in a patient with infected urine. If possible, a large dose of parenteral antibiotics should be given prophylactically if difficulty is anticipated and of course in every patient who is likely to be prone to systemic infection.

Whilst Catheter Indwelling

Inability to Retain the Catheter (Fig. 4.10)

The self-retaining balloon can deflate because of manufacturing defect, giving an incompetent valve on the balloon channel. Another cause of deflation is loss

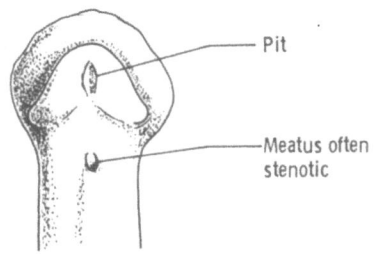

c

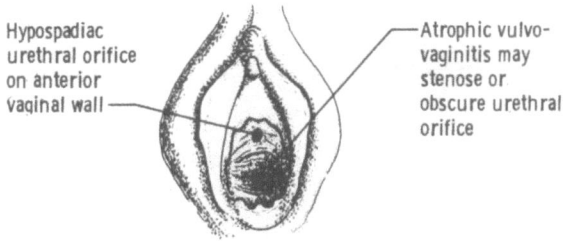

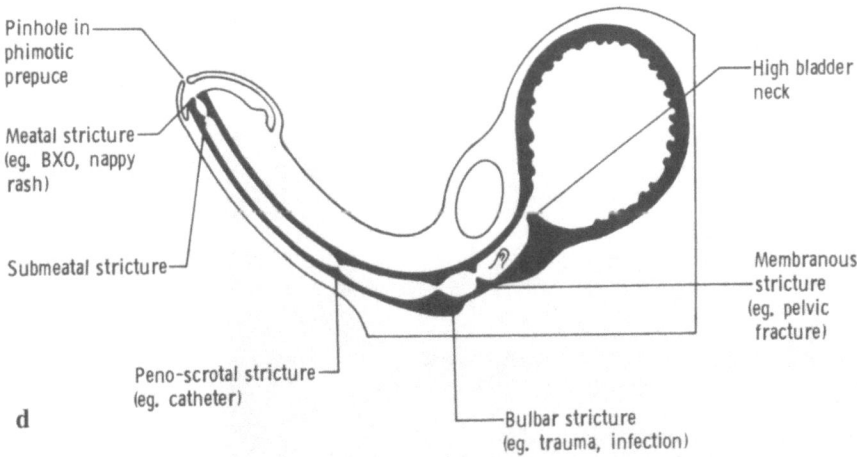

d

of water from a small balloon due to osmosis across the rubber membrane. This can be demonstrated experimentally and if a long period of catheterisation is expected it may be wise to fill the balloon with strong saline (Studer et al. 1983). Occasionally, urethral laxity is a problem, particularly in the neuropathic female, though if at all possible the natural inclination to recatheterise with ever larger catheters and more capacious self-retaining balloons should be resisted as these are more likely to increase the vicious circle in causing loss of

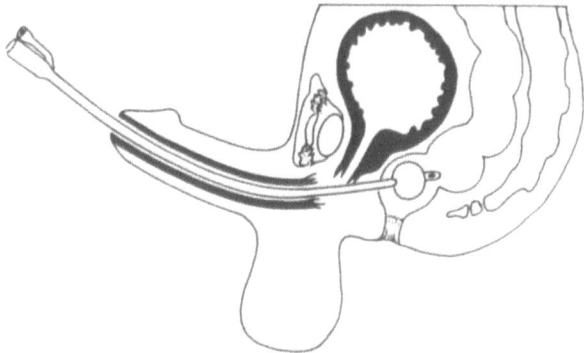

Attempted catheterisation after urethral injury may
result in perforation of urethra or perhaps other organs

a

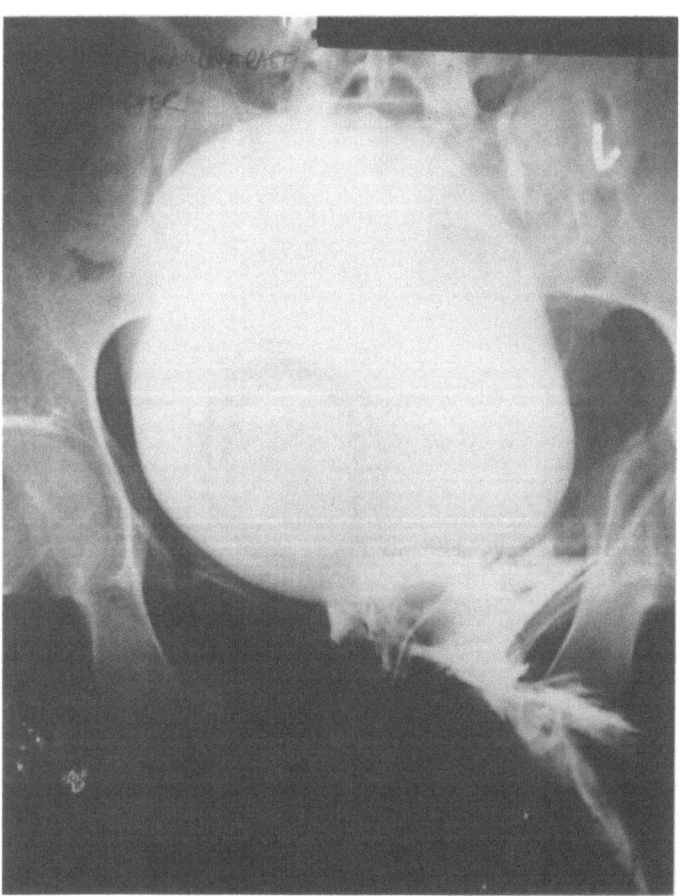

Fig. 4.9a–d. Perforation. **a** Partial traumatic urethral disruption completed by clumsy catheterisation. **b** Cystourethrography following catheterisation injury after pelvic fracture and membranous urethral injury: (i) in female, anterior perforation. Balloon lying in extravesical tissues. Bladder opacified by iv urography: (ii) in male, posterior perforation. Balloon lying in rectum. **c** Pattern of urinary extravasation after submembranous – bulbar – urethral injury. **d** Bladder perforation. (i) extraperitoneal; (ii) intraperitoneal.

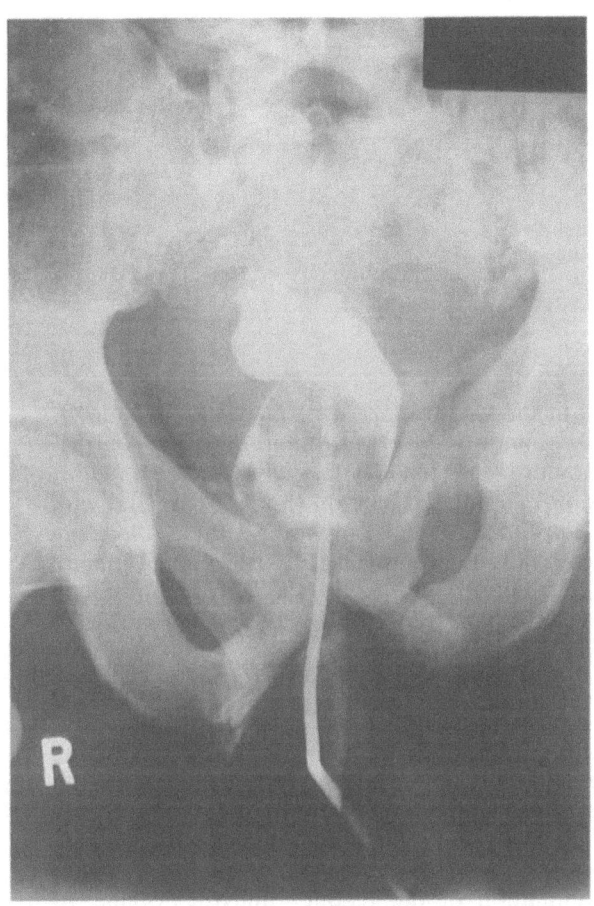

b(ii)

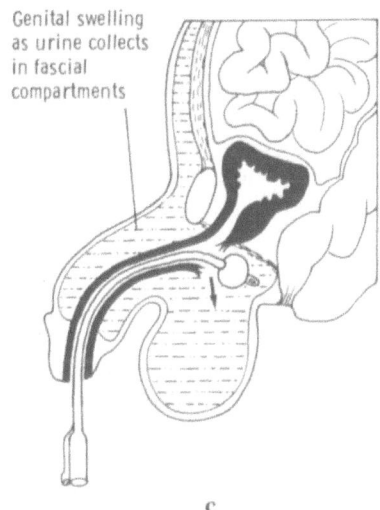

Genital swelling
as urine collects
in fascial
compartments

c

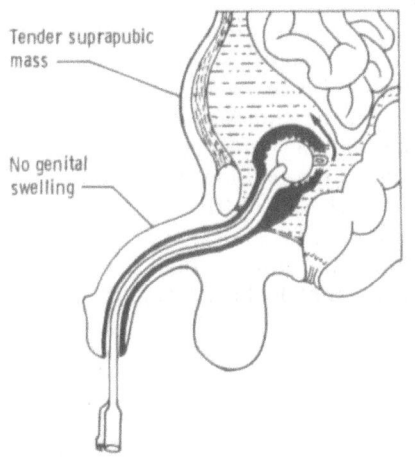

Tender suprapubic
mass

No genital
swelling

d(i)

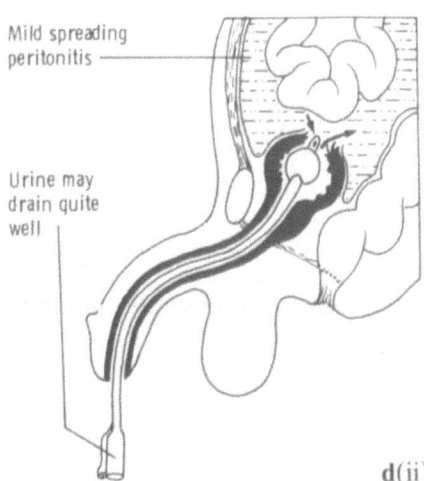

Mild spreading
peritonitis

Urine may
drain quite
well

d(ii)

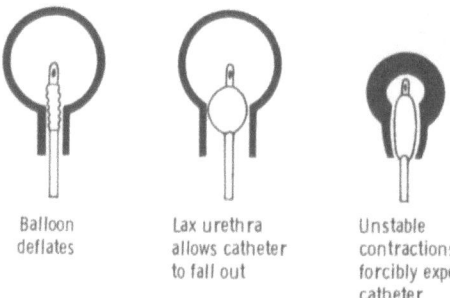

Balloon   Lax urethra   Unstable
deflates   allows catheter   contractions
                 to fall out   forcibly expel
                                   catheter

Fig. 4.10. Inability to retain catheter.

tone and even pressure necrosis in the urethra (*see Pressure necrosis*, below). Inability to retain a catheter is commonly due to unstable detrusor contractions, again, particularly in the neurogenic bladder (*see also Catheter spasm*, below). A tendency for expulsion of an inflated balloon should be treated with anticholinergic agents in the first instance, though only after catheter blockage has been excluded. Detrusor denervation accomplished by subtrigonal phenol injection is a more permanent solution (Ewing et al. 1982). More proximal denervation may be achieved by sacral nerve root block (Essenhigh and Ryan 1982; Torrens and Griffith 1974).

Leakage (Fig. 4.11)

As with the problem of catheter expulsion, so too is urinary leakage around the catheter commonly encountered during longterm indwelling catheterisation, particularly of the neuropathic female. It is also generally due to unstable detrusor contractions. These may be due to irritation by an over-inflated balloon or where there is inflammation of the bladder mucosa because of infection and/or debris. Occlusion of the catheter lumen will also lead to leakage if retention does not occur. Instability is probably present in almost every patient undergoing catheterisation, such that there is no point in documenting it by a urodynamic study. It can be extremely difficult to treat and may be resistant to large doses of anticholinergic agents. However, the use of a small volume (5–10 ml) balloon may minimise leakage as the "sump" of urine around the balloon is smaller than with the standard 30-ml. balloon. A Roberts' type of catheter may help as urine that has bypassed the end-aperture can enter the catheter via the hole proximal to the balloon. Other possibilities include Helmstein bladder distension and perhaps subtrigonal phenol injections. Very rarely, the situation in the female may be so desperate as to require some form of urinary diversion. It is commonly thought that a wider diameter catheter to obturate the urethra will prevent leakage. This is clearly an erroneous and hazardous concept.

Catheter "Spasm"

Not only do uninhibited detrusor contractions cause leakage but they may produce severe pain as the balloon is forced into the sensitive trigone. Typically

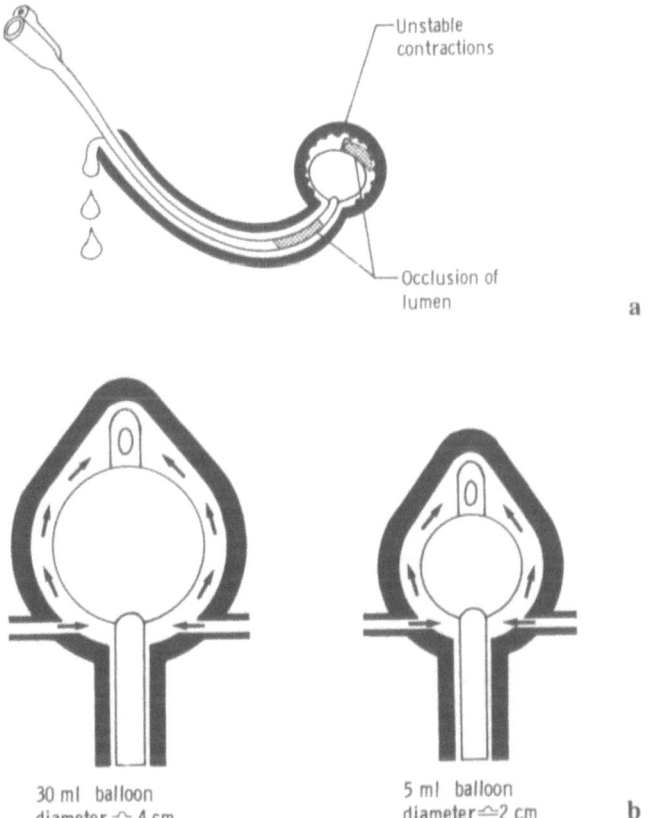

Fig. 4.11a,b. Causes of urine leakage around catheter. **a** Detrusor instability, luminal occlusion. **b** "Sump" effect, in proportion to balloon volume. Urine enters the bladder on the trigone distal to the balloon and will therefore need to flow "uphill" to enter the catheter drainage port. The 30-ml balloon will, therefore, create a larger potential reservoir for leakage and debris collection, giving rise to an increased risk of infection than with the smaller balloon.

the patient experiences bursts of suprapubic pain which radiate intensely to the tip of the penis. Sometimes only the penile pain is felt and may mislead the unwary to search for a local meatal problem. Treatment for catheter "spasm" is essentially the same as for catheter leakage. However, the urologist may be more inclined to use permanent sacral nerve block early on as the symptom can be so resistant that the only alternative for the patient with an indwelling catheter is supravesical diversion (Simon et al. 1982).

Erratic Drainage (Fig. 4.12)

Most of the causes are obvious. The catheter may not be fully in the bladder. This may be a particular problem after prostatectomy. Here attempted inflation of the catheter balloon in the membranous urethra causes pain. Furthermore the catheter does not move easily in the urethra after insertion. Another common cause is obstruction of the catheter aperture by the balloon. This can

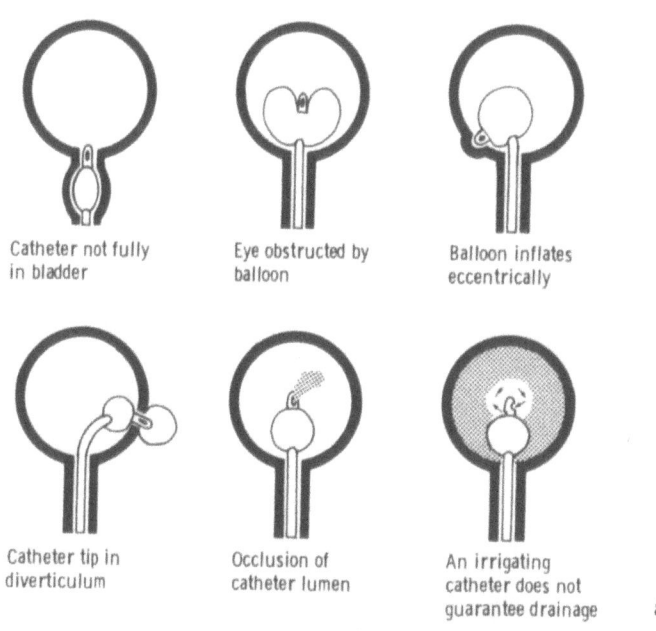

Catheter not fully   Eye obstructed by   Balloon inflates
in bladder   balloon   eccentrically

Catheter tip in   Occlusion of   An irrigating
diverticulum   catheter lumen   catheter does not
                                                       guarantee drainage   a

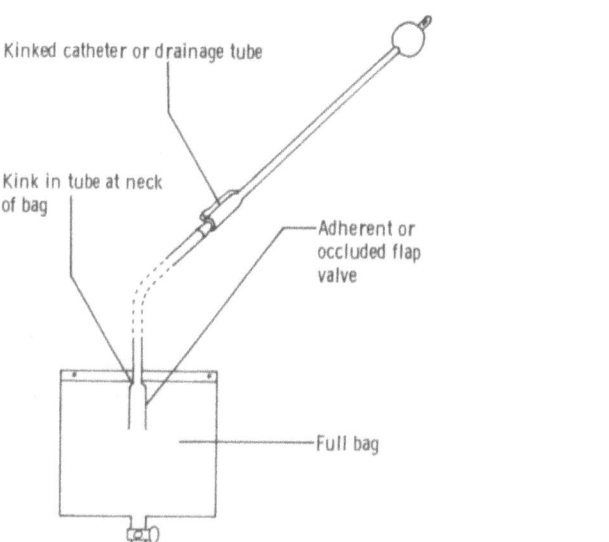

Kinked catheter or drainage tube

Kink in tube at neck
of bag
                                                       Adherent or
                                                       occluded flap
                                                       valve

                                                       Full bag

                                                                                 b

Fig. 4.12a,b.   Causes of erratic drainage. **a** Intravesical faults. **b** "Bag" faults.

be recognised and treated by complete deflation and reinflation to a smaller
volume. Sometimes the balloon may inflate eccentrically, deviating and perhaps pressing the catheter tip into the bladder wall. Occasionally the balloon
can be inflated inside a bladder diverticulum. More obvious causes include
occlusion of the catheter "eye" with blood clot, calculi, tumour debris or a
prostatic "chip". A three-way irrigation catheter can create special problems in

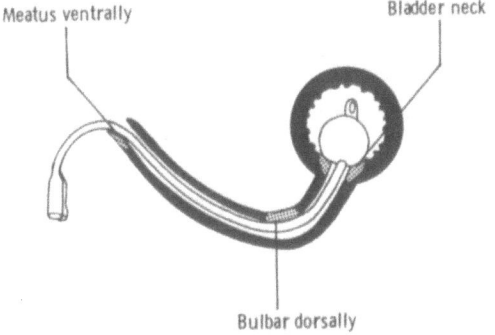

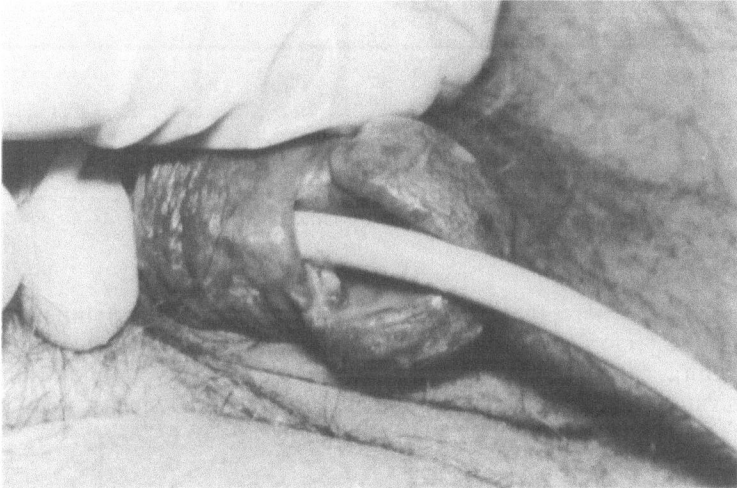

Fig. 4.13a,b. Pressure necrosis in the urethra. **a** Diagram of principal sites of pressure necrosis. **b** Erosion of distal urethra producing coronal hypospadias.

that it can apparently drain in the presence of acute clot retention. In these circumstances the effluent may be clear. The situation arises through irrigant entering and leaving the bladder without admixture with the organising blood clot.

Intermittent drainage can also be due to a selection of "bag" problems. These include a drainage bag held above the level of the patient's bladder, a kink at the neck of the bag, an adherent or occluded flap valve and finally a full bag.

Pressure Necrosis

Prolonged traction on the inflated catheter balloon can cause pressure necrosis of the bladder neck and proximal urethral sphincter mechanism (Fig. 4.13a). This is only likely to occur in two circumstances, namely where an attempt is made to appose the ends of the membranous urethra after rupture using the

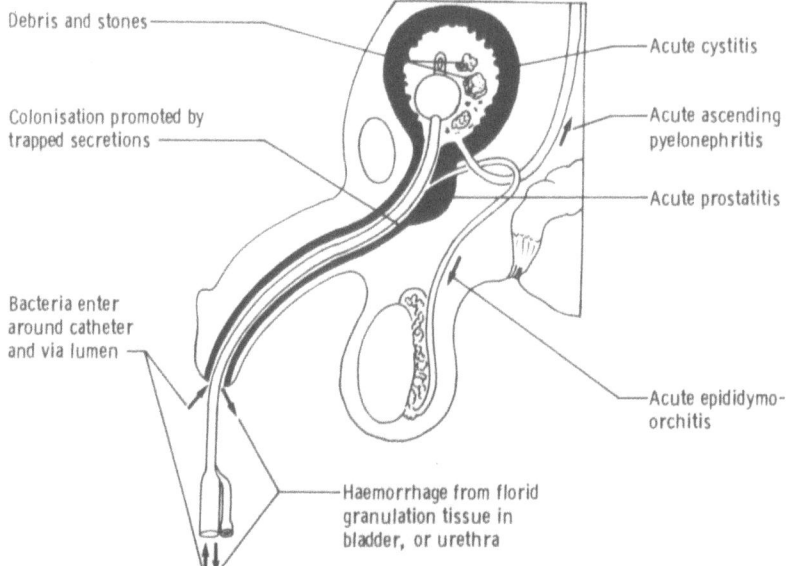

Fig. 4.14.   The consequence of infection in relation to the indwelling catheter.

catheter balloon and where the over-inflated balloon is used to tamponade
bleeding post-prostatectomy. In both situations incontinence may be the result.
The distal urethra can also undergo pressure necrosis from an indwelling
catheter. This can occur in both sexes producing in effect an acquired form of
hypospadias (Fig. 4.13b).

Infection (Fig. 4.14)

Urinary infections caused by indwelling catheters continue to be the most
common form of hospital-acquired infection (Slade and Gillespie 1985; Platt et
al. 1983; Turck and Stamm 1981; Kunin 1979; Drach 1976; Feingold 1970).
Among patients admitted as emergencies 10%–15% have a catheter left
indwelling and approximately 20% contract bacteriuria. Of patients who have
indwelling catheters for more than 10 days, 50% have infected urine and
catheterisation is probably unnecessarily prolonged in a significant proportion
of patients (Hartstein et al. 1981). It is an interesting fact that such nosocomial
urinary tract infection is commoner amongst patients being treated for non-
urological diseases. It is hoped that this reflects the awareness by experts of the
causative factors so that others can be educated in the correct technique of
catheter insertion and maintenance and are made aware of the importance of
limiting the period of indwelling catheterisation (Fincke and Friedland 1976).
   One of the most important factors in reducing infection is the use of the
closed sterile drainage system (Desautes 1974; Kunin and McCormack 1966).
Before this was instituted virtually every patient acquired an infection. The
modern closed-drainage system includes sterile disposable calibrated drainage
bags with a non-return valve and tap. Theoretically, if the catheter is inserted

Table 4.4. Organisms causing nosocomial UTI

	%
Escherichia coli	32
Klebsiella	14
Staphylococcus epidermidis	12
Pseudomonas	10
Streptococcus faecalis	9
Proteus	8
Enterobacter	8
Candida	2
Others, e.g., *Serratia, Haemophilus*	6

From Haase and Harding (1984).

and connected aseptically, there should be no reason why infection should occur at all provided the system is not broken. However, if vigilance is relaxed the infection rate will rise. Thus special care should be taken to avoid flow-back to the patient of either urine or even air bubbles in the tubing. Removal of samples for testing should be minimised and the practice of clamping the tubing to build up a quantity of residual urine for chemical or microbiological testing should be avoided.

One controversial aspect of catheter care concerns meatal cleansing (Burke et al. 1981). The earlier regimes insisted on obsessional perineal and meatal cleansing with germicidal solutions. Certainly it has been shown that extra-luminal migration of organisms can occur into the bladder via the periurethral mucous sheath. However, it is doubtful whether infections acquired in this way are clinically relevant. Retrograde *intraluminal* migration is less contentious and there seems little doubt that clinically relevant infection, often acquired by cross-contamination will occur in patients undergoing frequent intermittent irrigation or bladder washout. Localised infection can occur in the urethra involving the prostate and periurethral glands. Abscesses can develop and hence a paraurethral diverticulum.

Bacteria cultured from urine of patients with catheter-associated infections are derived from the faeces and are typically strains of *Escherichia coli* (Table 4.4). The longer the catheter becomes indwelling the more varied the urine culture. Infections acquired from the hospital environment rather than from the patient's own faecal flora are often by different organisms, which exhibit antibiotic resistance. These cultures may include yeasts if the patient is debilitated, has received immunosuppressive agents (e.g. after renal transplantation) or has been treated with longterm broad-spectrum antibiotics. Cross-infection of catheterised patients by hospital-acquired organisms sometimes occurs in epidemics. These tend to occur in high-dependency units, geriatric wards and urological departments. In the latter case, instruments or solutions used for meatal cleansing are often found to be contaminated (Garibaldi et al. 1974). Catheterised patients with persistent infection should be separated and barrier-nursed if a highly resistant organism is found.

The diagnosis of infection in the catheterised patient can be difficult. Symptoms of pyrexia, rigors, loin and abdominal pain and epididymitis may be self-evident. A clinical diagnosis may be supported by a pure growth of organisms on culture with a bacterial count of greater than 10^8 per l. However, microbiological evidence is often equivocal. The clinician should perhaps be prepared to accept that infection is present with much lower than conventional counts, particularly as serial cultures will reveal progressive rise in the count to significant values in the majority of catheterised patients, usually within three days of the initial culture (Stark and Maki 1984). The presence of leucocytes in the urine is unhelpful as these may arise through local irritation of the catheter in the bladder and a lower bacterial count may be relevant. In this respect it may be significant that in the non-catheterised patient with recurrent urinary infections urine culture may be negative according to accepted criteria but organisms can still be obtained by special techniques from the deeper layers of the urothelium (Elliott et al. 1984). Such organisms may have penetrated deeply beneath the surface due to persistent damage, presumably by bacterial toxin or enzymatic degradation of protective mucopolysaccharide on the surface. It is highly likely that a catheter could damage the all-important surface layers through local irritation, allowing penetration and deep proliferation of organisms which might not necessarily be revealed by urine culture.

The treatment of urinary infection in the catheterised patient depends upon whether the patient is asymptomatic and on the possibility of removing the catheter. Asymptomatic bacteriuria should not be treated if the catheter must remain, as it is highly likely that the bladder will become recolonised with resistant organisms. If treatment is to be given for septic complications a short course should be given of the appropriate antibiotic in high dosage. It is possible that changing the catheter might help and in this context it may be recalled that in patients with renal failure undergoing chronic ambulatory peritoneal dialysis who show recurrent bacterial peritonitis, infection can be ameliorated merely by changing the cannula. Alternatively replacement of the urethral catheter with a suprapubic catheter might also be effective.

In the past it was traditional to instil regularly a variety of antibacterial solutions (e.g., chlorhexidine, citrate) in patients with indwelling catheters (Thompson et al. 1984; Stickler et al. 1981; Warren et al. 1978). A variety of antiseptics have also been introduced into the drainage bag. None of these techniques has been shown to prevent infection.

There is no support for the use of prophylactic antibiotics in catheterised patients and drug-resistant organisms may be selected (Chodak and Plant 1979). However, it is generally agreed that the patient at special risk should be treated with high-dose broad-spectrum antibiotics for 2–3 days, covering the period of catheter introduction and withdrawal. Such high-risk situations include valvular heart disease, previous joint replacement surgery and the immunosuppressed patient. Patients who already have a catheter indwelling and are about to undergo urological surgery should certainly be treated for bacteriuria even if it is asymptomatic (Britt et al. 1977). Patients on a regime of intermittent self-catheterisation commonly have bacteriuria but again require no treatment except for symptomatic infections. It is, however, likely that treatment with an antibiotic in prophylactic dosage can in fact reduce the incidence of subclinical infection.

Urinary tract manipulation and, specifically, catheterisation, is a cause of bacteraemia and septicaemia. The distinction between the two is somewhat hazy and it is assumed that the former, if not treated promptly, will progress to the latter which still has a mortality of 50% or more. Proliferation of gram-negative organisms in the blood-stream is associated with septicaemic shock and profound effects on the peripheral circulation, lungs and clotting mechanism. Gram-negative septicaemia is more commonly due to urosepsis than other sources of infection. It may be significant that bacteraemia as shown by a positive blood culture is common in patients undergoing urological surgery, including catheterisation. In one early study the rate was as high as 20%. The fact that septicaemia is uncommon in such patients treated in urology wards is very likely to indicate the benefit of increased awareness and prompt treatment in any patient with early symptoms of infection. For most urologists this implies use of parenteral broad-spectrum antibiotics before the blood-culture results are available. An aminoglycoside is usually selected although a large variety of other drugs related to cephalosporin or penicillin, apparently having fewer side effects, are available.

Epididymo-orchitis

This specific form of ascending infection is said to occur in 6% of men undergoing prostatectomy (Drach 1976). The risk is increased considerably in men undergoing pre-operative catheterisation. Such conclusions have been drawn from older studies and the rates of infection are likely to be lower in the modern setting where very little open prostatic surgery is performed and there is a general tendency for catheters to remain for a much shorter period. When epididymitis was commoner the risk was reduced by performing a prophylactic vasectomy. Epididymitis is a most unpleasant condition which can be a cause of chronic ill-health and will ultimately only respond to orchidectomy. It is treated with antibiotics, perhaps local support for the scrotum and injection of local anaesthetic around the spermatic cord. Epididymo-orchitis may also be associated with prostatitis and very rarely with the development of prostatic abscess.

Encrustation

The production of free bladder calculi and encrustation are common complications of longterm indwelling catheterisation (Brocklehurst and Brocklehurst 1978). They cause occlusion of the catheter necessitating frequent bladder irrigation (Ruwald 1980). Catheter changes may be required more and more frequently and ultimately bladder washout and perhaps litholapaxy are required under general anaesthetic. The abrasive surface of the balloon coated with an eggshell calcification can contribute to chronic cystitis, squamous metaplasia, rarely leukoplakia and perhaps even frank carcinoma through chronic irritation.

The main inorganic constituent of catheter debris is magnesium ammonium phosphate (struvite) (Hukins et al. 1983). This is consistent with pathogenesis from chronic infection by urease-producing organisms and production of ammonium and a high urine pH (Griffith and Klein 1983). Chemical analytical methods as opposed to X-ray diffraction analysis have also demonstrated calcium phosphate (brushite and apatite), oxalate and uric acid (Hedelin et al. 1984).

Theoretically, infection need not be the sole cause of calcification. The presence of a foreign body in the bladder will invariably lead to epithelial damage. Specifically a breach of the glycocalyx or protective mucopolysaccharide layer with loss of the underlying superficial layer of urothelial cells can occur in association with trauma and inflammation. Crystal aggregates which are often present in normal urine adhere preferentially to the denuded basement membrane (Khan et al. 1984).

Prevention of catheter encrustation is difficult (Brocklehurst and Brocklehurst 1978). Total permanent eradication of infection is virtually impossible whilst the catheter remains. Treatment with urease inhibitors (hydroxamates) might be effective (Griffith and Klein 1983), but these drugs are toxic, being related to the cytotoxic agent hydroxyurea. Acidification is also difficult to achieve: oral supplements of ascorbic acid can help but the dosage is limited by gastric intolerance. Irrigation with acidic solutions (e.g., Renacidin can be helpful (Hukins et al. 1983) but the effect is only temporary. For patients with longterm catheters a weekly bladder washout is recommended to prevent excessive accumulation of debris. The chemical composition of the irrigant is probably unimportant as it is the mechanical action which produces the desired result. Claims have been made that allopurinol can of irrigation (Eddeland and Hedelin 1983). The mechanism is somewhat obscure. Urinary uric acid is diminished by the action of the drug as it is a xanthine oxidase inhibitor. However, uric acid is rarely a major constituent of the debris surrounding catheters, though a secondary action of allopurinol may be to diminish precipitation of oxalate and phosphate in urine. In practical terms allopurinol does not reduce encrustation but merely alters the constituents (Hedelin et al. 1984).

A novel approach to the problem of encrustation has been to utilise the so-called oligodynamic bactericidal property of silver ions. Coating the tip of a Foley catheter with fine silver powder has been shown to dramatically reduce the rate of urinary infection associated with longterm indwelling catheterisation (Akiyama and Okamoto 1979; Liedberg and Lundberg 1990). Prevention of infective stone formation might therefore be predicted.

Catheter Tumour (Fig. 4.15)

The tip of an indwelling catheter can lead to localised thickening in the bladder epithelium. To the uninitiated this can have the cystoscopic appearance of a broad-based tumour. The histological appearances show chronic inflammatory changes with no evidence of malignancy. Such "tumours" can be very vascular and the site of considerable bleeding. Haematuria can, however, arise elsewhere, particularly from generalised haemorrhagic cystitis and perhaps from friable vessels in the vicinity of the posterior bladder neck.

During Catheter Withdrawal

Difficulties may be encountered in removing a urethral catheter (Fig. 4.16). In particular the balloon can fail to deflate due either to a faulty valve at the point of aspiration or to an occluded inflation channel. Complete deflation may be prevented by mineral deposits.

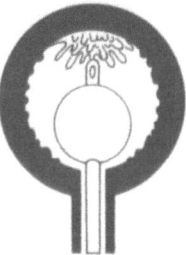

Fig. 4.15. The catheter "tumour".

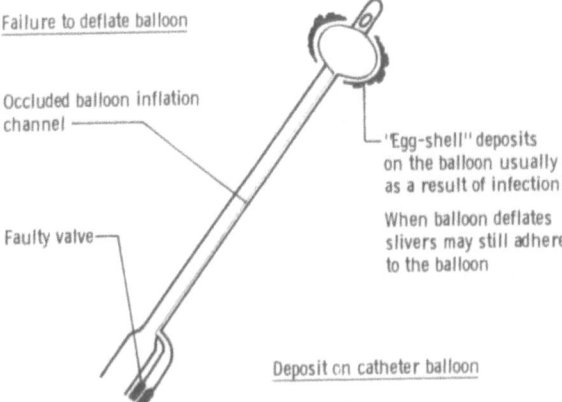

Failure to deflate balloon

Occluded balloon inflation channel

'Egg-shell" deposits on the balloon usually as a result of infection

When balloon deflates slivers may still adhere to the balloon

Faulty valve

Deposit on catheter balloon

Fig. 4.16. Causes of inability to withdraw the catheter.

There are various solutions to deflation problems: injection of a latex solvent (e.g., ether, acetone, liquid paraffin) into the balloon channel is usually successful. Alternatively the balloon can be over-inflated (above 80 ml) and then punctured by insertion of a suprapubic needle, perhaps aided by ultrasonography.

After Catheter Withdrawal

Stricture

Urethral stricture is a well-known complication following catheterisation (Sutherland et al. 1982; Anderson 1979; Edwards and Trott 1973). In general, symptoms of outflow obstruction develop within 6 weeks of catheter withdrawal. The site of stricturing corresponds to the regions of natural anatomical narrowing in the male urethra. The tendency to stenosis at these sites is promoted by the use of excessively large catheters. Avascular necrosis in the periurethral tissues due to pressure is more likely if tension is applied, producing "bow stringing" (Edwards et al. 1983). The greater the diameter of the catheter the more extensive the area of necrosis. Tissue damage is probably

Table 4.5. Effect of catheter material on cultured human cell lines (^{3}H uptake) and on rat urethra after 72-h exposure

Material	Cytotoxicity (cultured human cell lines)	Histological changes (rat urethra)
Silicone	<5%	Minimal, mild oedema
Plastic	25%	Mild oedema, some loss of surface epithelium
Latex	Variable 15%–100%	Moderate inflammatory infiltrate
		Epithelial loss, some haemorrhage
"Porges"		Increased inflammatory infiltrate
		More epithelial loss, some haemorrhage
Rubber		Increased inflammatory infiltrate
		More epithelial loss and haemorrhage

From Ruutu et al. (1985) and Edwards et al. (1983).

intensified by local infection in pooled secretions between the catheter and the urethral wall. Drainage of these secretions is of course inhibited with a wide catheter. If the sole purpose of catheterisation is to drain clear urine, a very small diameter catheter is quite adequate. An umbilical feeding tube will serve this purpose well although it has the small disadvantage that it must be sutured in position. The very high flow rate achieved with a larger catheter is only necessary if debris and clot are to be evacuated.

The list of causative factors of catheter stricture includes the inflammatory response in the periurethral tissues to compounds used in catheter manufacture. Animal experimentation can be used to check objectively the clinical impression that modern materials induce less local inflammation than those used traditionally. Implantation of such materials in the urethra of the dog (Engelbart et al. 1978) and rat (Edwards et al. 1983) demonstrates an order of irritability (see Table 4.5). However, strictures can develop after the use of carefully inserted silicone-coated catheters, left indwelling for only the briefest period. Pockets of incidence of high stricture have been identified, particularly in cardio-thoracic units (Abdel-Hakim et al. 1983; Ruutu et al. 1985; Sutherland et al. 1983; Ruutu et al. 1982) and occasionally in patients undergoing endoscopic surgery. In both groups it is unusual for catheters to remain in situ for longer than 48 hours. Here more subtle influences have been identified between batches of catheters. The microscopic appearances of the catheter surface (Axelson et al. 1977) and perhaps chemical irritants in the composition or contaminants are of potential importance. The problem has been carefully investigated by quantifying tissue reaction after subcutaneous implantation in animals (Wilksch et al. 1983). Another in-vivo test based on peritoneal foreign-body reaction in the rat may be easier to interpret and quantitate (Talja 1985). It is, perhaps, surprising that the degree of irregularity of the surface assessed by scanning electron microscopy appears to have rather little influence. Instead catheter irritability seems to derive from a soluble extract demonstrated in vitro on the viability of peritoneal macrophages cultured in a monolayer (Wilksch et al. 1983). This can also be demonstrated in other cell culture systems (Ruutu et al. 1985; Graham et al. 1983a,b; Wiluksch 1976). Although other appliances, such as endotracheal tubes, are subject to batch cytotoxicity testing, the same stringent quality control is not applied internationally to catheter manufacture (Ruutu et al. 1985; Engel 1983). In-vitro cytotoxicity testing should be instituted in addition to regular in-vivo assessment of tissue irritability.

Finally, the susceptibility of periurethral tissues expressed in their inflammatory response to foreign bodies might be idiosyncratic. The question of allergy has been carefully considered in connection with many implanted materials, e.g., those used in arthroplasty and heart-valve replacement, but not apparently in catheter manufacture.

Future Developments

There is clearly a need for improved quality control in catheter manufacture if sporadic episodes of complications reaching epidemic proportions are to be prevented. Less irritant materials must be developed and the incorporation of self-lubrication by the use of hydrophilic coating is an interesting innovation. It is hoped that advances will be made in the field of reconstructive urology, allowing natural voiding and obviating the need for longterm catheter diversion.

References

Abdel-Hakim A, Bernstein J, Teijeira J, Elhilali MM(1983) Urethral stricture after cardiovascular surgery, a retrospective and a prospective study. J Urol 130:1100–1102

Abrams PH, Dunn M, George NJR (1978) Urodynamic findings in chronic retention and their relevance to the results of surgery. Br Med J 2:1258–1260

Akiyama H, Okamoto S (1979) Prophylaxis of indwelling urethral catheter infections: clinical experience with a modified Foley catheter and drainage system. J Urol 121:40–42

Anderson RV (1979) Response of bladder and urethral mucosa to catheterisation. JAMA 242: 451–453

Axelson OH, Schonebeck J, Winblad B (1977) Surface structure of unused and used catheters. Scand J Urol Nephrol 11:283–287

Barrett DM, Furlow WL (1984) Incontinence, intermittent self-catheterisation and the artificial genito-urinary sphincter. J Urol 132:268–269

Binder CA, Gonick P (1969) Experience with the silicone rubber-coated Foley urethral catheter. J Urol 101:716–718

Bishop MC (1985) Diuresis and renal functional recovery in chronic retention. Br J Urol 57:1–5

Blandy JP (1975) Injuries of the urethra in the male. Injury 7:77–80

Borzyskowski M, Mundy AR, Neville BGR, Park L, Kinder CH, Joyce MRL, Chantler C, Haycock GB (1982) Neuropathic vesico-urethral dysfunction in children. Brit J Urol 54:641–644

Britt MR, Garibaldi RA, Miller WA (1977) Antimicrobial prophylaxis of catheter associated bacteriuria. Antimicrob Agents Chemother 11:240–243

Brocklehurst JC, Brocklehurst S (1978) The management of indwelling catheters. Br J Urol 2:102–105

Burchhardt P, Huland H (1978) Renal calculus dissolution in immobilised patients. Eur Urol 4:420–423

Burke JP, Garibaldi RA, Britt MR, Jacobsen JA, Conti M, Ailing DW (1981) Prevention of catheter associated urinary tract infections: efficacy of daily meatal care regimens. Am J Med 70:655–658

Chodak GW, Plant ME (1979) Systemic antibiotics for prophylaxis in urologic surgery: a critical review. J Urol 121:695–699

Crooks KK, Enrile BG (1983) Comparison of the ileal conduit and clean intermittent catheterisation for myelomeningocele. Pediatrics 72:203–206

Desautes KE (1974) Managing the urinary catheter. Geriatrics 29:67–71

Drach GW (1976) Diagnosis and management of infectious complications of urologic surger. In:Smith RB, Skinner DG (Eds). Complications of urologic surgery. WB Saunders, Philadelphia, pp 23–38

Eddeland A, Hedelin H (1983) Effects of allopurinol in patients with longterm indwelling catheters. J Int Med Res 11:116–119

Edwards LE, Lock R, Powell L, Jones P (1983) Post-catheterisation urethral strictures. A clinical and experimental study. Br J Urol 55:53–56

Edwards L, Trott PA (1973) Catheter induced urethral inflammation. J Urol 110:678–681

Elliott TSJ, Slack RCB, Reed L, Bishop MC (1985) Ultrastructure and bacteriology of the bladder in urinary tract infection. Journal of Infection. 11:191–199

Elliott TSJ, Slack RCB, Bishop MC (1984) Scanning electron microscopy of human bladder mucosa in acute and chronic urinary tract infection. Br J Urol 56:38–43

Engel G (1983) Adverse effects with catheters and toxicity testing. Med J Aust 1:444–445

Engel RME, Wise HA, Whitaker RH (1972) Otis internal urethrotomy with longterm urethral intubation: a comparison of latex and silastic catheters. South Med J 65:55–60

Engelbart RH, Bartone FF, Gardner P, Hutson J (1978) Urethral reaction to catheter materials in dogs. Invest Urol 16:55–56

Essenhigh DM, Ryan DW (1982) An appraisal of 53 blocks in the management of incontinence. Br J Urol 54:697–699

Ewing R, Bultitude MI, Shuttleworth KED (1982) Subtrigonal phenol injection for urge incontinence secondary to detrusor instability in females. Br J Urol 54:689–692

Feingold DS (1970) Hospital acquired infections. N Eng J Med 283:1384–1386

Ferrie BG, Glen EJ, Hunter B (1979) Longterm urethral catheter drainage. Br Med J 279: 1046–1047

Fincke BG, Friedland G (1976) Prevention and management of infection in the catheterised patient. Urol Clin N Am. 3:313–318

Garibaldi RA, Burke JP, Dickman ML, Smith CB (1974) Factors predisposing to bacteriuria during indwelling urethral catheterisation. N Eng J Med 291:215–218

Gibbon NOK (1976) The bladder in disorders of the nervous system. In: Blandy JP (ed) Urology. Blackwell, Oxford, pp 807–839

Graham DT, Mark G, Pomeroy A (1983a) Cellular toxicity testing. Med J Aust 1:444–445

Graham DT, Mark GE, Pomeroy AR (1983b) Cellular toxicity of urinary catheters. Med J Aust 1:456–459

Griffith DP, Klein AS (1983) Infection-induced urinary stones: In: Roth RA, Finlayson B (eds) Stones: clinical management of urolithiasis. Williams and Wilkins, Baltimore, pp 210–227

Guttmann L, Frankel H (1966) The value of intermittent catherenisation in the early management of traumas in paraplegia and tetraplegia. Paraplegia 4:63–83

Haase DA, Harding GKM (1984) The urethral catheter and infection. Surgery 3:1–6

Hartstein AI, Garber SB, Ward TT, Jones SR, Morthland VH (1981) Nosocomial urinary tract infection: a prospective study of 108 catheterised patients. Infect Control 2:380–386

Hedelin H, Eddeland A, Larsson L, Petersson S, Ohman S (1984) The composition of catheter encrustations including the effects of allopurinol treatment. Br J Urol 56:250–254

Herman JR (1973) Urology; a view through the retrospectoscope. Harper-Row, New York

Higson R, Ramsden PD, Smith JC (1978) Bladder rupture: an acceptable complication of distension therapy? Br J Urol 50:529–534

Hukins DWL, Hickey DS, Kennedy AR (1983) Catheter encrustations by struvite. Br J Urol 55: 304–305

Keitzer WA, Abreu A, Navarro I, Bernreuter E, Adams JS (1968) Urethral strictures: prevention with silastic catheters. J Urol 99:187–188

Khan SRN, Cockrell CA, Finlayson B, Hackett RL (1984) Crystal retention by injured urothelium of the rat urinary bladder. J Urol 172:153–157

Kunin CM (1979) Detection, prevention and management of urinary tract infections, 3rd edn. Lea & Febiger, Philadelphia

Kunin CM, McCormack RC (1966) Prevention of catheter induced urinary tract infections by sterile closed drainage. N Engl J Med 274:1155–1159

Lapides J, Diokno AC, Silber SJ, Lowe BS (1972) Clean intermittent self-catheterisation in the treatment of urinary tract disease. J Urol 107:458–461

Liedberg H, Lundberg J (1990) Silver-alloy-coated catheter reduce catheter-associated bacteria. Br J Urol 65:379–381

Lyon RP, Scott MP, Marshall S (1975) Intermittent catheterisation rather than urinary diversion in children with myelomeningocele. J Urol 113:409–417

Mauermayer W (1983) Transurethral surgery. Springer, Berlin Heidelberg New York, pp 402–403

Mulcahy JJ, James HE, McRoberts JM (1977) Oxybutynin chloride combined with intermittent clean catheterisation in the treatment of myelomeningocele patients. J Urol 118:86–90

Mundy AR (1984) Injuries of the lower urinary tract. Surgery 3:67–71

Murphy BF, Fairley KF, Birch DF, Marshall RC, Durman OB (1984) Culture of mid catheter urine collected via open-ended catheter: reliable guide to bladder bacteriuria. J Urol 131:19–21

Murphy L T (1972) The history of urology. Charles C Thomas, Springfield, Illinois

Nacey JN, Tulloch AGS, Ferguson AF (1985) Catheter-induced urethritis: a comparison between latex and silicone catheters in a prospective clinical trial. Br J Urol 57:325–328

Ohkawa M, Sugata T, Suwaki M, Nakashima T, Fuse H, Hisazumi H (1990) Bacterial and crystal adherence to the surfaces of indwelling urethral catheters. J Urol 143:717–721

Painter MR, Borski AA, Trevino GS, Clark WE (1971) Urethral reaction to foreign objects. J Urol 106:227–230

Pengelly AW, Stephenson TP, Milroy EJG, Whiteside, CG, Turner-Warwick R (1978) Results of prolonged bladder distension as treatment for detrusor instability. Br J Urol 50:243–245

Platt R, Polk BF, Murdock B, Plosner B (1983) Reduction of mortality associated with nosocomial urinary tract infections. Lancet 1:893–897

Poston GJ, Joseph AEA, Riddle PR (1983) The accuracy of ultrasound in the measurement of changes in bladder volume Br J Urol 55:361–363

Ramsden PD, Smith JC, Dunn M, Ardran G M (1976) Distension therapy for the unstable bladder: later results including an assessment of repeat distensions. Br J Urol 48:623–629

Ravichandran G, Fellows GJ (1983) The accuracy of a hand-held real time ultrasound scanner for estimating bladder volume. Br J Urol 55:25–27

Reuter HJ, Jones LW (1974) Physiologic low pressure irrigation for transurethral resection: suprapubic trocar drainage. J Urol 111:210–212

Rickwood AMK, Philp NH, Thomas DG (1983) Longterm indwelling urethral catheterisation for congenital neuropathic bladder. Arch Dis Child 58:310–314

Ruutu M, Alfthan O, Talja M, Andersson LC (1985) Cytotoxicity of latex urinary catheters. Br J Urol 57:82–87

Ruutu M, Alfthan O, Heikkinen L, Jarvinen A, Lehtonen T, Merikallio E, Standertskjold-Norderstam CG (1982) Epidemic of acute urethral stricture after open heartsurgery. Lancet 1:218

Ruwald MM (1980) Irrigation of indwelling urinary catheters. Urology 21:127–129

Savage JA, Birch DF, Fairley KF (1983) Comparison of mid-catheter collection and suprapubic aspiration of urine for diagnosis of bacteriuria due to fastidious micro-organisms. J Urol 129: 62–68

Schwartz BA, Wise HA (1982) Endourologic techniques for the bladder and urethra. Urol Clin N Am 9:165–167

Sherwood T, Davidson AJ, Talner LB (1980) Uroradiology. Blackwell, Oxford, 9: p47

Simon DL, Carron II, Rowlingson JC (1982) Treatment of bladder pain with trans-sacral nerve block. Anaesth Analg 61:46–48

Slade N, Gillespie WA (1985) The urinary tract and the catheter. John Wiley, Chichester

Smith PJB, Ball AJ (1984) Combined bladder and urethral drainage catheter. Urol 24:190–191

Stark RP, Maki DG (1984) Bacteriuria in the catheterised patient. What quantitative level of bacteriuria is relevant? N Engl J Med 311:560–564

Stephenson TP, Mundy AR (1985) Treatment of the neuropathic bladder by enterocystoplasty and selective sphincterotomy or sphincter ablation and replacement. Br J Urol 57:27–31

Stickler DJ, Plant S, Bunni NH, Chawla JC (1981) Some observations on the activity of three antiseptics used as bladder irrigants in the treatment of urinary tract infections in patients with indwelling catheters. Paraplegia 19:325–333

Studer UE, Bishop MC, Zingg EJ (1983) How to fill a silicone catheter balloon. Urology 22: 300–302

Sutherland PD, Maddern JP, Jose JS, Marshall VR (1982) Catheters and post-operative urethral stricture. Lancet 1:622–623

Sutherland PD, Maddern JP, Jose JS, Marshall VR (1983) Urethral stricture after cardiac surgery. Br J Urol 55:413–416

Talja M (1985) Rat peritoneal implantation test. Br J Urol. 57:329–333

Talja M, Korpela A, Järvi K (1990) Comparison of Urethral nuchion to full silicone, hyorryen conted and Siliconised later catheter. Br J Ural 66:652–657

Thompson RL, Haley CE, Searcy MA, Guenthner SM, Kaiser DL, Groschel DHM, Gillenwater JY, Wenzel RP (1984) Catheter associated bacteriuria: failure to reduce attack rates using periodic instillations of a disinfectant into urinary drainage systems. JAMA 251:747–751

Torrens MJ, Griffith HB (1974) The control of the uninhibited bladder by selective sacral neurectomy. Br J Urol 46:636–644

Turck M, Stamm W (1981) Nosocomial infection of the urinary tract. Am J Med 70:651–654

Turner-Warwick R (1973) Observations on the treatment of traumatic urethral injuries and the value of the fenestrated urethral catheter. Br J Surg 60:775–779

Vaughan ED, Gillenwater JY (1973) Diagnosis characterisation and management of post-obstructive diuresis. J Urol 109:286–290

Warren JW, Platt R, Thomas RJ, Rosner B, Kass EH (1978) Antibiotic irrigation and catheter-associated urinary tract infections. N Engl J Med 299:570–573

Wesley-James O (1982) Catheters and post-operative urethral strictures. Lancet 1:623

Whitaker RH (1973) Methods of assessing obstruction in dilated ureters. Br J Urol 45:15–20

Whiteside CG, Bates CP (1979) Synchronous video pressure-flow cystourethrography. Urol Clin North Am 6:89–93

Whitfield HN, Mayo ME (1975) Prolonged bladder distension in the treatment of the unstable bladder. Br J Urol 47:635–639

Wilksch J, Vernon-Roberts B, Garrett R, Smith K (1983) The role of catheter surface morphology and extractable cytotoxic material in tissue reactions to urethral catheters. Br J Urol 55:48–52

Wiluksch RE (1976) Quantitative cell culture biocompatibility testing of medical devices and correlation to animal tests. Biomaterials Med Devices, Artificial Organs 4:235–238

Wolk FN, Bishop MC (1981) Effectiveness of prolonged hydrostatic dilatation of the bladder. Urology 18:572–575

Chapter 5

Implantable Incontinence Devices

P.H.L. Worth

Many surgical techniques have been described to improve bladder neck and distal urethral function when they are either congenitally weak or have been ablated or damaged surgically. What can be done depends to a certain extent on the basic pathology and how much surgery has already been carried out. Techniques such as Young–Dees (Dees 1949) or Leadbetter procedures (Leadbetter 1964) do have their place although the overall results are not very satisfactory.

There are four approaches to the treatment of incontinence that I will discuss. The use of PTFE (Teflon) injections is applicable to both sexes, the evolution of the Kaufman procedure and the use of the Rosen prosthesis are both procedures applicable only to the male and, the most important, the use of the Brantley–Scott inflatable artificial urinary sphincter.

PTFE (Teflon) Injections

Injections of various substances have been used as an alternative to implantable devices to improve the function of the sphincteric mechanism. The theory is that fibrosis is caused in the tissues surrounding the sphincters or there is a reaction that increases the bulk of the tissues. There has been much interest shown over the years in the use of different substances and for the past decade Teflon (Polytef, PTFE) has been the agent of choice. The first substance to be used was sodium morrhuate. It was injected into the anterior vaginal wall (Murless 1938) but unfortunately it was a sclerosant and often a slough developed which caused a lot of pain and prolonged bleeding. However in 60% of patients there was some subjective improvement. Paraffin injections were also tried without producing much symptomatic improvement, but also not precipitating any major problems (Quackels 1955). A sclerosant was then used again, but although good results were obtained in 6 out of 7 women and 22 out of 24 men, 4 patients had pulmonary emboli and the technique fell into disrepute (Sachse 1963). The use of PTFE was introduced in 1973 (Berg 1973). Initially glycerine was injected to assess the possible benefit and if it was satisfactory PTFE was injected.

Polytetrafluoroethylene is a polymer made by heating tetrafluoroethylene, and is called, also, polytef and Teflon. This is then made up as a paste which contains in addition glycerine and polysorbate. The paste consists of particles 50–100 μm in size. When injected into the tissues the paste incites a foreign-body giant-cell response and eventually it is encapsulated by fibrous tissue and lymphocytes. There have been major worries about the continued use of PTFE because of reports of possible cerebral and pulmonary emboli. In experimental animals PTFE has been found in pelvic lymph nodes 50–70 days after injection into the periurethral tissues and 10.5 months later it was found in the lung, brain, kidney and spleen. Particles that migrate are usually less than 80 μm in size, but since the material that is injected consists of particles under 40 μm in size in 90% of cases, the theoretical risk of problems is quite big (Malizia et al. 1984). However no major morbidity has deen described, but the potential damage that could be produced suggests that the technique of PTFE injection should be used with caution. Politano (1982) reported no major complications in a series of over 300 cases.

Several manufacturers have produced instruments to make the injection of PTFE much easier. No-one should attempt to inject it without the right equipment, because the results will be unsatisfactory. It is necessary to use a small syringe in order to generate enough pressure and an insulin-type of syringe is ideal. If too fine a needle is used it will not be possible to generate enough pressure to get the PTFE into the tissues. Personal preference dictates the use of the syringe holder (Fig. 5.1), the Storz gun, the Wolf pressurised injector, or the Key Med instrument. As the latter two instruments are expensive and the number of PTFE injections done in any one unit will probably be quite small, it may be considered too extravagant to have an instrument especially for this technique. Whatever method of injection is used it is better to pass a long needle through a catheterising cystoscope and place the needle into the appropriate area under direct vision rather than to pass the needle vaginally, periurethrally, or through the perineum in the male. In the indirect methods it is very difficult to be sure exactly where the tip of the needle lies before one starts the injection. If the urethra or bladder neck is penetrated by the needle,

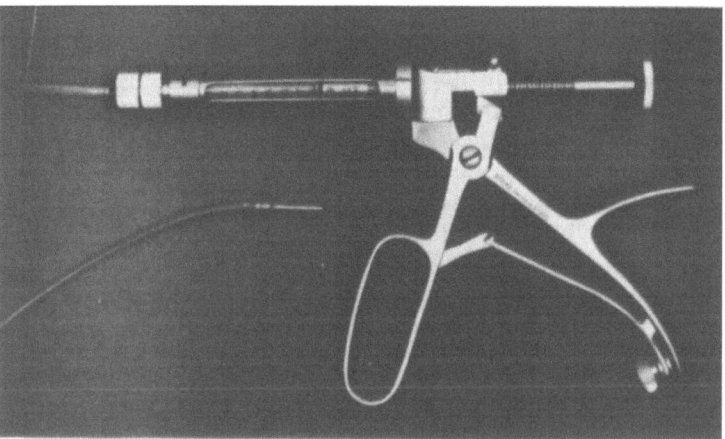

Fig. 5.1. One of the devices available for injecting PTFE.

it is more than likely that leakage of PTFE will occur into the bladder and it can be quite difficult to wash the pieces out.

The indications for use of PTFE in the female are stable stress incontinence with a low maximal urethral pressure and a good capacity bladder. If a major prolapse is present, this should be corrected surgically, probably first, because this will demonstrate the amount of incorrectable incontinence. In the male the major indication is post-prostatectomy incontinence. In treating females it is recommended that the needle should be introduced just below the bladder neck. An injection of 2–3 ml should be used in all four quadrants consecutively. A satisfactory result should be achieved if the mucosa has been raised so that the lumen looks occluded – an appearance not unlike a normal prostatic urethra in the male. If necessary the needle can be introduced a further 2–3 cm down the urethra and the procedure repeated, again in all four quadrants. Remember that the pressurised instrumental injection can insert 2–5 ml per fill, whereas the insulin syringe only holds 1 ml, so the whole procedure can be quite time-consuming. It also requires a very understanding theatre assistant, who may also be asked to do some of the injecting. In the male a similar sort of approach should be used starting at the bladder neck and working down the prostatic urethra to just below the verumontanum. Unfortunately, in patients with post-prostatectomy incontinence, there is very often significant scarring in the region of the distal sphincter and it may be impossible to produce any obvious change in the endoscopic appearance. However, the reaction to the PTFE periurethrally may be sufficiently good to produce a satisfactory result.

Patients may experience urethritis for 2–3 days and, therefore, some authors recommend the routine use of antibiotics. There is often a low-grade fever as well. At worst a perineal or periurethral abscess may result and in order to avoid this sort of problem, it is very important that the urine is sterile before the PTFE is injected. Although the technique can be done as a day-stay case, if the injections prove technically difficult it may be better to leave a catheter indwelling for 24–36 hours.

In recent papers the overall success rate is between 60% and 75%. Schulman et al. (1983a) treated 35 females with stress urinary incontinence with 74% success, 17% improvement and 9% failures. They have continued to use the technique with better longterm results. They are prepared to repeat the injection and have done so up to four times, injecting an average of 9.6 ml (Schulman et al. 1983b). Politano in his initial series had 62% satisfactory results (Politano et al. 1974). In 1982 he described his results in both sexes. In 54 females he had excellent results in 51% and good results in 20%, and in 111 men, some with post-prostatectomy incontinence and some with neuropathic problems, results were excellent in 45% and good in 35% (Politano 1982). In a further paper PTFE was used in 6 females with neuropathic problems and excellent results were obtained in them all. Continence was produced with the PTFE, and clean intermittent self catheterisation (CISC) was used for effective bladder emptying (Lewis et al. 1984). Lim et al. (1983) in a mixed group of 28 female patients with incontinence of various causes, had 21% cured and 53% improved, but results were considerably better in those who were found to have stable bladders on urodynamic testing, with 30% cured and 70% improved. Deane et al. (1985) had excellent results in females with normal resting anatomy, but only 50% success in those who had had previous surgery, or incompetence of the bladder neck at rest. Good results have also been obtained in children, 85% success in those with sphincter weakness and 50% success in those with neuropathic problems (Vorstman et al. 1985).

Kaufman Procedure

Several techniques of bulbar urethral compression have been described and there is no shortage in the ingenuity of ideas. Transposition of the gracilis, gluteus maximus, adductor longus or pyramidalis muscles have all been tried. The first person to try direct compression of the bulbar urethra was Lowsley. He placed sutures in the bulbospongiosus muscle on each side of the urethra and tied them together thereby narrowing the urethral lumen and compressing it with the bulbospongiosus muscle. Lowsley (1936) and Girgis and Veneema (1965) were the first to implant a foreign body, when they described the use of an absorbable collagen prosthesis which was placed deep to the bulbar urethra. It was attached to the ischiocavernosus and levator ani muscles which, when tied, both compressed and angulated the urethra. Berry (1961) placed a piece of acrylic impregnated with bismuth between the urethra and the bulbospongiosus muscle. It was held in place by suturing steel wires through the device and through the fascia covering the ischiocavernosus muscle. His initial results produced about a 50% improvement, but they were not sustained. Various modifications of the compressive device were introduced over a 10-year period, but a critical analysis of the results showed that at best only 15% were improved (Berry and Dahlen 1971). Hinman then modified the procedure by compressing the bulbar urethra and bulbospongiosus with a piece of rib which was screwed into the ischial tuberosity on each side. He achieved early success in about 60% of patients (Hinman et al. 1970).

Kaufman (1970) described the first of his many procedures for the treatment of urinary incontinence in the male. He felt that it was better not to use buried foreign materials, but due to lack of success with his earlier methods he later introduced a silicone-gel prosthesis. The first procedure – the crucifaction operation – involved separating the posterior ends of the crura from their origins and then crossing them over the bulbar urethra and fixing them to the rami of the ischial bones on the opposite side. The second procedure, which was also described by Puigvert, involved leaving the posterior ends intact, but separating the mid portions off the bone and sewing them together over the bulbar urethra (Kaufman 1972; Puigvert 1971). To improve the results of this procedure additional compression was obtained by insinuating a small piece of Marlex (polypropylene mesh) between the crura and the bulb. At this time an operation was described which involved wrapping six layers of Marlex laid over the bulbar urethra and fixed to the fascia over the ischiocavernosus muscle and periosteum (Salcedo 1972). The introduction of a silicone-gel prosthesis gave much better results and these continued to improve as the prosthesis was also improved (Kaufman 1973a). The original model was a silastic capsule covered in a velour of polyurethane but, because the incidence of urethral erosion was high, the model was changed so that the part that compressed the urethra consisted of the silastic capsule only and the velour was confined to the base and part of the sides. This was later strengthened by incorporating a plate of

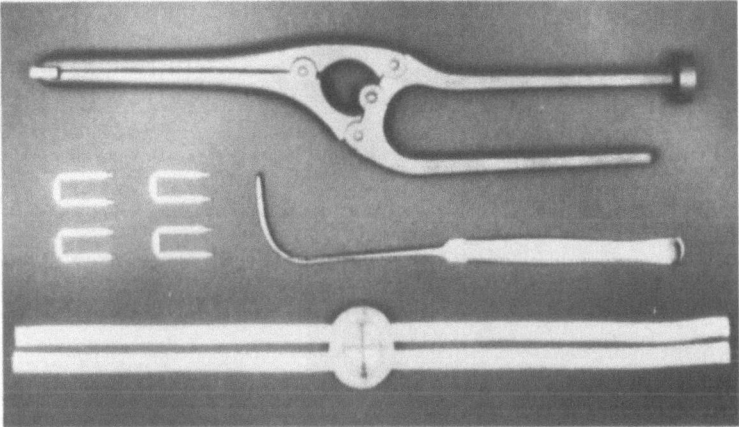

Fig. 5.2. The equipment necessary for implanting the Kaufman prosthesis. The staples are to be recommended, but the aneurysm needle can be used to put the tapes round the crura.

Marlex which supported the silicone capsule. Dacron tapes were attached to each side for fixation of the device. The device comes in four sizes, small, medium, large and extra large, which range from 2.5 × 2.0 × 1.7 to 5.0 × 2.7 × 2.0 cm (Fig. 5.2). The size to be implanted can only be determined at the time of the implant operation (Kaufman 1973b).

Having established that the patient is a good candidate for the implantation of the prosthesis (Reid et al. 1980), the actual surgical technique is not difficult (Kaufman and Raz 1979). It is important to be certain that there is no residual prostatic tissue present and that the urethra is free of stricture. Pre-operative preparation consists of sterilising the bowel and treating any urinary infection. The perineum should be shaved at operation and the area washed with aqueous Betadine (providone-iodine) at least 3 times a day for 2 days. An aminoglycoside and flagyl (metronidazole) are given to cover the operation and for 3 days post-operatively. An additional antibiotic may be indicated if there was initially a urine infection.

A mid-line incision is made in the perineum overlying the bulbar urethra. The subcutaneous fat is divided and the bulbospongiosus muscle exposed. The neurovascular bundles on each side are carefully preserved. An important step is to separate the bulb from the central perineal tendon. The posterior tapes are fixed with staples to the ischial bones deep to the attachment of the crura. Anteriorly, depending on the space available, either the tapes are passed round the crura or staples are placed deep to the crura and the tapes passed through them. The device is soaked in an antibiotic prior to insertion and once in situ is washed with more antibiotic and the wound is sprayed with providone iodine prior to closure. The tapes are then joined diagonally over the device, leaving a small knot which is usually palpable through the skin and is the point to aim for if, at a later date, the device needs injecting. The subcutaneous tissues are closed with sutures and the skin is closed with either a subcuticular stitch or interrupted Dexon (polyglycolic acid) or its equivalent. It is wise to drain the bladder with a suprapubic catheter and it is better to put it in at the start of the operation so that nothing is put into the urethra either during or after the

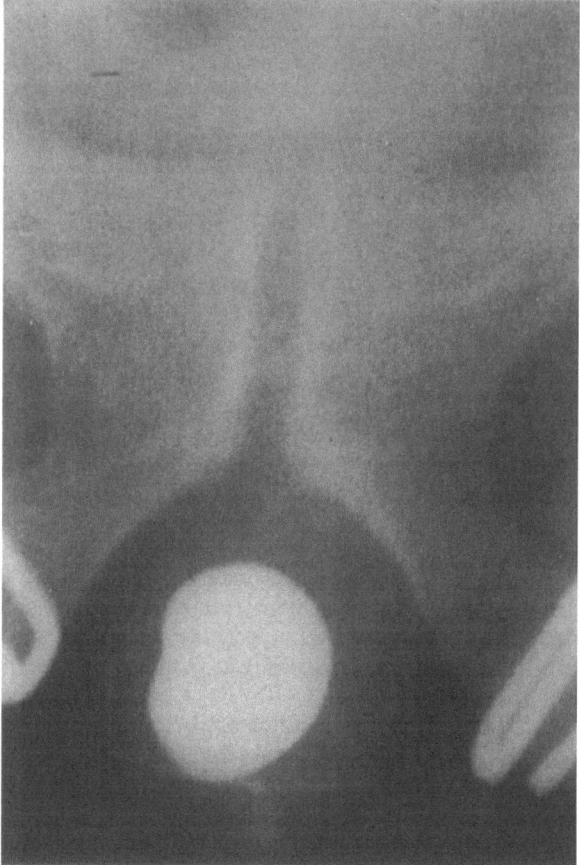

Fig. 5.3. X-ray of a Kaufman device injected with contrast.

operation. The catheter can be clamped at 3 days and once the residue is less
than 100 ml it can be removed. Occasionally the patient has difficulty voiding
because the bladder is relatively atonic – a fact that may be difficult to pick
up preoperatively if the incontinence is very bad. It is better to leave the
suprapubic catheter in place until the patient can void, even though it may take
4 weeks, rather than to loosen the device prematurely. Some authors suggest
measuring the urethral pressure at the time of insertion and adjusting the
compression accordingly to get a better result (Fowler and Auld 1985).

The initial results may be very good, but once the oedema from the operation has settled the urethral compression may diminish and some incontinence
may reappear. This can be helped by injecting the device. This is best done
in the radiology department. Although the device has a radiopaque marker
incorporated into the base plate, it is easier to aim the needle at the knot that
was left at operation. Intravenous contrast should be used, but it does tend to
diffuse away and so I often use an oily solution which is more difficult to inject,
but which tends to stay in the device. It is important to use a fine needle to
reduce the chance of leakage, but if an oily solution is used it is difficult to

inject it. Up to 10 ml can be used in the medium and large devices, but an extra large one can take 20 ml although it is probably wiser not to exceed 10 ml at a time and to be prepared to repeat the injection (Fig. 5.3).

Of the complications that can occur, urethral erosion is the most serious (Kaufman and Ritchie 1974). This is uncommon with the latest prostheses, but occurs if the device is fitted too tightly. Provided it does not happen in the early post-operative period it is rare to get a fistula. What the patient notices is local perineal pain when voiding and a post-micturition dribble. The device has to be removed and the bladder drained suprapubically. A urethral catheter should be used for 10 days, but it is not necessary formally to mend the urethra and, in my limited experience, it mends without a stricture. Since the device is a foreign body, the other serious complication is infection and if this does occur it is likely that the device will have to be removed. Before the use of staples the back tapes occasionally cut through the crura so that compression on the urethra was lost. The device can be repositioned by fixing a Dacron tape across it and putting staples in the ischial ramus to hold the tape.

Kaufman reported on 184 patients – 164 with post-prostatectomy incontinence and 16 with neurological problems (Kaufman and Raz 1979). At 6 weeks post-operatively 169 (92%) were better, but by 6 months this figure had fallen to only 71 (40%). Following injection of the device 112 (61%) were still very good after a year, but 72 (39%) were considered failures. Because of erosions 12 were removed and 8 had serious infection. However, the overall experience in Britain, where 38 surgeons had implanted 143 devices showed excellent results in 44%, and a good result in 32%. There were failures and, in addition, 23% had to be removed on account of infection or erosion (Worth 1982). These results were also achieved by Cox and Worth (1986) who had good results in 45% of patients.

The Kaufman device has proved very satisfactory and the results are accept-able. In the USA it has been discarded in favour of the Brantley Scott prosthesis which, it is claimed, gives superior results. This cannot be denied. However, as will be seen, there are problems with this device. For the elderly patient extremely disturbed by post-prostatectomy incontinence a Kaufman prosthesis also gives excellent results and creates very few problems for the user: it will still have a place in the management of these cases when surgical relief is deemed necessary.

The Rosen Device

A theoretical improvement on the Kaufman prosthesis is the device designed by Rosen (1976). This consists of a 3-pronged clamp, with two arms on one side, parallel to each other, and opposite them a base plate with an inflatable balloon. The urethra is placed between the two components. The balloon is connected to a reservoir bulb which has a special release valve (Fig. 5.4). The balloon is inflated by compressing the reservoir, the urethra is then pushed up by the balloon against the two arms and as a result urine cannot pass down the urethra. The balloon is deflated by manipulating the release valve. The urethra is not surrounded by the device and when the balloon is inflated it is angulated

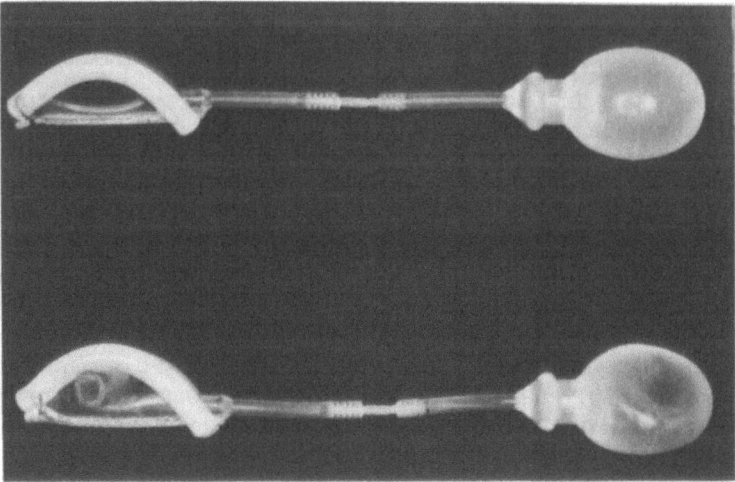

Fig. 5.4. The Rosen device. The lower part shows how the device compresses the urethra.

and compressed, but because this is not circumferential the blood supply to the distal urethra is maintained. In addition micturition does not have to occur against a fixed resistance when the balloon is deflated. This has certain advantages when the bladder has lost its power of contraction and abdominal straining is required. The device is made of a silicone elastomer and comes in three sizes.

The same careful preparation as for insertion of the Kaufman prosthesis is required. A mid-line perineal incision is made. The bulbar urethra is mobilised, leaving the bulbospongiosus intact and a tunnel made large enough to take the base plate of the device. This is then anchored to the perineal membrane with non-absorbable sutures and the arms are also fixed to the base plate. Before inserting the device all the air is removed and the reservoir filled with saline. The reservoir is then buried in the subcutaneous tissue of the scrotum. The two portions are then joined together with a special connector to prevent kinking, and the wound closed. The device should be left deflated for about 7 days and the patient should be allowed to pass urine through the urethra without catheter drainage.

The three major complications are infection, urethral erosion and mechanical failures. If the balloon is overinflated it will predispose to urethral erosion and sometimes an aneurysmal dilatation of the balloon may occur. This predisposes to rupture and also stops the device compressing the urethra satisfactorily. Rosen himself has quite limited experience with his device in terms of numbers (post-prostatectomy incontinence in Australia must be a rare event). In his first series he had good results in 60%, but in a later series of 30 patients he had good results in 77% (Rosen 1976, 1978). In addition there have been four main reports on the Rosen device discussing the results and problems. Small (1980) put the device into 16 patients and obtained good results in 11 (68%). However he did have a lot of mechanical problems and one urethral erosion. Augspurger (1981) operated on 17 patients with good results in 9 (53%). However on account of mechanical failures, aneurysmal dilatation and urethral erosions the rest had to be improved. In all Augspurger carried out 27 operations in 17 patients. Giesy et al. (1981) operated on 19 patients, but had a successful result in only 6: on account of mechanical failures he did 26 further operations. One patient in this series died because he failed to deflate the device for 5 days and succumbled to septicaemia. Worth (1982) collected the combined experience of British urologists. Good results were obtained in 73%, but 80% of the devices had to be removed because of erosion or infection.

From these results it can be said that, although the Rosen device is quite simple and easy to use, the problems that are associated with it such as mechanical failure, infection and urethral erosion make its continued use unacceptable.

The Brantley Scott Artificial Urinary Sphincter

The concept of a circumferential pressure-controlling device is not new. Foley (1947) designed a system which involved making a tunnel around part of the penile urethra, covering it with skin and then surrounding it with a cuff which could be inflated via a piston. This proved unsuccessful (Fig. 5.5). It was not

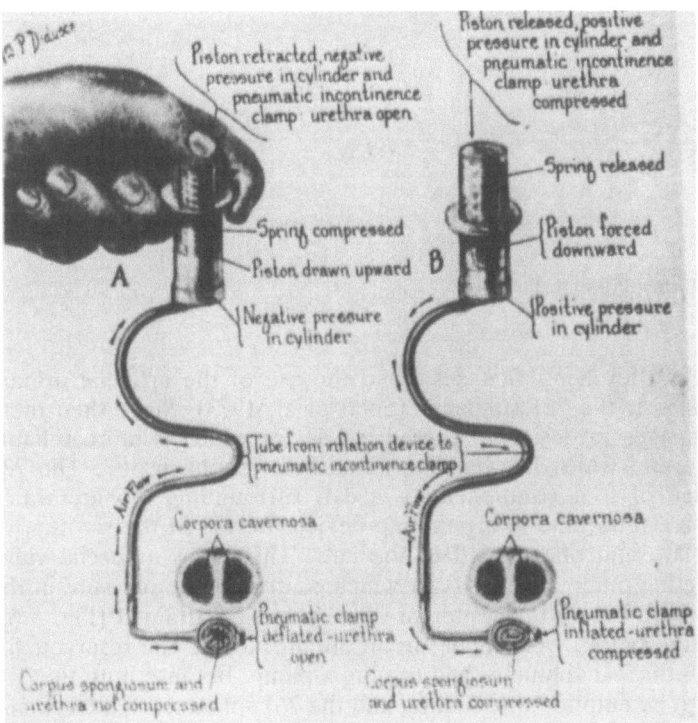

Fig. 5.5. The Foley device showing how the isolated urethra was compressed. Reprinted with permission from Foley FEB (1947) An artificial sphincter. J Urol 58:250–259.)

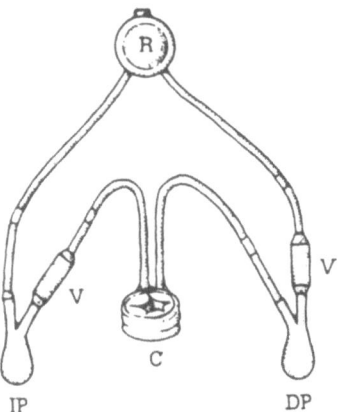

Fig. 5.6. AS 721. IP, inflating pump; DP, deflating pump; V, valve; C, cuff; R, reservoir.

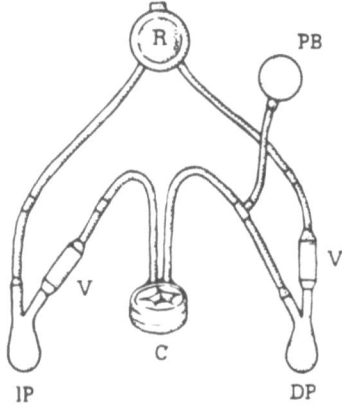

Fig. 5.7. AS 761 PB pressurising balloon.

until 1973 that Brantley Scott first described the use of the artificial urinary sphincter and called it the 721 sphincter (Scott et al. 1973). Since then there have been six changes in design to produce a device which is more reliable and easier to use and which has become much more sophisticated. The 721 sphincter consisted of four components – a cuff surrounding the urethra, a reservoir containing fluid, and two pumping devices buried in the scrotum or labia, one to inflate and one to deflate the cuff. There was a special valve between the deflating pump and reservoir which controlled the pressure in the cuff so that not more than 90 cm water pressure could be attained (Fig. 5.6). Modifications to the design were made, in an attempt to use the reservoir for pressure control – the 741 sphincter had too big a pump, because both the cuff and balloon had to be emptied for voiding, and the 761 sphincter had too many components (Fig. 5.7). The 742 sphincter had a resistor between the cuff and balloon and allowed automatic closure of the device (Fig. 5.8). Miniaturisation of the resistor and the valve allowed them to be combined into one unit and

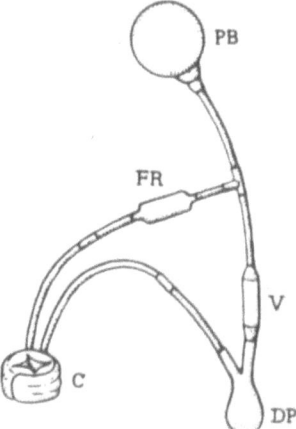

Fig. 5.8. AS 742 FR resistor.

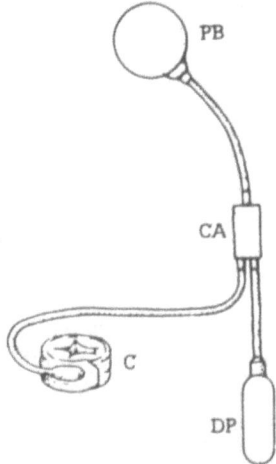

Fig. 5.9. AS 791 CA control assembly. This device is placed round the bulbar urethra.

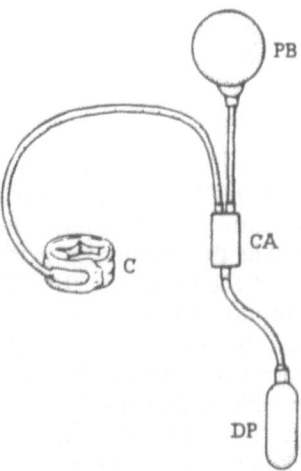

Fig. 5.10. AS 792. This device is placed round the bladder neck.

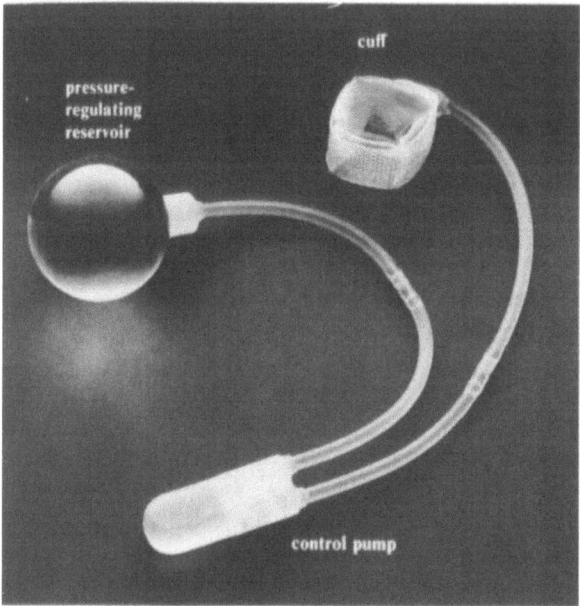

Fig. 5.11. AS 800.

the 791 (Fig. 5.9) and 792 (Fig. 5.10) devices were created. The difference between the two was that in the 791 sphincter the cuff was placed round the bulbar urethra, and in the 792 it was round the bladder neck. The cuff closed automatically which had disadvantages. The latest device is the AS 800 (Fig. 5.11) which has a deactivation feature in the pump unit which allows activation and deactivation to be carried out externally. The design of the system, the quality of the material used, better welding of the cuff to its inflatable component and twist-proof tubing to prevent mechanical twisting all make for a great reduction in device failure.

Surgical Principles and Techniques

Meticulous antisepsis is important and surgery should not be undertaken if there is an infection in the urinary tract (Scott et al. 1981). Any infection should be treated with the appropriate antibiotics preoperatively and prophylactic antibiotics given to cover the operation. Careful skin preparation is performed preoperatively, but shaving is left until the time of the operation. It is important to position the patient in a modified lithotomy, Lloyd–Davies position so that the lower abdomen and perineum can be approached easily. The abdominal incision when the cuff is being placed around the bladder neck should be as close to the top of the pubis as possible, either using a deep "V" incision or dissecting the recti insertion from the bone. This allows good exposure of the bladder neck area. Previous surgery may make it difficult to dissect around the bladder neck in the female. Brantley Scott has designed a special "cutter clamp" to make this easier. Since it is most important not to damage the posterior wall of the upper urethra it may be better to open the bladder to be certain that this area is not damaged. Alternatively the area can be inspected endoscopically while the dissection is taking place. When the sphincter is placed around the bladder neck, and especially if associated with bladder augmentation or substitution cystoplasty, the use of the mobilised omentum is to be recommended. The omentum can be placed round the suture line and then the cuff can be surrounded by it. To obtain adequate omentum it should be carefully separated from the greater curve of the stomach (and transverse mesocolon) by dissecting the branches from the gastroepiploic artery to the stomach and going as far as its origin from the gastroduodenal artery. The omentum can then be placed retroperitoneally in the paracolic gutter. If difficulties are encountered making the tunnel round the bladder neck or an abscess cavity surrounded by dense scar tissue is found following previous reconstructive surgery, it is probably best to place the omentum round the reconstructed area and delay putting in a cuff until a later date. The presence of the omental wrap makes this secondary surgery very much easier. When major reconstructive surgery has been undertaken and it is not certain whether or not a sphincter will be required it is legitimate to put in a cuff (wrapped in omentum) round the bladder neck. This may produce enough continence without the necessity for putting in the reservoir or pump.

In the male the bulbar urethra is exposed in a midline perineal incision and a 2 cm tunnel made round the urethra on the outside of the bulbospongiosus muscle. Schreiter (1985) prefers to put the cuff high up by mobilising the urethra off the perineal body and making a tunnel superfical to the superficial perineal membrane. The pump is carefully placed low down in the labia major in the female and anterior to the testicle in the male. The reservoir is placed in the prevesical space using a small groin incision when the cuff is placed perineally and the tubes are correctly connected without kinks using the quick connectors (Figs. 5.12, 5.13).

Choice of Cuff Size and Pressure Balloon

The circumference of the bladder neck or urethra is measured with the special cuff measurer with the aim of having quite a tight fit. It is usually not necessary to have a cuff size greater than 4.5–5 cm for the bulbar urethra. In the female the bladder neck cuff is usually between 6.5 and 7.5 cm, whereas in the male it will vary between 6.5 and 10 cm. The width is usually 2 cm.

As far as the balloon is concerned, one with the lowest practical pressure is used. This will help to reduce the risk of erosion, but may be associated with a high incidence of stress incontinence. Therefore in the older male age group, with a bulbar cuff, a 51–60 cm reservoir would be used and 61–70 cm in the younger age group. With a cuff round the bladder neck in young men, 71–80 cm or 81–90 cm reservoir would be used, but in women 61–70 cm or 71–80 cm size would be used. The higher pressure is reserved for those patients who have a lot of scar tissue. There is a higher risk of erosion with pressures of 80 cm, even when a cuff has been in situ for a long time, without problems, or when the reservoir is changed. It is suggested that the blood flow should be

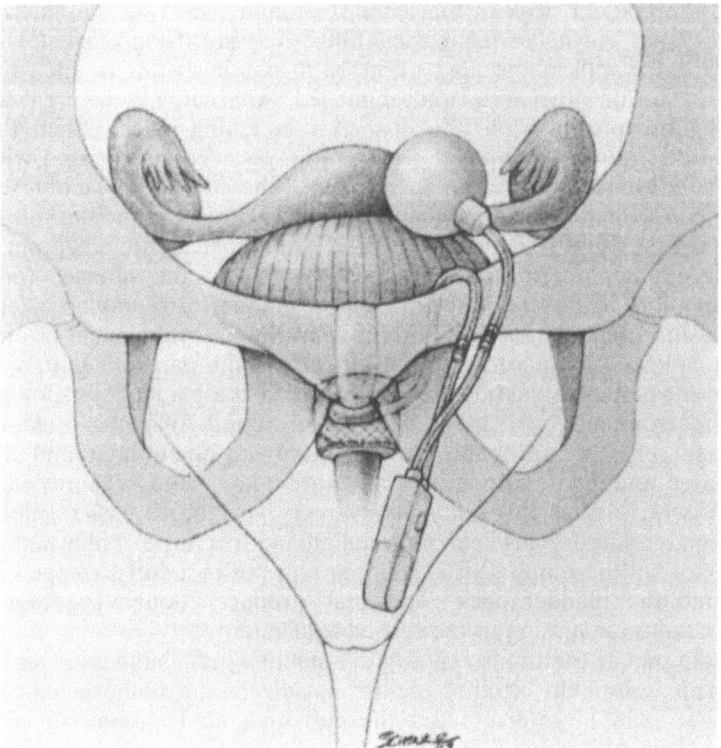

Fig. 5.12. Bladder neck placement of the AS 800 in the female.

measured with a Doppler and the reservoir pressure kept below it in order to avoid erosion, but at the expense of stress incontinence.

Activation and Deactivation

With the advent of the self-filling cuffs there was a risk of urethral erosion occuring in the early post-operative period, either because of damage to the urethra at the time of the cuff placement or by the continuous local pressure on the urethra. Furlow (1981) suggested the concept of primary deactivation – when the three components were implanted, but not connected – in order to reduce the chances of erosion as well as making sure that the cuff size is currently selected and as low a reservoir pressure as possible is used. In a series of 47 patients in whom the 742 sphincter device was used there were 8 erosions out of 42 which were activated from the time of the operation, but no erosions in 5 patients when the device was primarily deactivated. However, in a group of patients in whom the 791 sphincter was used there was a decreased incidence of erosion with deactivation although it did still occur in 4 of 34 cases. A particularly strong adverse factor was when a patient had had radiotherapy for carcinoma of the prostate and erosion occurred in both the activated and deactivated groups.

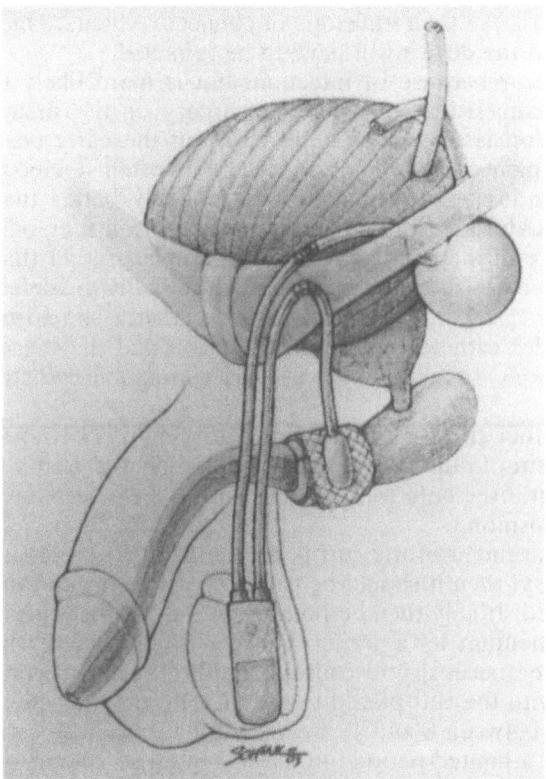

Fig. 5.13. Bulbar urethral placement of the AS 800 in the male.

These arguments are not so relevant now that the AS800 allows primary deactivation of the device without the need to carry out secondary surgery. However the AS792 still has certain advantages for young girls because the pump is smaller and fits in the labium more comfortably.

Another advantage of the AS800 is that a number of patients can deactivate their own device at night, because they do not need it to be functioning when they are recumbent.

Complications

There are a number of problems that may occur with the device and it is important to establish accurately what is wrong (Furlow and Barrett 1985; Webster and Sihelnick 1984).

Implanting a foreign body will inevitably result in infection in a small percentage of cases, however meticulous one has been in the pre-operative perparation and with the surgery and subsequent management. If a patient develops pain related to the device, antibiotic treatment should be reassessed or started immediately and the infection may be controlled. In the early post-operative period one is more likely to control it because the components of the device have not yet been enclosed in their envelope of connective tissue. Once the infection is well established the device will have to be removed.

Erosion of the cuff may occur because of infection, but is more likely to happen if the urethra was damaged at the time of surgery or the tissues are relatively avascular. Erosion is diagnosed quite easily in the early post-operative period because of pain and swelling and there is often a bloody urethral discharge. Careful endoscopic examination is probably better than ascending urethrography at establishing the diagnosis. Late erosion may only be diagnosed because of failure of the device causing incontinence rather than infection. Once diagnosed, the cuff will have to be removed. Usually the defect will heal without local surgery. A 14–18F gauge silicone catheter should be used for 7–10 days, the smaller catheter for urethral erosion and the bigger catheter for bladder neck erosions. In addition the use of a suprapubic catheter is useful.

It is better not to insert another cuff for at least 3 months, and it is better to reinsert the cuff at a different site. In the male if the bladder neck was used it is easy to insert a bulbar cuff, but if the bulb was previously used the device must be put in a slightly different position.

In the female, secondary placement of the cuff is very difficult. If omentum was used at the primary surgery, then it should be carefully placed around the defect when the cuff is removed. It may then be possible to put another cuff in the same place using the omentum as a buffer between the cuff and the urethra. Alternatively it may be necessary to consider urethral reconstruction using a laterally placed tube with the cuff placed round this. Primary deactivation should be mandatory for between 8 and 12 weeks and when the device is activated it should be done for a limited period of time, for instance 2 hours on and 2 hours off with deactivation at night.

If incontinence occurs at the time of activation it may result from cuff erosion, wrong sized cuff, mechanical dysfunction, wrong pressure reservoir or improper filling volume, urinary infection and detrusor instability or tissue rigidity. Inability to squeeze the pump may mean the tubing is either blocked by debris or is kinked. If the pump is collapsed there may be mechanical blocking or there may be fluid loss. In addition, blockage may occur because incorrect fluid was used to fill the device and crystallisation of the fluid has occurred. If antibiotics get inside the device, crystals may also form. An X-ray taken with the cuff deflated and inflated will show if there is any mechanical or user problem; it will show the distribution of the fluid and will exclude any kinks or fluid leaks (Fig. 5.14). It is also important to check that the bladder is emptying completely.

Urinary infection, although not responsible for detrusor instability, will make it worse and make it difficult to manage medically. If the cuff size was wrongly assessed at the primary surgery, it will be noted that it holds too much fluid because to empty it may take 4–5 pushes of the pump. Once the reservoir is more than 4 ml below its filling volume the pressure will fall. In late incontinence, the cuff may also be found to be too small because the tissue beneath it has atrophied. In both situations the problem can be remedied by putting in the correct sized smaller cuff. If leakage has occurred surgery will be needed and the reservoir tested first, by instilling 18 ml of fluid and measuring the volume again after 5 minutes. Low reservoir pressure may also be due to hypotonic fluid. Pump leakage is very rare, but may be tested electrically with

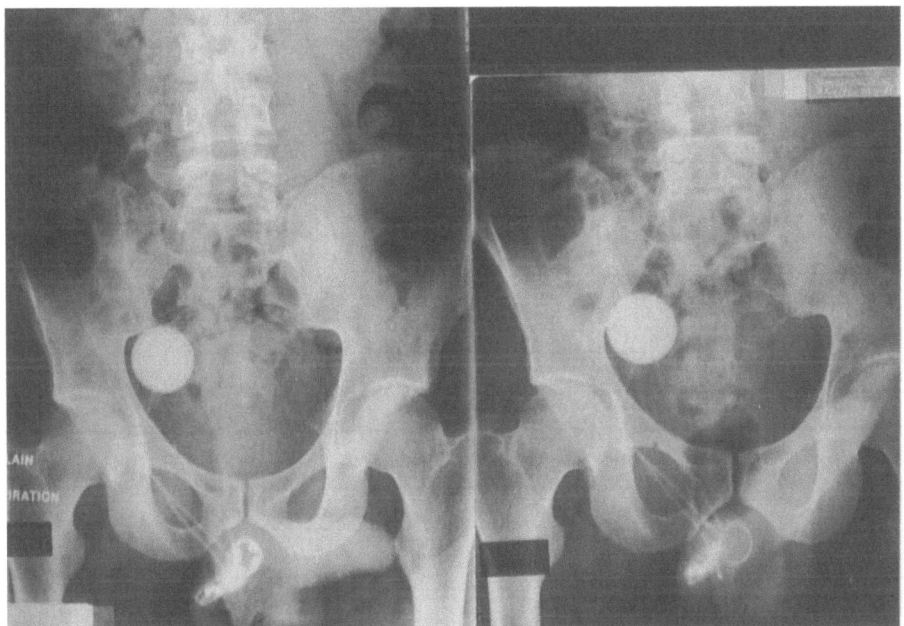

Fig. 5.14. X-ray showing an implanted activated AS 800.

the pump in situ. The cuff should also be tested electrically, but can be taken out and inspected. Electrical testing is dependant on the fact that silicone is non-conductive and there is therefore infinite resistence between the fluid in the device and in the tissue outside, unless a leak is present. Each component can be isolated and checked.

Exploration will also be necessary if part of the device is occluded by debris and each part should be tested in situ to determine the site of the problem. When it is obvious which part is causing the problem it can be changed, but occasionally it is not obvious what is the primary problem and all three components will have to be changed.

Indications for Use of the Sphincter

The indications for the use of the Artificial Urinary Sphincter (AUS) have widened considerably since it was first introduced in 1972 (Scott et al. 1973a, 1974). The two common conditions originally considered were congenital neuropathic bladders and post-prostatectomy incontinence (Scott et al. 1973b; Bruskewitz et al. 1980). Since the sphincter is now used in association with bladder substitution and augmentation, more complex neuropathic conditions can be considered, both congenital and acquired (Brown and Morales 1984; Mundy and Stephenson 1984; Stephenson et al. 1983). Bladder extrophy, which is now more frequently reconstructed and closed is a relatively common indication in the paediatric age group (Light and Scott 1983a). Stress incontinence in the female remains a small group (Tables 5.1, 5.2) in any series (Light and Scott 1985).

Table 5.1. Age of patients receiving AMS incontinence sphincters

Age (years)	Percentage of implants
0–10	11
11–20	20
21–30	8
31–40	9
41–50	6
51–60	13
61–70	21
71–80	11
81–90	1

Table 5.2. Aetiology of incontinence in 197 patients receiving AMS sphincters

Condition	Number (%)
Myelomeningocele	53 (26.9)
Post-prostatectomy	48 (24.5)
Post-TURP	34 (17.3)
Spinal trauma/tumour	11 (5.6)
Exstrophy/epispadias	10 (5.0)
Pelvic trauma/tumour	10 (5.0)
Other post surgery	7 (3.6)
Other	7 (3.6)

The minimum investigations to perform are full video-urodynamic studies, assessment of the upper tracts, cystoscopy and measurement of bladder capacity. It is necessary to exclude a urethral stricture and other bladder pathology.

In the ideal situation there should be absence of detrusor hyper-reflexia, absence of infravesical obstruction, including sphincter dysnergia, absence of ureteric reflux or upper tract stasis, absence of urinary tract infections and an adequate bladder capacity. In addition, manual dexterity is essential and the patient, or parents, must be motivated and intelligent. If the patient is immobile and has decubitus ulcers these should be treated before implantation of a sphincter is contemplated.

Neuropathic Bladders

The primary treatment is usually to try and keep the patient dry by the use of anticholinergic drugs and clean intermittent self catheterisation (CISC). If this fails full urodynamic investigations are necessary as it is important to classify the detrusor function into contractile, intermediate or acontractile (Mundy et al. 1985). Following sphincter insertion the intermediate group may markedly change their function to high-pressure, high-frequency contractions and as a result incontinence may occur (Bauer et al. 1986; Churchill et al. 1987; Light and Pietro 1986; Roth et al. 1986). It is therefore necessary to consider substitution or augmentation cystoplasty at the time of sphincter insertion to prevent apparent sphincter related problems later on. The cystoplasty will also be needed to reduce the pressure – a detubularised ileo-caecocystoplasty (Mainz pouch) or if the bladder capacity is adequate a "clam" type of cystoplasty using small bowel or colon (Bramble 1982). A decision also has to be made whether complete bladder emptying should be achieved by surgical ablation of the external sphincter, or by relying on CISC (Stephenson and Mundy 1985). Barrett and Furlow (1984) showed that using CISC was a perfectly safe procedure, although they favoured placing the cuff at the bladder neck and favoured patients with an adequate bladder capacity. In a series of neuropathic bladder patients they had 92% success with only three on CISC (Barrett and Furlow 1982). In an excellent review Light et al. (1983) compared the use of the sphincter to other established techniques, such as different types of diversion and concluded that good results could be achieved with the sphincter in 77% of cases, but with 1.66 operations per patient. However with CISC 66% of patients were socially continent without any complex surgery. If notice is not taken of the bladder behaviour less good results will be obtained (Gonzales and Sheldon 1982). Light and Scott (1984b) in a series of 132 children, the majority of whom had neuropathic problems, had excellent results in 90% using the AS792.

Raezer et al. (1980) accept that the sphincter has a place in the management of this group of patients and had 79% success, but ultimately had to remove the device in 32% of patients. Duckett (1983) in an editorial comment still felt that the complication rate was unacceptably high.

Acquired Neuropathic Bladders

Provided the condition is non-progressive there is a case for using the AUS, but the results will depend very much on the behaviour of the bladder and how it is treated in combination with sphincter insertion. Light and Scott (1983b) found that 90% of patients with acontractile bladders were dry, but only 50% in the intermediate group, and in the contractile group 70% were dry, but in some a cystoplasty was performed.

Exstrophy and Epispadias

This is now an important group because with the AUS a case can be made for using the sphincter primarily rather than undertaking complex bladder neck reconstruction, which if unsuccessful makes subsequent implantation of the sphincter very difficult. Burbige et al. (1987) had a high rate of complications – 15 in 8 patients with 13 secondary procedures. They had bowel shrinkage under the cuff but they rarely used the omentum. Light and Scott (1983a) had excellent results with 10 out of 11 children dry when they used the sphincter alone without bladder neck reconstruction. Hanna (1981) also had good results with exstrophy.

Undiversion

There is a group of patients who have been diverted, not because they have poor control, but because there is a problem with their upper tracts. If these can be resolved they are candidates for undiversion and will not need a sphincter. A more common group to consider is those patients with myelodysplasia who were incontinent before diversion. If these children are undiverted, major reconstructive procedures will be necessary to obtain adequate bladder capacity and a sphincter will be needed to produce continence. Surgery may be needed to obtain satisfactory emptying or CISC can be used (Mitchell and Rink 1983). Light et al. (1983a) also had good results in a small number of patients. Light and Scott (1984a) put the sphincter around the bowel in reconstructed patients, but had better results with the ileo-caecal segment. Light and Engelmann (1985) showed that ureteric reflux was more common. There is still considerable debate about putting the sphincter around the bowel, but a particularly poor prognostic problem is the patient who has had pelvic irradiation and is a candidate for reconstruction rather than diversion.

Post-prostatectomy Incontinence

Unfortunately this condition occurs all too often, but has proved an ideal group to treat with the sphincter after careful selection. No patient should be considered too soon after the primary surgery because improvement in the incontinence can be expected. Mundy and Stephenson (1984) found that only 11% of patients with post-prostatectomy incontinence were suitable for implantation because of the high incidence of detrusor instability. Very often there is a combination of sphincter weakness and detrusor instability but if the latter cannot be controlled medically a sphincter should not be implanted. Barrett and Furlow (1983), using the AS791 sphincter, achieved a success rate overall of only 74%, but if the group who had had radiotherapy for carcinoma of the prostate were excluded 93% were dry. When primary deactivation was not used the incidence of urethral erosion was very high at 82%, even when the lowest pressure reservoirs were used. It is probably better to exclude patients who have had radiotherapy from sphincter implantation, because of the poor results. The ideal patient should be totally incontinent, have no instability and have a normal bladder capacity and compliance. Schreiter (1985), using the higher position of the bulbar cuff, had 92.7% success in 41 patients, failure being due to erosion and infection in 2 patients.

Lindner et al. (1983) reported a series in which post-prostatectomy incontinence predominated and most had had previous surgery. Primary deactivation improved the results, but in fact the erosion rate was lower with activation, but probably reflected the poorer risk patients in the deactivated group. Bruskewitz et al. (1981) had 50% failures because of erosion.

Stress Incontinence in Females

There can be few indications for primary implantation of this sphincter for this condition. Provided the patients with significant detrusor instability are excluded good results from conventional surgery can be expected. Currently the popular procedures are the Burch colposuspension (Burch 1961), the Marshall Marchetti Kranz suspension (Marshall et al. 1949), the Stamey endoscopic bladder neck suspension (Stamey 1980), the Pereya–Raz suspension (Pereya 1959; Raz 1981), various bladder neck slings and their modifications.

Overall, good results will be obtained in 90% of cases; although some authors claim almost 100% success, the length of the follow-up and critical analysis of what constitutes a success is important. The AUS is therefore likely to be reserved for the patients with failed surgery, when by definition they are likely to have the "drain pipe" urethra and in whom the implantation will be difficult. It is very important to place the cuff round the bladder neck without damage to the urethra.

Light and Scott (1985) operated on 39 women who had had an average of 2.2 operations (range 1–5). Previous surgery had been successful technically in that the bladder neck was correctly sited anatomically but the urethral function was inadequate. Of the patients 87% were totally dry and 92% overall were satisfied with the result.

There have been many papers describing the results of sphincter implantation and not all of them have been mentioned. Some of them refer to small numbers of patients but the results obtained by Brantley Scott (1989) in adults and Barrett and Parulker (1989) in children are worth studying. The more experience an operator has, the better his selection of patients and the results to be expected. Continence in excess of 90% should be achieved, but reoperation is a likely event in up to 15% of cases, so all patients with an implanted sphincter need very careful longterm follow-up.

References

Augspurger RR (1981) Pitfalls of the Rosen anti-incontinence prosthesis. J Urol 125:201–203

Barrett DM, Furlow WL (1982) The management of severe urinary incontinence in patients with myelodysplasia by implantation of the AS 791/792 urinary sphincter device. J Urol 128:484–486

Barrett DM, Furlow WL (1983) Radical prostatectomy incontinence and the AS 791 artificial urinary sphincter. J Urol 129:528–530

Barrett DM, Furlow WL (1984) Incontinence, intermittent self catheterisation and the artificial genito-urinary sphincter. J Urol 132:268–269

Barrett DM, Parulkar BG (1989) The artificial sphincter (AS-800): Experience in children and young adults. Urol Clin North Am 16:119–132

Bauer SB, Reda EF, Colodny AH, Retik AB (1986) Detrusor instability: a delayed complication in association with the artificial sphincter. J Urol 135:1212–1215

Berg S (1973) Polytef augmentation urethroplasty. Arch Surg 107:379–381

Berry JL (1961) A new procedure for correction of urinary incontinence, preliminary report. J Urol 85:771–775

Berry JL, Dahlen CP (1971) Evaluation of a procedure for correction of urinary incontinence in men. J Urol 105:105–106

Bramble FJ (1982) The treatment of adult enuresis and urge incontinence by enterocystoplasty. Br J Urol 54:693–696

Brown J, Morales P (1984) Artificial urinary sphincter 800. Urology 23:479–483

Bruskewitz R, Raz S, Smith RB, Kaufman JJ (1980) AMS 742 sphincter. UCLA experience. J Urol 124:812–814

Bruskewitz R, Raz S, Kaufman JJ (1981) Treatment of urinary incontinence with the artificial sphincter. J Urol 126:469–472

Burbige KA, Reitelman C, Olsson CA (1987) Complications of artificial sphincter around intestinal segments in reconstructed exstrophy patients. J Urol 138:1123–1127

Burch JC (1961) Urethrovaginal fixation to Coopers ligament for correction of stress incontinence, cystocele and prolapse. Am J Obstet Gynecol 81:281–290

Cox R, Worth PHL (1986) Results of treatment of post-prostatectomy incontinence using the Kaufman prosthesis. Eur Urol 12:154–157

Churchill BM, Gilmour RF, Khoury AE, Mclorie GA (1987) Biological response of bladders rendered continent by insertion of artificial sphincters. J Urol 138:1116–1119

Deane AM, English P, Hehir M, Williams JP, Worth PHL (1985) Teflon injection in stress incontinence. Br J Urol 57:78–80

Dees JE (1949) Congenital epispadias with incontinence. J Urol 30:34–42

Duckett JW (1983) Editorial comment. J Urol 129:740

Foley FEB (1947) An artificial sphincter: A new device and operation for control of enuresis and urinary incontinence. J Urol 58:250–259

Fowler JW, Auld CD (1985) The control of male stress incontinence by implantable prosthesis. Br J Urol 57:175–180

Furlow WL (1981) Implantation of a new semi-automatic artificial genitourinary sphincter: Experience with primary activation and deactivation in 47 patients. J Urol 126:741–744

Furlow WL, Barrett DM (1985) Recurrent or persistent urinary incontinence in patients with the artificial urinary sphincter: diagnostic considerations and management. J Urol 133:792–795

Giesy JD, Barry JM, Fuchs EF, Griffith LD (1981) Initial experience with the Rosen incontinence device. J Urol 125:794–795

Girgis AS, Veenema RJ (1965) Perineal urethroplasty: A new operation for correction of urinary incontinence in the male patient. J Urol 93:703–708

Gonzales R, Sheldon CA (1982) Artificial sphincters in children with neurogenic bladder: longterm results. J Urol 128:1270–1272

Hanna MK (1981) Artificial urinary sphincter for incontinent children. Urology 18:370–373

Hinman F, Schmaelzle JF, Cass AS (1970) Autogenous perineal bone graft for post-prostatectomy incontinence. Technique and results of prosthetic fixation of urogenital diaphragm in man. J Urol 104:888–892

Kaufman JJ (1970) A new operation for male incontinence. Surg Gynecol Obstet 131:295–299

Kaufman JJ (1972) Surgical treatment of post-prostatectomy incontinence: use of penile crura to compress bulbous urethra. J Urol 107:293–297

Kaufman JJ (1973a) Treatment of post-prostatectomy urinary incontinence using a silicone gel prosthesis. Br J Urol 45:646–653

Kaufman JJ (1973b) Urethral compression operation for the treatment of post-prostatectomy incontinence. J Urol 110:93–96

Kaufman JJ, Raz S (1979) Urethral compression procedure for the treatment of male urinary incontinence. J Urol 121:605–608

Kaufman JJ, Ritchie JP (1974) Urethral erosion: Complications of Kaufman anti-incontinence operation. Urology 3:218–220

Leadbetter GW (1964) Surgical correction of total urinary incontinence. J Urol 91:261–266

Lewis RI, Lockhart JL, Politano VA (1984) Periurethral polytetrafluoroethylene injections in incontinent female subjects with neurogenic bladder disease. J Urol 131:459–462

Light JK, Engelmann UH (1985) Reconstruction of the lower urinary tract: observations on bowel dynamics and the artificial urinary sphincter: diagnostic considerations and management. J Urol 133:594–597

Light JK, Scott FB (1983a) Treatment of epispadias exstrophy complex with AS792 artificial urinary sphincter. J Urol 129:738–740

Light JK, Scott FB (1983b) Use of the artificial urinary sphincter in spinal cord injury patients. J Urol 130:1127–1129

Light JK, Scott FB (1984a) Total reconstruction of the lower urinary tract using bowel and the artificial urinary sphincter. J Urol 131:953–956

Light JK, Scott FB (1984b) The artificial urinary sphincter in children. Br J Urol 56:54–57

Light JK, Scott FB (1985) Management of urinary incontinence in women with the artificial urinary sphincter. J Urol 134:476–478

Light JK, Pietro T (1986) Alteration in detrusor behaviour and the effect on renal function following insertion of the artificial urinary sphincter. J Urol 136:632–635

Light JK, Flores FN, Scott FB (1983a) Use of the AS792 artificial sphincter following urinary undiversion. J Urol 129:548–551

Light JK, Hawila M, Scott FB (1983b) Treatment of urinary incontinence in children: the artificial sphincter versus other methods. J Urol 130:518–521

Lim KB, Ball AJ, Feneley RCL (1983) Periurethral Teflon injections: a simple treatment for urinary incontinence. Br J Urol 55:208–210

Lindner A, Kaufman JJ, Raz S (1983) Further experience with the artificial urinary sphincter. J Urol 129:962–963

Lowsley OS (1936) New operation for the relief of incontinence in both males and females. J Urol 36:400–413

Malizia AA, Reiman HM, Myers RP, Sande JR, Barham SS, Benson RC, Dewanjee MK, Utz WJ (1984) Migration and granulomatous reaction after periurethral injection of polytef (Teflon). JAMA 251:3277–3281

Marshall VF, Marchetti AA, Krantz KE (1949) The correction of stress incontinence by simple vesicourethral suspension. Surg Gynecol Obstet 88:509–518

Mitchell ME, Rink RC (1983) Experience with the artificial urinary sphincter in children and young adults. J Pediatr Surg 18:700–705

Mundy AR, Shah PJR, Borzyskowski M, Saxton HM (1985) Sphincter behaviour in myelomeningocoele. Br J Urol 57:647–651

Mundy AR, Stephenson TP (1984) Selection of patients for implantation of the Brantley Scott artificial urinary sphincter. Br J Urol 56:717–720

Murless BC (1938) The injection treatment of stress incontinence. J Obstet Gynaecol 45:67–73

Pereyra AJ (1959) A simplified procedure for the correction of stress incontinence in women. West J Surg Obstet Gynecol 67:223–226

Politano VA (1982) Periurethral polytetrafluoroethylene injections for urinary incontinence. J Urol 127:439–442

Politano VA, Small MP, Harper JM, Lyncee CM (1974) Periurethral teflon injection for urinary incontinence. J Urol 111:180–183

Puigvert A (1971) Surgical treatment of urinary incontinence in the male. Urol Int 26:261–268

Quackels R (1955) Deux incontinences apres adanomectomiegueries par injection de paraffine dans le perinee. Acta Urol Belg 23:259–262

Raezer DM, Wein AJ, Duckett JW, Cromie WJ (1980) A clinical experience with the Scott genitourinary sphincter in the management of urinary incontinence in the pediatric age group. J Urol 123:546–547

Raz S (1981) Modified bladder neck suspension for female stress incontinence. Urology 17:82–85

Reid GF, Fitzpatrick JM, Worth PHL (1980) The treatment of patients with urinary incontinence after prostatectomy. Br J Urol 57:532–534

Rosen M (1976) A simplified artificial implantable sphincter. Br J Urol 48:675–680

Rosen M (1978) The Rosen inflatable incontinence prosthesis. Urol Clin North Am 5:403–414

Roth DR, Vyas PR, Kroovand RL, Perlmutter AD (1986) Urinary tract deterioration associated with the artificial urinary sphincter. J Urol 135:528–530

Sachse H (1963) Sclerosing therapy in urinary incontinence: indications, results, complications. Urol Int 15:225–244

Salcedo H (1972) Surgical correction of post-prostatectomy urinary incontinence using marlex mesh: preliminary report. J Urol 107:440–441

Schreiter F (1985) Bulbar artificial sphincter. Eur Urol 11:294–299

Schulman CC, Simon J, Wespes E (1983a) Injection endoscopique de teflon dans le traitement de l'incontinence urinaire femine d'effort. Rev Med Brux 4:95–97

Schulman CC, Simon J, Wespes E, Germeau F (1983b) Endoscopic injection of teflon for female urinary incontinence. Eur Urol 3:246–247

Scott FB (1989) The artificial urinary sphincter: Experience in adults. Urol Clin North Amer 16:105–118

Scott FB, Bradley WE, Timm GW (1973a) Treatment of urinary incontinence by an implantable prosthetic sphincter. Urology 1:252–259

Scott FB, Bradley WE, Timm GW, Kothari (1973b) Treatment of incontinence secondary to myelodysplasia by an implantable prosthetic urinary sphincter. South Med J 66:987–990

Scott FB, Bradley WE, Timm GW (1974) Treatment of urinary incontinence by an implantable prosthetic urinary sphincter. J Urol 112:75–80

Scott FB, Light JK, Fishman I, West J (1981) Implantation of an artificial sphincter for urinary incontinence. Contemporary Surgery 18:11–14

Small MP (1980) The Rosen incontinence procedure: a new artificial urinary sphincter for the management of urinary incontinence. J Urol 123:507–511

Stamey TA (1980) Endoscopic suspension of the vesical neck for urinary incontinence in females: report on 203 consecutive patients. Ann Surg 192:465–471

Stephenson TP, Mundy AR (1985) Treatment of the neuropathic bladder by enterocystoplasty and selective sphincterotomy or sphincter ablation and replacement. Br J Urol 57:27–31

Stephenson TP, Stone AR, Sheppard J, Saburry RY (1983) Preliminary results of AS 791/792
  artificial sphincter for urinary incontinence. Br J Urol 55:684–686
Vorstman B, Kaufman MR, Lockhart J, Politano V (1985) Polytetrafluoroethylene injection for
  urinary incontinence in children. J Urol 133:248–250
Webster GD, Sihelnick SA (1984) Trouble shooting the malfunctioning Scott artificial urinary
  sphincter. J Urol 131:269–272
Worth PHL (1982) Assessment and treatment of urinary incontinence. J R Soc Med 75:665

Chapter 6

Urinary Incontinence Appliances, Aids and Equipment

R.N.P. Carroll

Continence confers comfort and dignity whereas, by contrast, incontinence not only deprives the sufferer of these qualities but also reduces self-respect and confidence. The aim of treating people with incontinence is to improve the quality of their lives because only some can be cured. The management of incontinence of the chronically ill and disabled may be quite different from the management of a patient who is fully ambulant and able to work. Incontinence is often a taboo subject and many patients are reluctant to discuss the problem even with close relatives.

The term urinary incontinence has only recently gained respectability and consequently the subject is only now being spoken about without too much social stigma being attached to it. By virtue of this change in public attitude, the medical and nursing professions have taken the opportunity by writing in the press and by discussion on radio and television, of further enlightening the public about this health care problem and the services that are available to control it. In the past the management of urinary incontinence has been something of a Cinderella subject and in the words of at least one commentator, the problems have been swept under the carpet!

It is very difficult to assess the incidence of urinary incontinence in the community but McGrother and colleagues (1986) suggested that a general practitioner with about 2500 patients on his list would have at least 40 incontinent patients. The incidence increases with age and it is estimated that 12% of women and about 6% of men over the age of 65 years suffer from incontinence. Women suffer from incontinence at a younger age than men but by the age of 85 the incidence is the same in both sexes. Research carried out by the magazine *Woman* in 1985 showed that one-third of incontinence sufferers were under the age of 35 and most of these women first developed symptoms after childbirth. It is estimated that there are between three and four million adults in the United Kingdom who seek advice about their incontinence and probably an equal number who do not.

Urinary incontinence care is provided by the nursing and medical professions but the expertise is variable. Because of the lack of an information database there is no national policy about how the problems should be tackled. The number of medical meetings, symposia and publications on incontinence has increased enormously over the last few years and as a consequence young doctors are now being made aware that incontinence is a problem that they will have to understand. In the United Kingdom, the single most important advance has been the establishment in 1981 of the Association of Continence Advisors. Continence advisers are fully trained nurses who have developed an interest, commitment and expertise in the field of urinary continence and it is to be hoped that their number will increase greatly.

It has been said that the largest portion of the National Health Service budget is spent either directly or indirectly on incontinence. Manufacturers supply about 120 million bed pads (underpads) annually in the United Kingdom. The National Health Service contracts for body-worn pads are of the order of £17–20 million per year and this does not take into account the money spent in the private sector. A vast sum of money is written off each year because of the damage leaking urine does to clothes and bedding, not to mention the large cost of laundering such items while in use before they are discarded.

Embarrassment surrounds incontinence because the patients are wet, may smell and are aware that the protective clothing can be bulky. Many consider themselves to be social outcasts because of these factors. My experience is that those people who have undergone urinary diversion are much less self-conscious after they have come to accept their stoma and appliance than those who have to wear a device such as a leg bag or bulky pads between their legs. In choosing and recommending a particular appliance or pad for a patient, the patient's preference must be taken into account. In assessing which particular device to recommend it is important to ascertain from the patient whether the urine comes out in a gush or a dribble and whether there is also faecal incontinence and whether such incontinence is of the solid or liquid type. Patients' ambulatory status and whether they are bed-ridden or paralysed are factors which determine the recommendations that are made. In addition to mobility, the patient's dexterity, mental agility and physical function will influence the final decision about the options offered. It may be lack of dexterity in emptying a uribag or changing a pad which determines appliance selection unless the patient can readily call on a dependant or carer to assist in time of need. Some people who are not incontinent at night mainly suffer from vertical incontinence during the day while they are walking about. Others cope reasonably well during the day but their incontinence is dominant at night. This of course is particularly true of young children who suffer from nocturnal enuresis. It is obvious that time and effort have to be put into the assessment of each individual patient's needs before the appropriate advice can be proffered.

Appliance Choice

Below is an attempt to classify and subdivide the various appliances, aids and equipment which are available. Most of them can be classified in one category but some others overlap categories and a little licence has been taken in the classification. The manufacturers' literature and some articles on incontinence cannot be entirely relied upon for correct terminology and so I trust that nobody will be too offended if they feel that the categories do not fit entirely with their concepts. I apologise also if there have been significant omissions.

The market is changing all the time and this means that it would not be too difficult to omit a significant breakthrough in incontinence, particularly if the product has not been well advertised. In trying to assess the available products, one difficulty which I encountered was the restriction placed by purchasing authorities in the range of appliances bought within their area. This has meant that I do not have practical experience of all items mentioned below but I have tried to highlight the ones more commonly used on the basis that they have gained recognition through usage.

Patient attendance at incontinence clinics makes one realise that the choice available to the user is such that with very few exceptions such as with the all-in-one diaper type and nappy, it is uncommon to find two patients in the clinic who are using identical incontinence appliances. The problem is compounded by the anatomical differences of the male, female and children which demand separate designs. It is an almost impossible task to describe accurately the state of the art in urinary incontinence appliance manufacture.

Permanent Indwelling Catheters

The preference of the doctor, nurse or patient for dealing with any individual problem might be the use of a permanent indwelling catheter. Given that this decision has been made, the choice of the correct catheter may go some way to reducing or eliminating management problems. Although urinary catheters have been discussed elsewhere in this book, it is justifiable to make or repeat some comments in respect of the choice of catheter for permanent use in incontinent patients.

The Foley catheter was invented over 50 years ago and was intended as a post-prostatectomy catheter with the balloon intended to act as a tamponade in the prostatic cavity. In time, the balloon catheter came to be used as a self-retaining catheter for other purposes. In incontinent patients the smallest catheter, and balloon, consistent with functional requirements should be used. In patients who are paralysed, or suffer from multiple sclerosis, self-retaining catheters sometimes fall out, together with their inflated balloons intact. The poor musculature of the pelvic floor allows the urethra to dilate irrespective of the catheter diameter or size of balloon used. In time, the larger diameter catheters and hyperinflated balloons will be extruded spontaneously. In that situation another solution to the patient's incontinence problem will have to be found.

There is no aspect of catheter care about which greater confusion arises than the balloon size. When the balloon is inflated with 30 ml of water, the balloon will take on the configuration of a golf ball with the tip of the catheter emerging at the polar aspect. The catheter is therefore circumferentially surrounded on all parts by a cushion of water and the tip of the catheter will remain at a constant height above the trigone. This means that a reservoir of urine will pool around the lower hemisphere of the balloon and act as a medium for infection and debris collection. In addition when the catheter is deflated, the calcium phosphate encrustation on the balloon will flake off like egg shell and fall into the sump of urine. With repeated deflations the sump of urine containing calcium phosphate material and other debris can lead to stone formation or provide the sediment to block a renewed catheter.

A 10-ml balloon will inflate to the configuration of a small marble and because the catheter tip is raised only a small distance above the trigone, more urine is drained from the bladder than would have been the case if a catheter with a 30-ml balloon had been used. Until recently the 5-ml and 10-ml balloon size figure printed on the inflation channel represented the volume of the balloon and did not take into account the volume of the inflation channel. The British Standards Institute (BSI) have recommended that the figure on the inflation channel ought to be "fill volume," in other words the sum of the balloon volume and the inflation channel volume. The balloon should be filled with sterile water rather than tap water because the latter may pass through the wall by osmosis. Tap water may contain impurities and these could block the inflation channel and make deflation difficult. Saline is not advised because crystal formation can affect the inflation channel and air should be avoided because the balloon will float and the catheter not drain adequately. In addition, the tip of a floating catheter could irritate the dome of the bladder causing spasm and detrusor contractions resulting in bypassing of the catheter. Some manufacturers produce prefilled Foley catheters which already contain the appropriate volume of sterile water. These catheters are very easy to inflate and are excellent for domiciliary practice as they obviate the need for separate needles, syrings and sterile water.

Adult catheters come in two lengths, standard and female. The standard length catheter should be avoided for longterm use in a female with a permanent indwelling catheter. The smallest diameter catheter consistent with adequate drainage should always be used. The size of catheters is measured in Charriere (French) units and a unit is equal to one-third mm. Therefore, a number of 24F catheter has a diameter of 8 mm. The large diameter catheter should only be used if debris and encrustation are expected or if the urine is quite viscous. In longterm usage it is usually unnecessary to use catheters of a larger size than 18F. In those situations where bypassing occurs, particularly in men, it may be useful to use a Bi-Coude (Roberts) tipped catheter. This has an eye above and below the balloon and if the spasms produce detrusor contractions with bypassing of the urine through the bladder neck, the eye of the catheter below the balloon can very often drain this urine and minimise leakage. Bypassing is a feature in patients with multiple sclerosis and very often the insertion of a Roberts Bi-Coude catheter may improve the patient's comfort and reduce the need to change the catheter to a larger size together with a larger balloon.

It is not uncommon for permanent indwelling catheters to become blocked and there is no easy way to avoid this. A high fluid intake is desirable but some patients who are disabled or sick are unable to ingest large quantities of fluids. Irrigation through a three-way catheter is one option but in non-acute hospitals it is uncommon for patients with permanent indwelling catheters to be fitted with a three-way catheter. The blocking problem is usually managed by breaking the seal on the catheter to carry out wash outs. Noxyflex (n-oxythiolun) is the most effective solution and although it is several times more expensive than Hibitaine (chlorhexidure gluconate), it is still the preferred solution. Hibitaine should only be used when Noxyflex is not available. The breaking of the seal on the closed drainage system of a two-way catheter predisposes to infection whereas intermittent irrigation using a three-way system results in a lower incidence of infective problems.

About 5% of patients who have permanent indwelling catheters block their catheters within a few days of these being changed. Such patients are known as "blockers". No matter how often the catheter is changed, and irrespective of the size or type of catheter inserted, blockage occurs within a very short space of time. It seems as though these people have an abnormal biochemical make-up or, more correctly, they have a urine of a particular consistency of chemical make-up that facilitates blockage. At the moment there is no solution to the problem of "blockers" and ultimately permanent indwelling catheterisation is not the answer to their problems and other remedies have to be found.

Self Catheterisation

The discipline of patient self catheterisation has been widely practised for many years but not all incontinent patients are suitable for this form of self treatment. It is usually applicable to those patients who have little or no bladder sensation. In practice, it means that they are unable to empty their bladders and when their bladders are full they become incontinent. Some of these patients manage reasonably well by day but at night, despite evacuating their bladders before retiring, they are incontinent. Others have to catheterise themselves regularly by the clock throughout the day and again last thing at night. Most of these patients are ambulant but some are wheelchair-bound. It is particularly difficult for wheelchair-bound female patients to practise self catheterisation but some of them do succeed. It is very much easier for the wheelchair-bound male patient to practise self catheterisation.

The catheterisation can be sterile intermittent self catheterisation or clean intermittent self catheterisation. In the first instance the catheters come prepacked, are sterile and discarded after use. The clean intermittent self catheterisation technique allows each catheter to be used several times. They are merely washed and dried but some patients immerse them in an antiseptic solution such as Hibitaine. Some people prefer to use one catheter for a day and others use the same catheter for several days before changing it. The nealton catheter is usually used by the male whereas in the female, the preferred type is a short straight catheter such as is used in obstetric practice to empty the bladder before delivery.

Female catheters and the catheters used for children are usually about 10 cm in length and those for men up to 30 cm. The catheter sizes for children are 6–10F and for adults 10–12F. Patients are encouraged to empty their bladders four to six times a day, last thing at night and first thing in the morning.

Clean Intermittent Self Catheterisation

The practice of clean intermittent self catheterisation has been with us for a decade and is mainly performed by females and children. It is not necessary for the patient to take antibiotics but some do because of a history of recurrent urinary tract infection. A high fluid intake is by far the most important deterrent to urinary infection. After use the catheters are merely washed and dried until required.

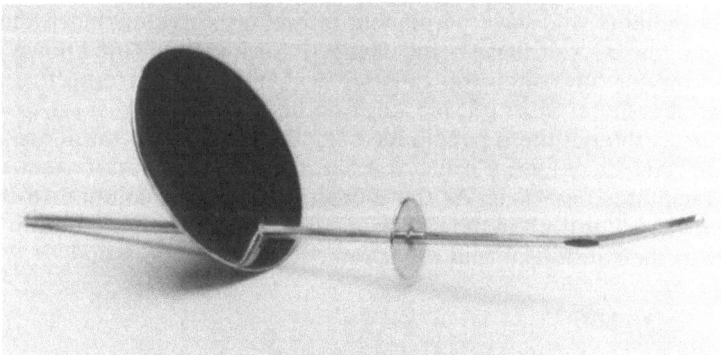

Fig. 6.1. Female metal catheter with built-in mirror for intermittent self catheterisation (Chas Thackray & Co Ltd.).

It is not uncommon for the patient to become disenchanted with clean self catheterisation but some patients manage to catheterise themselves successfully over many years without the urine ever becoming infected or any significant problems developing in the urethra. This is much more common in children and females than in the male. There are not many longterm hazards associated with clean intermittent self catheterisation but we have recently encountered one patient who has developed a squamous cell carcinoma on the back wall of the bladder – possibly due to the trauma caused by using a fairly rigid short catheter for self catheterisation. In addition to the commonly used PVC catheters there is also a female catheter with built-in mirror to facilitate self catheterisation (Fig. 6.1).

Sterile Intermittent Self Catheterisation

Many general practitioners are unhappy with the concept of clean intermittent self catheterisation and much prefer their patients to use sterile catheters. Many women themselves insist on sterile catheters being available and the development and marketing of the Swedish Lofric catheter (Astra Meditec) has been a significant advance. The Lofric catheter contains polyvinylpyrrolidone (PVP) which absorbs water by binding water molecules and sodium chloride (NaCl) giving the water saline properties. When the Lofric catheter has been immersed in water for 30 s, the water coating ensures that no friction will be produced during its passage through the urethra. This firmly-bound water coating comes into direct contact with the urethra and produces a protective layer which minimises friction. The passage of the catheter is almost a painless procedure and there is minimal discomfort with this variety of catheter as it does not require local anaesthesia, lubricant or gel for its use.

The catheter itself is made out of medical PVC which is non-toxic and pyrogen free. The tip of the catheter is rounded and the hydrophilic layer consists of a polymer containing PVP. The manufacturers of the Lofric catheter have now developed a Lofric Catheter Kit. This is a disposable urinary catheter with disposable collection bag which is made of medical PVC and can hold about 700 ml of urine. The appliance is supplied sterilised in its own individual wrapper which is peeled apart to allow the appliance to be removed. About 30 ml water is poured into the system, the catheter is passed into the bladder and urine drains directly into the collection bag. At the end of the procedure the catheter is returned to the bag, the long tube is tied off and the entire kit disposed of. This device is a neat, convenient, safe way of performing sterile self catheterisation.

Male Collection Devices and Drainage Bags

Some men complain of the loss of small quantities of urine intermittently and there is another group who dribble constantly and are very wet. The needs of the two groups are quite different and an attempt is made to clarify the wide variety of appliances and aids that are in common usage.

Intermittent Male Incontinence

Men may be incontinent after a prostatic resection and they usually complain of the loss of small amounts of urine. This type of incontinence may occur in the first few months following surgery and usually is self limiting. The loss of a few drops of urine may be sufficient to come through the outer clothing and leave a wet patch which is found to be embarrassing. These men otherwise pass their urine well and with good control. They are able to start the stream and feel satisfied that the bladder is empty but at some later stage a few drops of urine are lost. There are also patients who suffer from a urethral stricture who complain of a small loss of urine at the end of micturition irrespective of how long they wait for the dribbling to stop after shaking themselves. In these patients a column of urine is trapped between the sphincter mechanism and the stricture. When the penis is dependent urine trickles down the urethra under the influence of gravity and dampens the clothes. There is another small group of patients who have minor degrees of instability, whose bladders contract from time to time and jet out a small quantity of urine which again can be enough to show as a wet patch on their trousers.

Male Dribble Bags or Pouches

Those patients with intermittent dribbling can easily be fitted up with a dribble bag or pouch to prevent their clothes becoming dampened. The pouches are so constructed that they fit over the end of the penis and can be placed inside Jockey/Y-type underwear without causing a bulge. Some of them can be strapped to the penis and others secured by drawstrings. Most of the pouches have a waterproof exterior and contain an absorbable material inside to soak up the urine. For men who suffer from retraction of the penis, there is a drop shield variety which contains their scrotum and penis and is manufactured by LIC Ltd. There are not less than 10 manufacturers of such dribble bags and pouches in the United Kingdom but not all the products are available on prescription. One of the most effective dribble pouches is called the Dibbs

Male Drip Shield. The absorbing material is concentrated in the lower part of the pouch and so there is no unnecessary dissemination of urine. The pouches absorb up to 60 ml of urine and there is an overnight variety which holds 120 ml. The absorbent is cellulose fibres combined with super absorbents (see below) and the exterior has a polyethylene-coated microporous polyester non-woven fabric while the inner coating has a semi-permeable polypropylene non-woven fabric.

Some devices come fitted with a belt for security and others incorporate a diaphragm and belt (Ward Surgical Appliance Company Ltd., Surrey, England). The Aquadry Male Incontinence Pouch (CF Thackray Ltd., Leeds, England) incorporates a PVC bag with a drainage tube to which a collection bag can be fitted. The non-reusuable variety is the Alexa Dribble Bag which has a non-return valve (Henleys of Hornsey Ltd.). There is, in addition, a rubber sheath drip-catcher which is marketed by the Genito Urinary Manufacturing Company (London, England) and this comes with or without tape understraps.

Appliances for Constant Dribbling

Paul's Tubing (Penrose). The time-honoured conventional method of dealing with male urinary incontinence is to apply Paul's (Penrose) tubing over the penis and secure it by whatever system the nursing staff can dream up. The tubing is connected to a uribag which is attached to the patient's leg. This device remains in common use in hospitals for patients who are bed-ridden and who may be on the neurological (usually after a stroke), geriatric or urology wards. The main problem with the tubing is that because of its flimsy nature it may twist and become blocked. The urine then builds up in the tube between the end of the penis and the block and in time the Paul's tubing becomes disconnected. Repeated dislocation of the Paul's tubing may have a demoralising effect which results in the search for another system to deal with the incontinence. Sometimes difficulty is encountered in securing the Paul's tubing to the penis and to this end Velcro or tapes are utilised. Paul's tubing comes in two widths and connecting it to the uribag can cause even bigger problems than securing the tubing around the penis. The tubing has to be pleated to fit around the connector of the uribag and it is often difficult to make this junction leak-proof. The development of the condom urinal over recent years has rendered the Paul's tubing almost obsolete although it is still used for longterm bed-ridden patients in some institutions.

Penile Clamp. The penile incontinence clamp which is covered in latex rubber comes in four sizes – large, medium, small and infant. It has a sponge rubber insert and a spring ratchet fastening device. Patients usually acquire these clamps from retail outlets and use them indiscriminately without knowing the damage that they may cause. In people with sensory loss they can traumatise because the patients do not know how much pressure to apply to the urethra when closing it. There may well have been an indication for using these clamps in the past but it is now not acceptable to prescribe or advise a patient to try such a device for urinary incontinence without strict medical supervision.

Condom Urinals

Arguably the biggest advance in male collecting devices has been the development and perfection of the condom urinal. This device has gone a long way to displacing the older types of urinals although it is not possible to fit them to every penis. This may be because the penis may be considerably shrunken or shrivelled and in that situation a condom urinal may be difficult to keep securely in place. Some patients develop sensitivity to the condoms whilst others find the condom aesthetically unacceptable. When a condom urinal works well, it can be the most acceptable of all the urinals available. Many of the patients who use condoms do so only by day and are able to dispense with them at night. The advantage of this situation is that the penis is allowed at night to "recover" from the contact with material on the penile shaft. This intermittent use makes utilisation by day more acceptable with reduction in skin problems. There are 24 manufacturers listed in the United Kingdom's Department of Health tariff list and seven of these manufacturers market at least two distinct varieties. These 31 types are manufactured with or without adhesive strips and in sizes varying from small, medium and large to extra large. Many manufacturers market five sizes as opposed to four. This means that there are not less than 120 penile sheaths available for selection and such a variety has the effect of causing confusion when it comes to making a choice.

Superficially, the condom urinals made by different manufacturers may look quite similar but some of them have quite distinct and discrete differences which can confer an advantage. The condom urinals can be kept in place usually for several days before there is a need to change them. Most are kept in place by adhesive strips and others have rubber straps, buttons or Velcro to secure them. Some are self retaining such as the Aquadry penile sheath (CF Thackray Ltd.). This is an easily-applied adhesive-coated sheath and is simply rolled onto the skin of the penis and squeezed to the tissues. The adhesive coating holds the condom in place and it forms a water-tight seal. A uriseal liner (Simpla and CR Bard Ltd.) is made of hypoallergenic material which is sympathetic to the skin and is easily removed leaving no residue on the skin. CR Bard (Crawley, England) market Crixilene which expands and contracts with the wearer thereby eliminating penile constriction.

The condoms themselves are usually made of soft latex rubber and many of them have bulbous stems which minimise the possibility of urine back flowing or pooling in the condom. The outlets of the condoms are usually reinforced to prevent kinking. The InCare self adhesive incontinence sheath is designed to prevent soreness and laceration caused by back flow of urine along the penile shaft. It comes with a unique disposable plastic collar with special finger cuts which allow correct positioning and easy application. It has a one-way flap which prevents back flow of urine and keeps the penile shaft dry and also has the advantage of preserving the integrity of the adhesive. The wide bore outlet has a double row of convolutions allowing a maximum flow rate of urine and this also prevents kinking and twisting. An innovation is the Bard Uriplan self sealing penile sheath (Fig. 6.2a,b). This comes with its own applicator which is fitted over the end of the glans penis; the glans is grasped between the windows in the applicator and the protective strip of adhesive is removed from the open end of the applicator. The applicator is pushed towards the base of the penis whilst drawing the tip of the penis towards the closed end of the applicator.

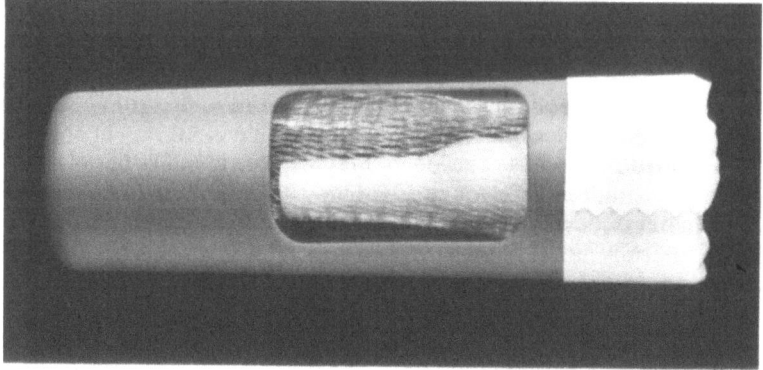

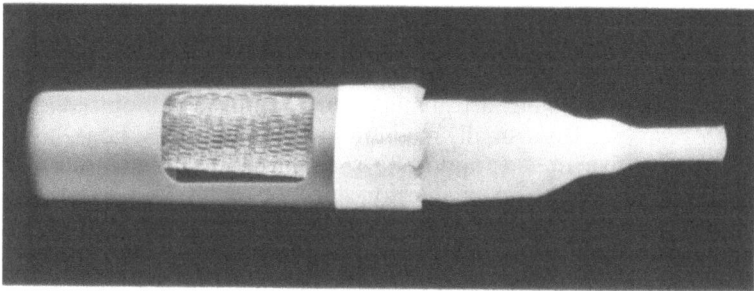

Fig. 6.2. **a** Bard Uriplan self-sealing penile sheath within applicator (CR Bard Ltd.). **b** Bard Uriplan self-sealing penile sheath withdrawn from its applicator.

The applicator is removed and the sheath is pressed gently around the penis to activate the adhesive. This device can easily be applied by patients with dexterity problems.

It is very difficult to make an assessment of the relative merits of the different types of penile sheaths. At the moment there are no British Standards for penile sheaths nor indeed for the material which goes into them. Latex is the commonest material used, but it can be an irritant to the skin. Patients with increased sensitivity find the correct application of a penile sheath can be quite critical and problems arise from applying the sheath too tightly. The Bard sheath-applicator may go some way to overcoming the difficulties of applying the condom.

Drainage Bags

Urine collection bags are subdivided into body-worn bags and those larger bags for night-time use. The drainage bag described below can either be attached to a urethral catheter, a condom urinal as described in the section above, or the other type of body-worn urinals described below. Most of the body-worn bags are made of plastic but some patients have a preference for rubber bags (kipper). Of the 24 manufacturers who produce plastic leg bags, seven make rubber bags in addition. Plastic bags can be used for about 5–7 days on average and rubber bags, if properly cared for, will last for between 4 and 6 months. The night bags are usually of plastic and are designed to hold about 2 l and some, but not all, have a drainage outlet and are equipped with non-return and anti-reflux valves. One of the problems is that there are no British Standards for these appliances.

The body-worn bags usually come in volumes of 350, 500 and 750 ml and the bags are attached to the thigh, knee or leg. They can be used with equal facility by males or females. The bags are fixed to the limb by latex straps, foam straps, fabric tapes or Velcro fasteners but the latter damage ladies' stocking or tights. The length of inlet tube will vary according to the intended position for wearing the bag and the height of the patient. The shortest inlets are about 5 cm in length and are suitable for thigh wear. A medium length is 10 cm for knee wear and longer inlets are for calf wear. The outlet tap is either a removable rubber cap or a removable rigid spigot. Other varieties of outlet include a twist-and-pull valve, a screw-off cap and a push-pull valve which lies horizontally. Extension tubing connects the urinal with the bag and comes in two sizes, short and long. In practice, a 750-ml bag has little appeal because it becomes too heavy in use. It has the advantage that it can be used as a night bag simply by detaching it from the leg and placing it on the mattress to one side of the body or alternatively between the patient's legs.

The rubber kipper bag has been available for many years and is still used by some male patients as a body bag in preference to plastic bags because it can easily be attached to some of the harness urinals described below. Night bags usually hold 2 l of urine. Some, but not all, have an outlet tap, and bedside hangers are available from which the night drainage bags may be suspended. Night-bag connectors are made by several manufacturers to facilitate the attachment of the night drainage bag to either the urethral catheter or urinal.

Suspensory Systems for Drainage Bags

Bag slippage is a problem for many patients, particularly if they are mobile, and some patients have a preference for a suspensory system which is designed to take the weight of a filled bag. Most of the bags used with this type of drainage system are of the plastic disposable variety but the suspensory system itself is designed to last very much longer. The variety favoured by male patients is the Shepheard Sporran Belt (EMS Medical Ltd.). There are only three other manufacturers of suspensory systems. They include the Urisac Portabag Belt (Seaton Products Ltd.), the Legbag Holster which comes in three sizes (HG Wallace Ltd.) and the Portabelt (Warne Franklin Medical Products). For female use, Simpla market the Barnstable Pattern Legbelt Holster. This is a leg-bag garment made from hard-wearing polyester and cotton and comes with an adjustable nylon belt with Velcro fastenings. The holster is worn on the outside of the hip and thigh and in addition to being suspended by a nylon belt, it is secured around the thigh by soft jersey fabric. This unobtrusive garment is shrink-resistant. A pouch is fitted on the outside of the holster to accommodate the drainage bag. The outlet of the bag projects through an aperture at the bottom of the pouch and such a bag can be emptied without the need to remove the bag from its pouch. In practice these leg-bag holsters are used for females with permanent indwelling catheters.

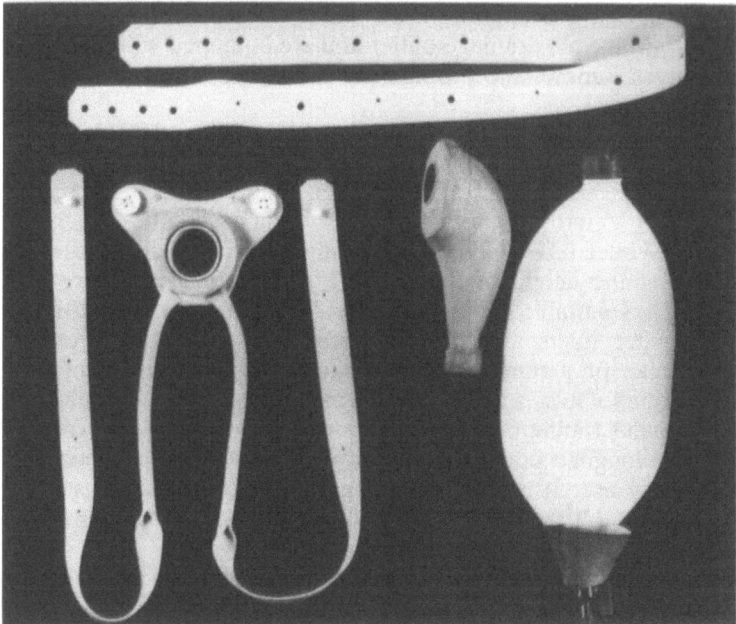

Fig. 6.3. Male pubic pressure urinal showing component parts (Downs Surgical Ltd.).

Male Body-worn Urinal Systems

The drug tariff supplement published by the Department of Health devotes 21 pages to itemising the products of 15 manufacturers of urinal systems. In addition to this published list, there are many other urine-collecting devices which are not available on prescription but are produced by other manufacturers. It is, therefore, extremely difficult to ascertain which particular urinal devices are the most effective.

Pubic Pressure Device. Fig. 6.3 illustrates an example of a pubic pressure device (Downs Surgical Ltd., Leeds, England). It consists of a rubber pubic plate which contains a central hole through which the penis is fitted. The plate is held close to the body by a waistband and leg understraps which have to be fitted tightly. A rubber cone is fitted over the flange of the pubic plate and the penis hangs down inside this cone. The white rubber bag (hot-water-bottle shaped) is attached to the cone and there is a tap at the bottom for the release of urine. Alternatively, a length of rubber tubing can be inserted between the cone and the bag and in that situation the bag is then strapped to the thigh with the rubber straps provided. This particular device is widely in use; it has been on the market for many years and is particularly suitable for men with a retractile penis or who are deemed not suitable to use a condom urinal. Fig. 6.4 shows the completely assembled appliance. The white bag is of the kipper variety and is made by more than one manufacturer. These kipper bags can be either attached to the leg or hang free inside the patient's street clothing because they are suspended by the harness.

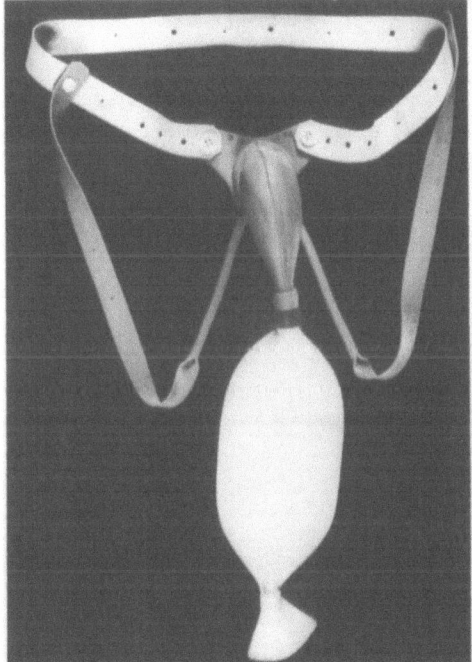

Fig. 6.4. Male pubic pressure urinal assembled.

Diaphragm Type Device. The diaphragm type device is shown in Fig. 6.5. It is similar to the pubic pressure urinals except that it is not held so tightly to the pubis. The penis hangs through the diaphragm which has a feathered arrangement for a comfortable fit. A condom urinal can than be applied over the penis and attached to a uribag which is secured to the leg.

Sheath Type Device. Sheath type devices are of two types. The Stoke Mandeville variety is shown in Fig. 6.6; it has been available for about 30 years and formerly a standard contraceptive condom was used as the sheath. To assemble the parts, a 2-mm hole has to be cut at the end of the condom which is then stretched over a nylon stud so that the rim of the stud protrudes to allow the stud and the sheath to be inserted into the rubber tube. Some dexterity is required to assemble this part of the appliance. The tube is then connected to the kipper bag which is applied to the leg and the bag is given extra support by a fabric strap which is attached to the waistband. This device is commonly used and has stood the test of time. Compared to the original device of 30 years ago the present appliance has been much improved. Fig. 6.7 shows the assembled device which is manufactured by the GU Manufacturing Company Limited.

Fig. 6.8 shows another type of sheath device. Here a corrugated rubber sheath is fitted over the penis, sometimes with an internal separate sheath. It is held to the body by means of a waistband and, ordinarily, leg straps are not used. The detachable corrugated sheath fits inside the cone which in turn is attached to a collection device. In the example shown there are two collecting chambers, both of which can be attached by leg straps to the thigh.

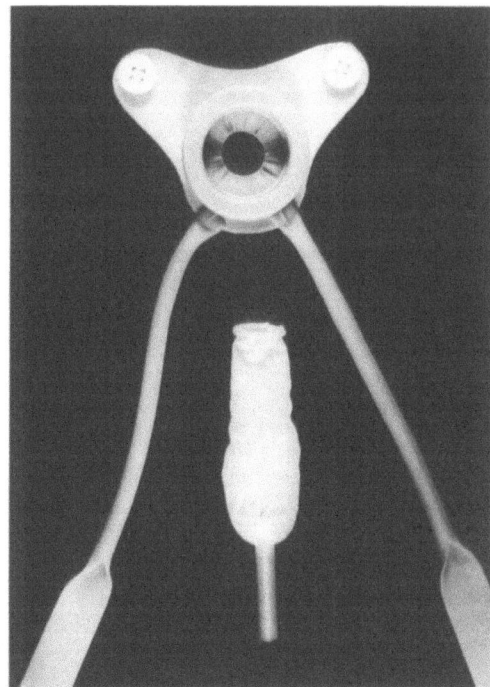

Fig. 6.5. Diaphragm-type device with condom urinal shown separately.

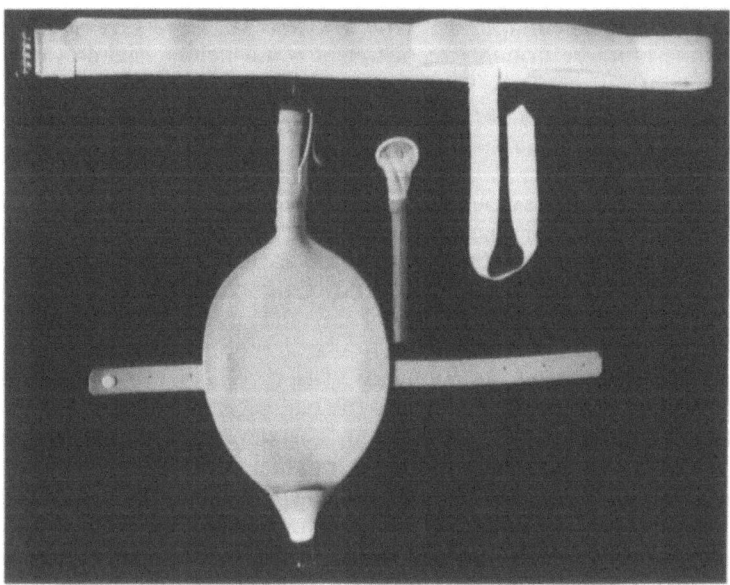

Fig. 6.6. Stoke Mandeville sheath type device showing component parts (GU Manufacturing Co. Ltd.).

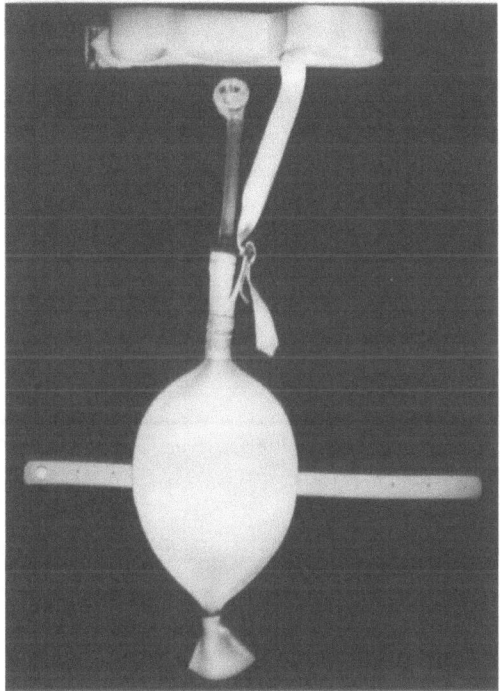

Fig. 6.7. Stoke Mandeville sheath type device assembled.

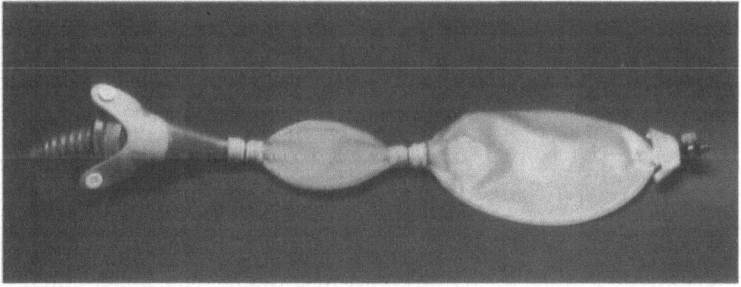

Fig. 6.8. Male urine collecting device with corrugated rubber sheath which fits over the penis, and has two collecting chambers (Leyland Medical Ltd.).

Penis and Scrotal Type. For those men who are unable to keep on a sheath because of penile retraction there is an appliance available whereby the penis and scrotum fit inside a rubber cone supported by waist and leg understraps and attached to a kipper collection bag.

Drip Type Urinal. The drip type urinal is an extra large sheath on a diaphragm type urinal. There is no drainage bag except as an optional extra. The small amount of urine which collects within the sheath can be emptied by a screw cap at the distal end. These urinals collect between 50 and 100 ml of urine and are

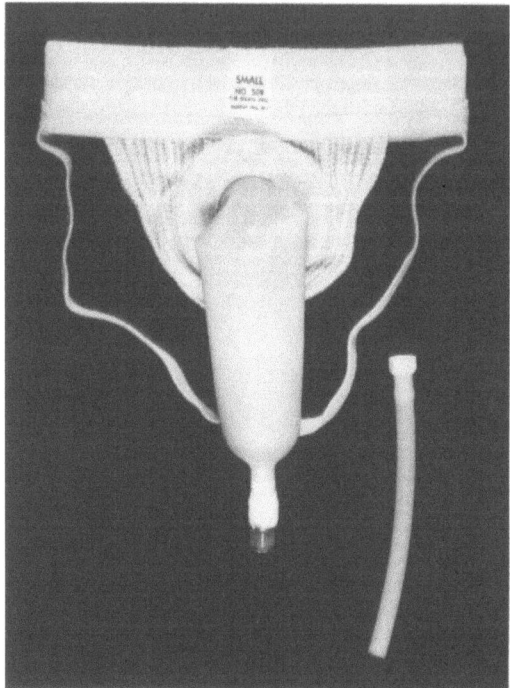

Fig. 6.9. Uriplan and Maguire drip type urinal (CR Bard Ltd.).

suitable for men with post-micturition dribbling or mild dirbbling incontinence. At night-time a collection bag can be attached to the device. An example is shown in Fig. 6.9 which is similar to an athletic support, the pouch of which acts as a support and attachment for the urinal device.

Body-worn Garment Incorporating Urinal. Fig. 6.10 shows the Payne Mark 8 Male Incontinence Appliance. This consists of plasticated underpants with an aperture into which a rubber flange is fitted. A plastic collection bag is fitted over the flange. The collecting devices come in varying sizes, all of which have an outlet at the end of the bag so that it can be hung free inside the street clothing or, alternatively, attached by straps to the thigh. The penis emerges through the garment aperture and flange before hanging inside the inner part of the collecting bag, which also acts as a non-return valve. Fig. 6.11 shows the assembled appliance. It is particularly applicable for a patient with a retracted penis and is also useful for a very large person, particularly when chairbound. There is no need for understraps, which might cause pressure sores in somebody who is not mobile. The body-worn garment is also useful for those people who have difficulty with gait or hip problems. Such a person might have difficulty in keeping a conventional harness in place. Fig. 6.12 shows a similar device which is the Payne Mark 7 appliance. This differs from the Mark 8 in that there is a reinforced cone top available in various sizes, which can be fitted to either a rubber bag or a semi-disposable plastic bag. The flange of the Mark 7 has a wing device for security and this fits inside the garment.

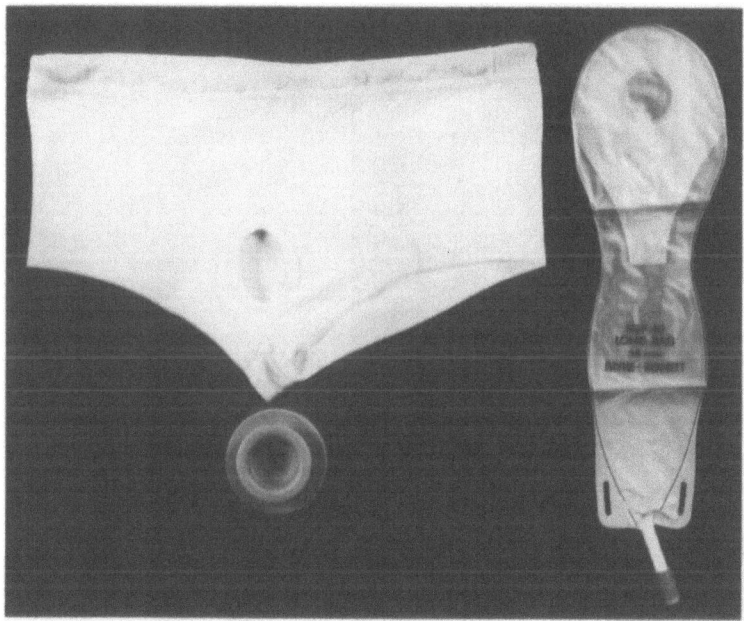

Fig. 6.10. Body-worn garment incorporating urinal showing component parts of the Payne Mark 8 Male Incontinence Appliance.

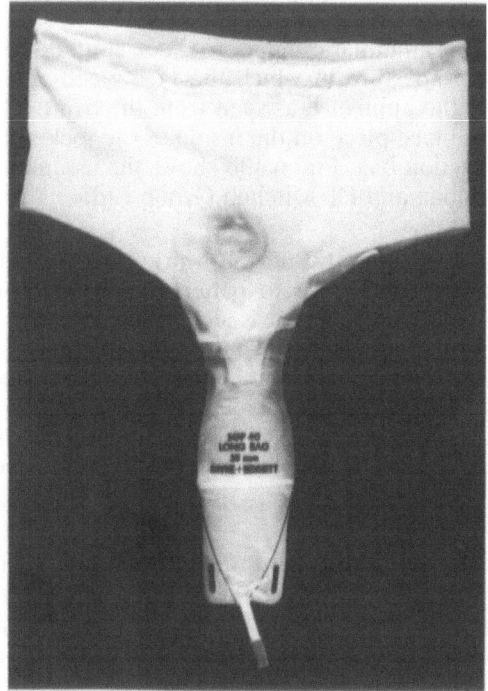

Fig. 6.11. Payne Mark 8 Male Incontinence Appliance assembled.

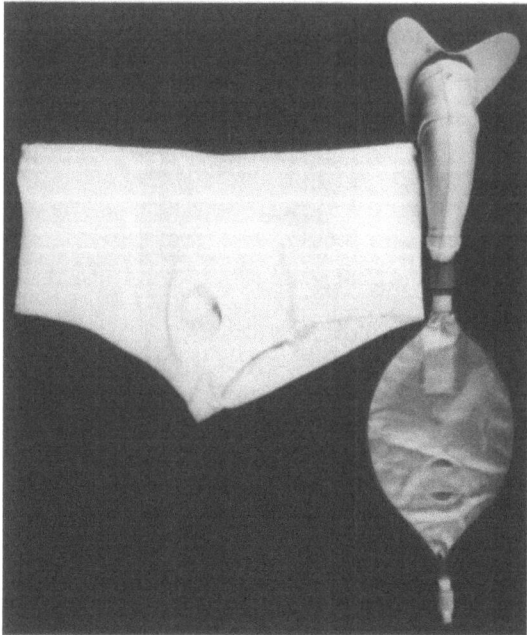

Fig. 6.12. The Payne Mark 7 Male Incontinence Appliance showing reinforced cone top which is available in various sizes.

Jock Strap Appliance. Fig. 6.13a shows an athletic support or jock strap device. The pouch on the jock strap has an aperture in which the face piece of the appliance is fitted. The figure shows the appliance as seen from the front. The coned rubber fitting is attached to the face piece on the inside of the jock strap and this in turn is attached to a collection bag. Fig. 6.13b shows the assembled device which is manufactured by Kinpax and FT Mitchell Group Ltd.

Lightweight Plastic Appliance. Fig. 6.14 shows the Payne Mark 4 Lightweight Plastic Appliance, which is particularly applicable to patients suffering from short-term incontinence who are allergic to rubber. It is simple to apply and is ideal for patients who only need to use an appliance to go out in public. It consists of a material face piece and belt loops, foam pad and plastic bags. A foam leg-strap attaches the bag to the thigh. The aperture in the material face piece comes in two sizes and a measurement card is available with the appliance. This material face piece is also available with a scrotal support as an optional extra.

Child-sized Male Urinals. Child-sized male urinals tend to be of rubber and are manufactured by Downs Surgical Limited. There is the Chailey child-sized urinal which is a rubber one-piece with curved top and integral sheath. It has understraps, rubber belt and standard child-sized rubber bag. There is also the Mini-Mitcham urinal which has a Downs pubic pressure flange to which the Mini-Mitcham bag is attached. This bag is disposable.

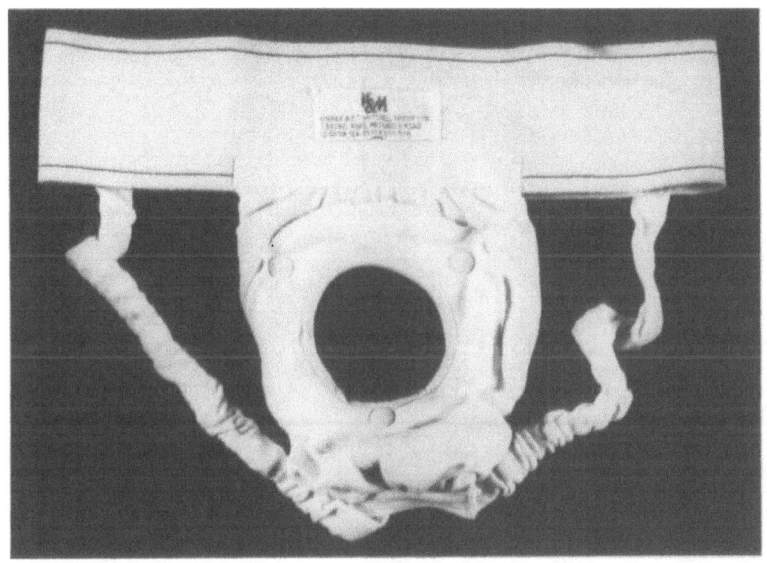

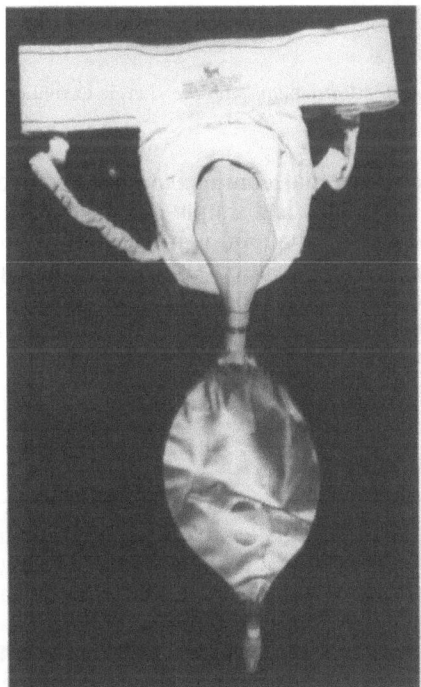

Fig. 6.13. **a** A jockstrap appliance (Kinpax and FT Mitchell Group Ltd.). **b** A jockstrap appliance assembled showing coned rubber fitting and connection bag (Kinpax and FT Mitchell Group Ltd.).

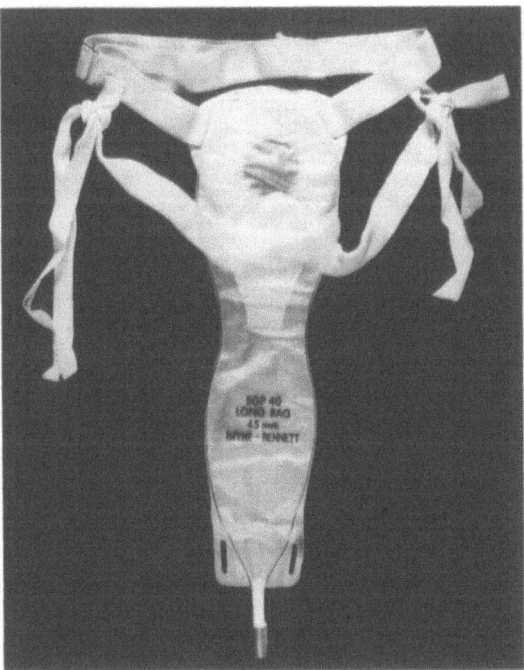

Fig. 6.14. Lightweight plastic appliance, Payne Mark 4 for patients who are allergic to rubber.

Male Adult Continence Cuff. Recently an external continence cuff has been marketed which is illustrated in Fig. 6.15a,b. This is a simple cuff fastened by Velcro which contains an inflatable balloon. The balloon is inflated by means of a syringe which the patient can use himself to occlude the urethra. The cuff is placed at the peno-scrotal junction and would seem to be a useful adjunct in the continence equipment field although it will probably be effective only in people with mild incontinence.

Female Collecting Devices

The female anatomy is not conducive to the application of body-worn collecting devices. Although there have been many attempts at inventing, developing and perfecting devices for collecting leaked urine in the female, none of them are universally successful. The products have either not been accepted by the wearer or have given rise to unexpected problems or failed to correct the problems that have been anticipated. Some recent advances have shown the way ahead and may, in time, lead to an acceptable principle which, combined with developments in the plastics industry, might allow the acceptance of a satisfactory female collecting device.

There are many appliances on the market and some female patients have found a device which they find acceptable, even if it has to be modified for their own particular requirements. In general, women prefer a pants-and-pad arrangement to a collecting device, which is in contrast to their male counter-

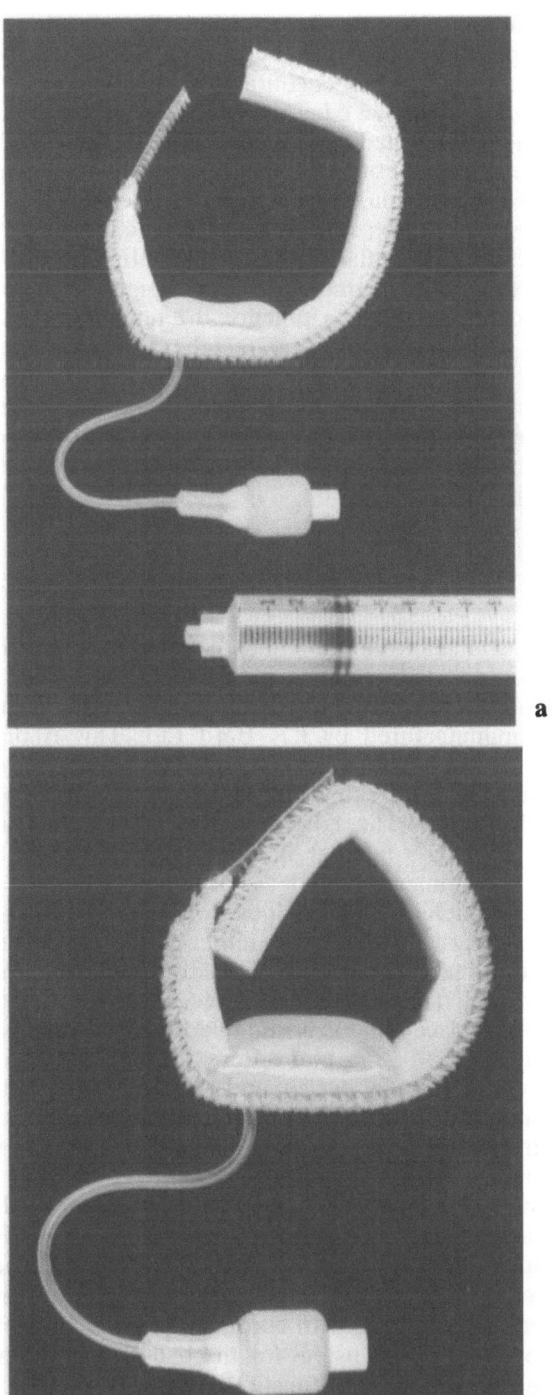

Fig. 6.15a,b. Cook Continence Cuff before and after inflation.

parts who prefer a collecting urinal. Perhaps the female familiarity with the use of sanitary towels predisposes them to accept pants and pads whereas in the male familiarity with the contraceptive sheath encourages them to prefer the condom urinal. Twenty years ago it would have been true to say that there was no female collecting device available that had been marketed to any extent. In the early 1970s the Edwards Female Incontinence Device was produced. This device, which was placed partly in the vagina, depended for its effectiveness on the application of upward pressure on the urethro-vesical junction thereby occluding the urethra. It was designed essentially for stress incontinence but in practice was tried for both stress and urge incontinence. The design was simple and in theory should have worked, although in practice the tendency of the upward pressure on the vaginal mucosa gave rise to mucosal erosions and even ulceration, thereby precluding universal acceptance and usage. There have been other devices, both before and since the development of the Edwards appliance, which have depended upon the occlusion of the urethra by some form of vaginal tamponade but unfortunately these devices have been no more successful and have been abandoned.

Female Body-worn Urinals

There are at least four devices available, none of which compress the urethra or act as a tamponade in the vagina. The principle is that the leaked urine is collected into a device which transfers the urine to a collection bag. One of the oldest on the market is that manufactured by CR Bard Ltd. This is only applicable for day-time use and is available in one adult size. It is made of latex and consists of a central banana-shaped catheter with an opening on its upper surface which is applied to the vulva. The edges of the catheter opening incorporate an inflatable cushion which is inflated by a bulb inflator, similar to that used for inflating a sphygmomanometer. The device is applied to the body by means of a band from the catheter to which loops on a waist belt are attached. The inflatable bulb is worn by the body, either inside or outside underwear. The collection device is further secured by tie straps and the urine drains from the catheter into a kipper leg bag which is secured to the leg by straps. This device can easily be displaced and is unsuitable for night-time use. The Kinpex and FT Mitchell Group have a range of different devices which are similar in concept but slightly different in design and have tie straps and understraps and sponge rims in the night model. These pressure applicators are attached to light-weight bags and fittings which are available in three sizes to fit children, adolescents and adults.

In Care Medical Products have developed a female urinary collector in the from of a pouch made from barrier film which acts as a urinary conduit in the non-ambulant patient. It is held in place by an anatomically shaped skin barrier which protects the skin and holds the collecting device in place. There is one size but the precut skin barrier can be enlarged to accommodate variations in anatomy. This device may prove to be very useful for the bed-ridden patient and its use may help to reduce the laundry bill of institutions.

The most significant advance in female external urinary drainage systems has come from Holland. Mandhy Products BV market a system which depends on some of the principles already described but has an innovative design which might prove to be more acceptable than anything hitherto manufactured. This female external urinary drainage unit consists of a panty, external catheter, absorbent pad insert, drainage tube and drainage bag. It is a compact, easy-to-fit and easy-to-wear device. The principle depends on removing the urine from the body, as in the Bard device, but differs from the latter in that a sanitary napkin is inserted into the catheter device. The innovation provides more protection, security and comfort than the simple catheter collecting device. The disposable panties are manufactured in varying sizes. The waist band has an adjustable Velcro closure that requires minimal dexterity for use. There is a soft, flexible external catheter which is positioned over the vulval area like a sanitary towel and is attached to the front and the back of the panty by means of adjustable button holes. There is a soft absorbent insert pad, very similar to a sanitary towel, which is placed in the catheter. The surface of the pad is covered with a stay-dry material which minimises skin irritation. The pad is made of highly absorbent cellulose filling that directs the flow of urine away from the body and into the drainage tube attached to the flexible external catheter. The drainage tube is made of a corrugated design which allows the uninterrupted flow of urine, regardless of the wearer's position. A collection bag is attached to the thigh with conventional leg straps. The device can be used by day or by night and gives a high level of protection and comfort. It also allows for freedom of movement and the panty can be replaced by a more conventional panty if required. This device may well become the yardstick by which further developments are judged.

Protective Clothing

There can hardly be an area in health care more in need of standardisation than the field of urinary incontinence particularly with regard to underpads and body-worn pads. In recent years there has been a mushroom-like explosion in the number, variety, quality, effectiveness and also unsuitability of pads for the incontinent. The British Standards Institute is attempting to lay down basic recommendations and guidelines for the minimum acceptable rate of absorbency in the body-worn pads. Unfortunately there is no uniformity as to what tests should be applied to absorbency and a number of different countries, appliance firms and purchasers have their own tests which they apply to assess the pad in terms of "value for money".

Mattress and Bedding Protection

Very often mattress protection is used simply as a precautionary measure when there is the possibility of urinary or faecal incontinence. In other situations, it is used because it is known that there will be soiling and many of the people who require mattress and bedding protection are not ambulant and may be confined to their beds for large parts of the day and all night. Consequently there is a range of products depending on the anticipated amount of soiling that might take place. These products are divided into those for domestic and those for institutional use. The former are of the light-weight short-term variety and sometimes the middle-weight when longer term use is required for people who do not sleep properly but who move around and are restless. In institutional use, the middle-weight range can be quite useful but a heavy-duty mattress cover is certainly required for double incontinence, particularly in people who are very restless at night.

A mattress protector fitted completely over the mattress has fitted ends which prevent slipping. It is waterproofed and designed to cover and protect the top and sides of the mattress. The waterproofing itself can cause a certain amount of discomfort to the patient. Fitted covers are preferable to loose sheeting where full-length covering of the mattress is essential. It is necessary to be able to launder these protective coverings, otherwise the odour of the excreta will become impregnated in the non-disposable mattress protector. A mattress cover envelopes the mattress and usually contains a zip, Velcro fastening or studs to secure it in place. This has the advantage that the cover is turned with the mattress and so one surface is not constantly exposed to soiling and the associated odour. In addition there are mattress sheets or draw sheets, duvet and pillow covers which can be hand or machine washed. Most of the protectors and the sheets can be either cleaned or cleansed with a damp cloth and a mild detergent to which disinfectant solution is added.

Pads for Beds and Chairs

Disposable underpads for bed or chair use constitute the largest single item purchased by the NHS in the United Kingdom for the management of incontinence. These underpads are designed to be placed underneath the patient and do not cover the whole of the mattress but merely an area which in size represents the part of the body encompassed by the lumbar area, buttocks, perineum and upper thighs. They are not designed for use with protective pants, because they are ineffective when used in such a way. The pads are usually made from cellulose wadding which is sealed on both sides with a waterproof backing. As these pads are designed for use without protective body-worn pants, great care must be taken of the patient's skin. The patient's hygiene is important and the skin must be washed and dried before placing an incontinence pad in position.

The disposal of these pads has not been a great problem – the soiled pad must be placed directly into a suitable container for disposal. A new consultation document from the Department of the Environment recommends a change in the disposal practice of incontinence pads. Previously they were disposed of in the domestic garbage can and in institutions are frequently incinerated. There is now a feeling that clinical waste should be regarded as industrial waste as applied under Part 1 of the Control of Pollution Act 1974 and legislation may be introduced to ensure that disposable underpads will have to be incinerated at municipal sites. Disposable pads have the major share of the market but it may be that the new legislation may force manufacturers, carers and users to move towards the reusable or non-disposable pads. This will put a greater emphasis on the laundry service and washing-machine facilities but may be more cost-effective than using the disposable pads, especially if they have to be packaged for incineration at a municipal site.

Reusable Pads

The Kylie Absorbent Bed Sheet probably provides a universally acceptable reusable pad. The pad separates the patient from the urine by means of a hydrophobic upper layer and any urine voided is absorbed by the underlayer. This allows a certain amount of comfort and the sheet is guaranteed for about 200 washes. The new Terrymac by Wetsafe (Neptumer Ltd.) drawsheet is on trial by the Department of Health and may provide a break-through in this area because it has a highly durable waterproof backing, can be boiled, machine washed and even sterilised. The fabric is stretchable, highly durable, can be washed at high temperatures and is shrink-resistant. It has good thermal properties and optimum water absorption.

Henleys Medical Supplies market Alegra Reusable Underpads which can withstand at least 300 commercial launderings. They are made from synthetic fabrics and the quilted brushed nylon surface of the pad provides comfort and a feeling of warmth while airflow helps to keep the patient cool. Polyester padding protects delicate skin and can be used over pressure points. The waterproof backing is bonded to a non-woven material which is non-slip.

Body-worn Pants and Pads

Arguably the most popular system for containing urinary, faecal or both types of incontinence is the use of body pants and pads. There are literally hundreds of different types of pads available but the pants and pads should be personally fitted and tailored to meet the individual need. Individual patients' requirements may vary. Some prefer to have a high absorbency pad which may or may not be comfortable and others attach more importance to the design factor. Whichever type is chosen the pad should be discreet and easy to use. Because there is such a plethora of available pads the advice of a Nurse Continence Advisor should be sought in order to give the patients the best possible advice. In assessing the best system it is very important to identify the type and degree of incontinence, the patient's physical ability and dexterity as well as their mental function.

Pants

1. Traditional plastic or rubber pants may be bought in many stores without any reference to the medical or nursing professions. This has been the time-honoured way in which patients seek succour for their incontinence and usually do so while trying to hide their problem from relatives and friends. These pants are worn outside the normal underwear and some people do not use an incontinence pad inside their own underwear or between the underwear and the rubber or plastic pants. This really is the "do-it-yourself" way of dealing with incontinence without seeking medical advice and one never ceases to be amazed by the number of people who turn up in clinics with such a device without ever having spoken to their own medical advisor about their problem.

2. The marsupial pouch has gained universal acceptance over the last decade or more. The Kanga pant-and-pad system has been the most popular and has

brought enormous comfort and relief to many sufferers. This pant has a waterproof pouch into which the pad is inserted. The fabric of the crotch (the angle formed by the legs where they join the human trunk) is a one-way polyester fabric which allows urine to pass through into the pad while keeping the skin of the genital area dry. This pad-and-pant system is basically for urinary incontinence and is not suitable for faecal and urinary incontinence in the same patient. The problem with the pad is that a certain amount of dexterity is required in order to insert and remove it. The Kanga pant can be worn by both male and female because the marsupial pouch is externally placed. However, it is possible to have the pouch internally placed. In the external marsupial pouch, there is a slight difference between the male and female variety in that there is a fly or overlapping opening in the male design.

3. A variation on the marsupial pouch is the drop-front pant. This pouch can be levered away from the underpant and when the pad has been changed the drop-front part is secured to the pant by Velcro or studs. Fastening can take place either at the front or the side of the pant. This front pant is in many ways probably easier to use by people with reduced dexterity.

4. The stretch pant is simply used to secure a pad. These pants are made by many companies by the Tenasystem marketed by Molnlycke (Sweden), and are, because of their effectiveness, proving popular. With stretch pants, a plastic backing pad must be used.

5. There is a plastic bikini tie pant which is self-explanatory.

6. The disposable pant pad. The Comfie Protector Pants (Vernon–Carus, Preston, England) can be used for either male or female, ambulant or bed fast patients. These are fully disposable and incorporate an absorbable integral pad and they are available in a wide range of sizes for children and adults. The Comfie range includes reusable regular stretch pants and short-life, lightweight pants, and the Comfie disposable incontinence garment which is designed for the semi-ambulant or bed-fast patient is suitable for doubly incontinent patients.

7. Disposable diaper or nappy. This may be trapezium-shaped and may contain an integral pad. The narrow part of the diaper is placed in the crotch and secured in the front of the body by wrapping the tie pieces in front of it which are secured by adhesive built into the fabric. Proctor and Gamble manufacture the Attends product. This consists of an absorbent, disposable brief and it is of considerable value to wheelchair-bound and bed-fast patients. Its main features are its high absorbency in the crotch area and the fact that it has a built-in wetness indicator which changes to blue indicating the level of wetness. This prevents the Attends from being worn too long and facilitates skin protection. It is a valuable adjunct for people who are skin sensitive in the perineal and pelvic area and are unable to feel wetness.

Apart from those identified as disposable, nearly all the pants can be machine or hand washed. They are made of a variety of fabrics including plastic, nylon, PVC and polyester.

Body-worn Pads

It is estimated that NHS contracts for body-worn pads amount to £17–20 million per annum. This does not take into account the body-worn pads that are sold over the counter or ordered through mail order firms by incontinent patients. There is an enormous market for such products, which seems to be increasing all the time. The purchaser is bedevilled by not knowing whether he or she is getting value for money because of the lack of standardisation and guidelines about what the products should be able to achieve.

Pad Types

1. Poly Inserts amount to 15% of the market and are used for the marsupial pouch type of plastic pants. They come in three sizes, small (20–25 g), medium (30–35 g) and large (40–45 g). They are marketed by, amongst others, Contenter Surgical Company Ltd. (Contenter Liners), Ganmill (Unitex Pads), Kanga Hospital Products (Kanga Pads) and International Disposables Incorporation UK Ltd (Urocare IDC Pad). The Contenter Liners are washable, the others are not.

2. Poly-backed Rectangular Inserts account for 18% of the market and are used with stretch pants. They have the facility of self-adhesive backing strips enabling them to be used with the user's own underwear or alternatively inside stretch pants. They come in three sizes, small (20 g), medium (45 g) and large (60 g). These are marketed by Ancilla (UK) Limited, and there are Molnlycke Products, IDC (Urocare polythene-backed pad), Smith and Nephew (Dandeliners) and Vernon-Carus Comfiepad, amongst others.

3. Shaped (Anatomique) pads were designed to cope with both faecal and urinary incontinence and they can be used with stretch pants. The pad weights vary from 60 to 135 g and they are marketed by Ancilla (Molnlycke), IDC (Celatose) and Smith and Nephew (Newcastle, England).

4. Wing Fold pads are similar in weight to the shaped (Anatomique) pads. They are marketed by Kanga and Robinsons of Chesterfield. The shaped and wing fold variety account together for 30% of the market.

5. Adult All-in-One pads account for 38% of the market. It is surprising to realise that this variety heads the list, particularly as this type of device is akin to putting someone in a large nappy with resulting lack of self respect. The all-in-one product is secured by sticking tapes. It has the advantage of being used without a garment for easier nurse management. These products are supplied by Ancilla (Molnlycke), IDC, Peaudouce (Slipad), Proctor and Gamble (Attends) and Vernon-Carus (Comfie-Disposable Incontinence Garment).

Pad Systems – Disposable

There are basically two systems for disposable pads. In the first variety the pad is kept away from direct contact with the skin as with the pouch type pants of Contenter, Kanga and Urocare. All the pads are held in a pouch with a polyester type fabric protecting the user's genitals and surrounding skin.

The second type of pad system is the kind kept close to the user's skin and held in place by stretch pants, plastic pants or in the case of the adult, an all-in-one by reusable tapes at the side.

Pad Systems – Reusable

Ganmill have developed a Butterfly Pad which is the first reusable shaped incontinence pad. It is designed so that it can be used by women or men. It can be hand or machine washed and can be used for diurnal or nocturnal incontinence. It comes in four sizes and is specially formulated with a waterproof backing which does not crinkle. The pads are made of pure cotton for maximum comfort and their asymmetrical design makes them suitable for men and women. The pads are silent in use and thereby carry a high discretion index. They can be used with stretch pants or normal underwear. Because they are reusable they should be cost effective. They need to be adequately presoaked before being washed and do not need high temperatures. They can be drip dried, tumble dried or spun. They must not be used with bleach or sterilising solutions as the waterproof liner can be affected by these chemicals.

Pad Contents and Absorbency

The standard pad consists of a plastic backing, an absorbent and a cover stock. Irrespective of the system in use the pads are made from tissue, pulp and non-woven fabric except for the reusable ones. Most pads are disposable. The plastic backing usually encroaches on the sides of the pad so as to minimise leaking. The cover stock is of viscous or polypropylene but there is no general agreement as to which fabric makes the better cover stock. The absorbent is either 100% chemical or chemical thermo-mechanical pulp (CTMP) or a combination of these. In essence the chemical absorbs quicker but CTMP absorbs more urine per gram of pulp. Some pulp suppliers are now starting to offer reels composed of a mixed chemical and CTMP pulp usually with a ratio of 80% cellulose to 20% chemical.

Pad absorbency is the amount of water that 1 g of pulp absorbs and in general this should be at least 10 ml of urine. The key for absorption is the rectangle of pulp in the centre of the pad and this is irrespective of whether the pad is rectangular or all-in-one. This rectangular part takes the flow of urine and then disperses it throughout the pad. If this dispersal does not take place, the pad may be ineffective although it may be heavy in total overall weight. Testing absorbency is carried out by all manufacturers but there is, as yet, no test that is universally accepted. This means that comparing the effectiveness of pads can be a futile exercise and a standard test ought to be applied to all pads.

Pad Design

Pad design and production is limited by the machine capabilities and the machines used in production may cost from £350 000 to £750 000. A manufacturer will need some sort of assurance that the pad will find a market to justify his investment in the machinery. There is clearly reluctance to take risks in machine purchase and this means that in practice many of the pads on the market are copies of other manufacturers' products. There is, therefore, not too much individuality in the design of pads. Another difficulty is that machines cannot be modified to take account of new ideas and research developments and innovations may not be so attractive because of the risk factor in designing a new machine, especially as the profit margin on pads is quite small.

Super Absorbents

Super absorbents are used world-wide for baby diapers, the Japanese leading the way in this respect. Super absorbents are up to ten times more absorbent than fluff pulp when used with water, but their absorbency performance is drastically reduced when used with urine. Super absorbents have been tried over the years with some adult products but they cost between seven and ten times more than the equivalent pulp weight. The wearers complain that when the super absorbent is wet and the granules have expanded, it is like sitting on a cold jelly or carrying one between their legs. There is also a design difficulty in finding the best place to put the granules in the pad for maximum performance. It is possible for the granules to form a block on expansion and thereby not allow urine to pass through to other absorbent areas in the pad. The balance between super absorbent and pulp is also critical: if the pad has too little pulp the integrity can be affected with the result that it may fall apart in use.

However, there seems to be little doubt that the future development of incontinence pads will be with the use of super absorbents. In time, with the introduction of more products and higher sales, the unit cost of super absorbents should reduce.

IPS Hospital Services have introduced their Super Strola incontinent pad which is made with a super absorbent polymer core with a capacity superior to fluff pulp. The absorbent core is ensured by a network of interlocking thermoplastic fibres which eliminate its breakup. The pads are worn with stretch pants or conventional underwear and there is an adhesive strip to keep the pad in place. The Conveen pad, which is marketed by Coloplast Ltd., is also available in high-street outlets and is used for mild incontinence in females.

Stress incontinence pads are thin and discreet and are quite attractive to women because they do not distort the contour of the figure and give high absorbency in addition to comfort. Despite their higher cost it is distinctly possible that in time, patient preference will determine what is demanded in the market.

Most manufacturers are carrying out trials; research with super absorbent products and super absorbent polymers is now producing better results with urine and having a "drier" feel, so the user is not so aware of the wet jelly effect.

Pad Performance

As yet there are no standards for pad performance laid down by the British Standards Institute or equivalent European bodies. This means that pads are changed at the whim of the user and not necessarily in relation to how much urine has been absorbed. This makes assessment of absorbency in field trials very difficult because individual preference, standards of hygiene and ideas of comfort or discomfort determine when the pad will be changed. The choice of pad for any individual patient will really be determined by the degree of incontinence and so again the assessment of the patient is critical. There are patients whose incontinence may improve and who may have to use an all-in-one pad initially, then try the Molnlycke Tenaform range as the incontinence improves and finally rely on a simple insert pad as the problem resolves. Quite apart from the pads mentioned above, many women with mild stress incontinence use sanitary towels or Kleenex tissues to mop up the involuntarily voided urine. A survery of high-street outlets revealed that many post-menopausal women were buying sanitary towels in bulk. A survey of their buying habits revealed that the sanitary towels were used for urinary incontinence but not by themselves but rather by their husbands. If the purchase price of sanitary towels for incontinence and Kleenex tissues were added to the existing cost of £17–20 million which we know is spent by the NHS on incontinence the real expenditure figure might be doubled.

Odour Control

Excreta odour occurs when urine or faeces come in contact with the air thereby causing bacterial decomposition. To minimise or reduce this problem, detergents or disinfectants should be used to destroy the odour or alternatively nebulisers or counteractants can be used to combine chemically with the odour to eliminate it. It is important when using these products not to use too strong a solution because these in turn may have an adverse chemical effect and create problems of their own.

Fresh air sprays or perfume sprays, which are masking agents, minimise the offending smell by creating another odour that is acceptable. However, under certain conditions, the smell can become associated with the offending odour and the combination becomes unacceptable.

Odour is more of a problem with the bed-ridden or wheelchair-bound patient than it is with the ambulant patient. The bed-ridden and chair-bound patient should be changed as soon as the incontinence occurs but unfortunately this is not always possible. The need for changing the patient is in order to protect the skin. Soiled bed linen or clothing should be soaked in a mild antiseptic solution or cold water before laundering and then placed in designated laundry containers. The bed linen and clothing should not be allowed to touch the floor or furniture because, over a period of time, the excreta odour will permeate the fabric and no amount of cleaning will remove it. The concept of using a charcoal pad between the disposable pad and pant might be useful to counter the smell of intractable incontinence.

Enuresis Alarms and Trainers

Nocturnal enuresis affects many families in the community. Most children become dry by day before the age of 2 years and many will have contol at night by the same age. It is not uncommon for boys to lag behind girls in gaining continence. I do not offer enuretic alarms or training systems to children under the age of 7 years as I do not feel that such young children can cope with them. Alarms can have a disquieting effect as some children are terrified by them. Sometimes the parents and siblings, together with the family animals, are all woken but the incontinent child continues to sleep through the alarm and ensuing disruption. It is probably more important to counsel the mother and father about the alarm than it is the child. We usually advise the parents that in the first instance the alarm will not work and they are not to expect the desired results for some time. We explain that the alarm should trigger off a signal in the child to which the child has been previously oblivious. The urine will set off the alarm and with any luck the child will wake and evacuate the bladder. Counselling of the child is important because it is necessary to explain that if the child wakes up it is necessary to practice the discipline of getting out of bed, going to the toilet and going through the motions of evacuating the bladder even if, in fact, the bladder is empty. It is only by carrying out this discipline that the child, in time, comes to recognise the signal that the bladder is full and actually wakes up before becoming incontinent.

It is also important to tell the parent that the child must be warm in bed as the chances of enuresis are higher if the child is cold. We frequently find that children wake up at night and recognise the signal as coming from their bladders but, because of fear of the dark, they wet themselves rather than make the journey to the toilet. In these situations it is sensible to leave a landing light on throughout the night to help allay fears. The problem with an alarm is compounded if children share a bedroom and it is distinctly possible that all the children in the same room will then be woken up by the alarm with the resulting difficulty that parents will have in getting the children back to sleep. For these reasons, alarms only have a limited practical application.

Alarm Design

Most enuresis alarms consist of a control unit which contains the batteries and electronic circuitry and a urine sensor. The urine sensor is usually a pair of mats, or just occasionally a single mat, positioned beneath the bottom sheet of a bed. If two mats are used, a piece of linen or old sheet should be placed between them, and a waterproof sheet should be placed beneath the bottom sensor to protect the mattress. Even if the child is cold in bed, it is counter-productive to wear underwear and pyjama bottoms because these garments delay the transport time of urine to the sensor. When the urine comes in contact with the sensor, the electronic circuit is triggered and the alarm is sounded which wakes the child. It is very important for the child to turn the alarm off himself because this ritual is part of the strict discipline the child must follow if the technique is going to be successful. In practice it takes about 6 weeks for a child to become dry using an enuretic alarm.

In most equipment the alarm is audible but there are devices where a flashing light or vibrator can be used instead. Alternatively, extension alarms or extra loud alarms are available but these have the effect of waking the rest of the household. The sensor can be body-worn, in which case it will need to be secured by underpants, and this particular type of sensor has the advantage that it can be used either by day or by night. The control box is usually small with these devices and can be placed in a pocket or, alternatively, attached to the body by means of a harness.

A recent development has been the bed-wetting alarm produced by Nottingham Medical Aids Ltd. This consists of a control box which is pinned to the pyjama top or shirt and a central pad which is worn inside the underwear and fixed by means of a clip. This device is neat and considerably less cumbersome than most of the conventional designs.

The control box usually outlives the sensor mats which have to be replaced from time to time. Sometimes we find that the parents are reluctant to return the enuresis alarm to the hospital and this may be because the mats have become damaged and the parents are too embarrassed to bring them back. The parents need to be strongly reassured that the mats are easily replaced and that they are not as robust as the control box. The parents, however, do have to be reminded that the batteries in the control box need to be changed from time to time and the onus is on them to ensure that the control box is working.

Potty Trainers

Many manufacturers sell potty trainers which consist of a potty or toilet bowl insert with a urine sensor in the bottom. This produces an audible alarm or a musical reward. The box can be either the external variety or it can be incorporated in the potty base.

Toileting Aids

Some patients' incontinence has less to do with the function of the lower urinary tract and more to do with immobility or disabilities. There are toileting aids to facilitate independence and privacy of such patients and the most significant feature of these is securing the correct position of the person on the lavatory seat. They need to be seated comfortably with the trunk well supported, slightly tilted forward with the feet firmly on the floor.

Hand rails can be wall- or floor-mounted on one or both sides of the pan. Their height should be adjusted and fixed to the sitting position and/or standing position for a man if he chooses to urinate in that manner. Vertical hand rails are either forward for pull-off or horizontal for the pushing up movement. These are placed at elbow level when the person is seated. The hand rails can be angled for personal preference.

A toilet frame or surround can be secured to the floor to provide stability when sitting down or getting off the pan. Lavatory seats can be obtained with adjustable clips to secure and fit the pan and they are easily removed for cleaning. They slope from back to front and usually have an opening or groove at the front to facilitate personal cleansing of the crotch. For the severely disabled, spring-loaded seats are available. Washable seat covers are available for added comfort.

A commode is nothing more than a chair with a hinged flap concealing a chamber pot. They are available as free-standing models or they can be mobile for use over an existing toilet. They can be of adjustable height with splayed legs to provide stability and the padded arm is removable for transfer of the patient. The container (for urine) should be easy to clean and to carry. It is usually removable from the back. A policy should be decided upon with respect to responsibility for emptying commodes and such a policy is very important in institutions.

HG Wallace have recently marketed Femicep. This is a device which can be used by females who are immobile and is placed on the bed or couch between their legs and allows them to micturate into a container, the urine then draining away into a uribag. It can be used by females either sitting or lying down without any assistance. Discomfort is reduced to a minimum and hygiene is maintained through easiclean surfaces and attachable bed reservoirs. Additional reservoir bags are easily obtainable.

Hand-held Urinals

Hand-held urinals are an aid to continence when mobility is restricted and toilet facilities are not amenable. Female urinals are made in a variety of designs to meet the requirements of different individuals. Hip abduction, dexterity and the quantity of urine voided go some way to determining a patient's preference. The patient's clothing, such as wrap-round skirts and open-crotch pants facilitate use of the urinal. For bed-bound patients it is not uncommon to use a pad underneath the patient to aid continence, but usually when confidence is established the pad can be discarded. The common type of hand-held urinal is in the form of a conventional bed pan. There is another variety which is oval-shaped; one half of the top surface is closed over, which is the part that the patient's buttocks sit upon. There is also a type not unlike the male standard urinal, except that it has a much wider opening to facilitate the vulval fit.

For the female patient who can stand up there are three varieties of urinal. There is the boat-shaped, hand-held version which can be inserted between the legs. There is also an elongated variety which fits over the vulva and pubis and has a detachable handle. The bottom end of this urinal has a tube which drains urine away to a toilet bowl. The third type is another hand-held variety but is anatomically shaped to the vulval opening and in this variety the receptacle is composed of a polythene bag. All but the last urinal are non-disposable and need to be cleaned regularly to prevent odour occurring.

There are several varieties of male urinals, some of which are graduated and some of which have a lid that can be applied to prevent spillage. There is a stainless-steel variety which looks rather like a jug when stood upright and a PVC urinal with a non-return valve which has an integral wire closure to hold open during use. There is also a standard urinal, the funnel of which is fitted with a latex flutter valve and rubber seal to prevent spillage. This device of the non-spill variety is very useful for the confused patient or for those whose dexterity is impaired. Female types of urinals can be used by the male if he has a small or retracted penis although this type is not available with a non-spill adaptor.

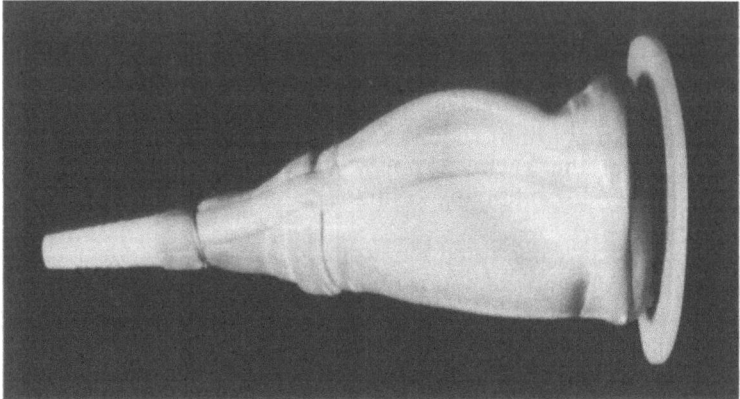

Fig. 6.16. Payne's urine director.

Urine Director

A urine director is a rubber device (Fig. 6.16) and is a convenient, easy to use, washable and reusable aid which, while not an incontinence appliance as such, is used by some men with physical mobility or dexterity problems who encounter difficulties in directing the urinary stream away from the clothes and surrounds irrespective of whether they stand or sit to urinate. After use it is rinsed and dried and kept inside a plastic bag or cover in a pocket. The device shown here is marketed by SG & P Payne.

Acknowledgements. I have received a great deal of help in the preparation of this chapter from Mr. Stuart Payne, of SG & P Payne, who was kind enough to provide me with all the material and samples that I required. I was also given considerable assistance from Sister Barbara Begg at the Urodynamic Unit of the Manchester Royal Infirmary and Mr. Gary Hay of Vernon–Carus, who was kind enough to arrange for me to be shown around the factory and provided me with information about super absorbents. I am grateful to the University Department of Medical Illustration at Manchester Royal Infirmary for producing the prints.

Bibliography

Department of Health and Social Security (DHSS) Drug Tariff Supplement. October 1987
Directory of Continence Appliances (1986) 3rd edn. Association of Continence Advisors, 346 Kensington High Street, London, W14 8NS
Hospital Equipment and Supplies Magazine. United Trade Press Ltd., 33–35 Bowling Green Lane, London, EC1R 0DA
McGrother CW, Castleden CM, Duffin H, Clarke M (1986) Provision of services for incontinent elderly people at home. J Epidemiol Community Health 40:134–138
Smith N (1988) Aids for urinary incontinence. Br Med J 296:772–773

Chapter 7

Prosthetic Urethral Substitution

P.J.R. Shaw

Introduction

The repair of the urethra once it has been affected by disease has always provided a challenge to urologists. Many procedures have been designed for urethral repair and have been in use for many years (Browne 1949; Nedelec and Auvigne 1966). Modifications of long-existing techniques and also their rediscovery still continue. The majority of these techniques use tissue from adjacent structures, scrotal or penile skin being the most commonly used grafts. The majority of reconstructive procedures were designed for the treatment of urethral strictures. As interest in urethral reconstruction has continued, innovative techniques are being tried in other situations in which urethral replacement is necessary, such as hypospadias, epispadias etc. Experience has shown that primary urethral reconstruction using homografts is associated with excellent functional results. The number of techniques for urethral reconstruction are as varied as their many authors: scrotal inlay (Turner-Warwick 1960), pedicled scrotal skin island patches (Blandy et al. 1968), pedicled prepucial island patches or tubes (Duckett 1981), free full-thickness and split-thickness skin grafts (Devine et al. 1963), tunica vaginalis testis (Kishev 1962) and bladder mucosal tube grafts (Memmelaar 1947; Thuroff et al. 1983) and endourethral split skin grafting (Gaur 1983) have all been successfully used for urethral reconstruction.

Most urethral abnormalities may be repaired with one of the techniques described above. Provided suitable graft tissue is available, using the patient's own tissue should provide the most successful results. It has been suggested that there is no urethral abnormality that may not be successfully reconstructed, with skill, patience and a combination of techniques. Where reconstruction has been tried and has failed, successive attempts at surgery may make an already difficult problem insuperable except to all but the most experienced of surgeons. A simple prosthetic tube graft could more readily be inserted to replace a urethra affected by disease. This may reduce the time and potential complications which may arise from complex urethral reconstruction.

De Nicola in 1950 was the first to successfully replace the human urethra with a silicone tube. His patient gave a history of 30 years of urethral stricture of gonococcal origin, with multiple episodes of fistula formation and extravasation. After bladder decompression De Nicola performed primary incision and drainage of huge penile and scotal masses and found that part of the urethra was missing. Two weeks later a 10-cm silicone tube was used to replace the damaged urethra and the patient was still voiding well 14 months later.

This historic event was followed by many experimental attempts to replace the urethra with synthetic materials. These attempts to replace the urethra have included venous patch and tube grafts, lyophilised human dura (LHD), silicone rubber patches, siliconised Dacron, and polytetrafluoroethylene (PTFE, Goretex) grafts. The majority of attempts to replace the urethra have taken place as experimental studies in animals with only few attempts at urethral replacement taking place in man.

The use of allografts is based on the premise that re-epithelialisation of the graft would take place with the formation of a neo-urethral lining within the graft. Consideration of the risk of infection, rejection, fistulation and calculus formation was also necessary.

Techniques of Prosthetic Urethral Replacement

PTFE-Patch Urethral Substitution

Felt made from polytetrafluoroethylene (PTFE; Teflon) was used by Kelâmi et al. (1970) in experiments on the urinary bladder of dogs, with encouraging results; the use of PTFE patches for the closure of surgically created defects in the dog urethra followed (Kelâmi et al. 1971). Oval defects created in the perineal urethra of 5 dogs were covered with oval PTFE felt patches. Early fistula formation in 2 of 10 dogs (5 treated with PTFE patches and 5 with lyophilised human dural patches – no comment was made into which group these fell) settled within 2 months spontaneously. Epithelialisation took place only very slowly, though the interstices of the graft were filled with connective tissue and there was no encrustation. Voiding was satisfactory in all the dogs. No rejections occurred.

Lyophilised Human Dura (LHD)

Kelâmi et al. (1972) were the first to use lyophilised human dura (LHD) for urethral replacement, first as an isolated patch of a urethral defect and then made into a tube for urethral replacement. The first study in 5 dogs (Kelâmi et al. 1971) used a LHD patch to cover a surgically created oval defect in the perineal urethra (see previous section). The patch had been completely absorbed and replaced by an epithelium-covered scar without urethral stenosis. This encouraging study led them to experiment with a LHD tube, a collagen tube and a collagen/Dacron tube (Kelâmi et al. 1972). Their results were not as encouraging as in their patch urethral substitution as Table 7.1 shows. They suggested further experimental studies but their results were not encouraging enough for this technique to be used in man.

Table 7.1. Results of replacement of the urethra in dogs (Kelâmi et al. 1972)

	Number of cases	Post-operative bleeding	Fistula	Infection	Stenosis	Success
LHD	5	1 (died)	2	–	–	2
Collagen	5	–	2	1 (died)	2	0
Collagen/Dacron	5	–	2	–	–	3

Siliconised Dacron

The Sparks mandril graft is made from a double-knitted siliconised Dacron mesh (Sparks 1973). Its use has been in vascular surgery for arterial substitution. A tube made from this material has been used in experimental studies in dogs for the replacement for a segment of excised urethra (Dubernard et al. 1976; Hakky 1976, 1977). Of 9 dogs only one developed a fistula in the early post-operative period. Urinary flow was poor after catheter removal but returned to normal within 4 weeks. Urethrograms demonstrated urethral narrowing. This was confirmed macroscopically by the loose attachment of the graft to the urethra. The graft was both covered and undermined by epithelium in different areas and supported by a fibrous tissue outer layer. Graft extrusion was seen to be taking place.

Eight mongrel dogs underwent urethral substitution by silicone prostheses lined by Dacron velour. The prostheses were covered by epithelium in each dog and it was suggested that this prosthesis could be used successfully in man (Palleschi and Tanagho 1978).

Polytetrafluoroethylene (PTFE)

PTFE or Goretex (reinforced expanded PTFE, Gore Flagstaff, Arizona, USA) grafts are commercially available for the replacement of arteries and veins. They have been successfully used for some years in vascular surgery after initial successful experimental studies in dogs by Matsumoto et al. (1973) and Campbell et al. (1975). Goretex is available in diameters ranging from 3 to 24 mm with a graft thickness of 0.5 mm.

The complete replacement of the urethra has been carried out in experimental studies in dogs. Dreikorn et al. (1979) reported the successful replacement of the urethra in 12 male dogs. During a follow-up period of up to 12 months they recorded only 1 temporary fistula. Anwar et al. (1984) reported the results of 12 urethral replacements in 10 dogs. Although their early results were encouraging (only 1 dog with a fistula at 2 months), late complications were seen in all of 4 dogs followed for 3–6 months.

The only comment made about the histological changes in association with the graft (Anwar et al. 1984) was of calcification of the prosthesis but no epithelialisation of its lumen.

The complications encountered were those which could be anticipated; of fistula formation, stenosis, extravasation and calcification.

The conclusions from these studies were contradictory. Dreikorn et al. (1979) reported encouraging results but mentioned the short-term follow-up period and Anwar et al. (1984) was unable to recommend the use of PTFE for urethral replacement.

Vein Grafts

The use of vein as a substitute for diseased arteries has become popular in vascular surgery and has been in use since 1894 (Gluck). Interest in substitution of both the urethra and ureter by the use of vein homo- and hetero-grafts has continued for many years (Kjaer et al. 1976). To date the use of vein replacements of the urethra have been confined to animal studies (Kjaer et al. 1976; Frang et al. 1982).

The replacement of segments of canine urethra has been performed in experimental studies. Lyophilised femoral vein (Kjaer et al. 1976) was used in 9 dogs to replace 3 cm of surgically excised perineal urethra. They reported a successful outcome in 8 of their animals. One developed a fistula and infection and 1 a haematoma which spontaneously resolved.

Satisfactory voiding occurred in all the successful implants. They found that the graft was completely lined by transitional epithelium in 4–8 weeks. The lyophilised veins were felt to have produced no immune response and minimal inflammatory response.

The use of autologous vein grafts was not accompanied by the same success in initial studies by Frang et al. (1982). The use of the long saphenous vein of the same diameter as the removed 3 cm of urethra (again in dogs) was associated with considerable tension at the anastomosis which was associated with graft failure (though no results were quoted for this early research). Frang et al. then used everted autologous external jugular vein grafts of a larger diameter. Of 10 dogs so treated, 2 developed marked stenosis but none showed fistula or graft rejection. The vein structures had been completely replaced by connective tissue lined by transitional epithelium (the same result as found by Kjaer et al. 1976). One innovation that Frang et al. employed was the application of tissue glue to the anastomotic lines. All the anastomoses were splinted with polyethylene tubes.

General conclusions from these studies were that replacement of the human urethra with vein grafts may be possible provided the vein graft is of larger diameter than the urethral diameter and the anastomosis is not under tension.

Silicone Rubber Tubes

Following the first report of urethral replacement by artificial materials in man (De Nicola in 1959) several animal studies have been carried out using silicone-elastomer urethral replacements with either tube or patch grafts (Heller 1965; Gilbaugh et al. 1969). The diameter of the silicone tube appeared to be the most important factor to reduce the incidence of both fistulae and stenosis, the larger diameter tubes being associated with no complications. Replacement of the dog urethra with a silicone tube of 15F diameter was not associated with complication in 3 dogs, whereas, where the urethral segment was replaced with a 10F tube (3 dogs) all developed fistulae, stenosis and prosthetic displacement. In the successful replacements the prosthesis was

Table 7.2.   Results of urethral replacement with silicone prostheses in human adult males

Author	Number of patients	Prosthesis	Post-operative result	Complications
Sankey and Heller (1967)	9	Patch	9/9 normal voiding	2 patches displaced, 3 reoperations
Moulonguet and Jaupitre (1973)	2	Tube	2/2 normal voiding	1 migration of tube and calculus
Court et al. (1973)	3	Tube	3/3 normal voiding	1 leaked and prosthesis replaced
Vincent and Anquetil (1976)	1	Tube	1/1 normal voiding	None

surrounded by a fibrous capsule lined by transitional epithelium and there was a small gap between the prosthetic tube and the "neo-urethra" which was demonstrated on urethrography.

Human urethral replacement with a silicone-tube prosthesis has been performed in 6 males and with a silicone-rubber patch in 9 males for either inflammatory urethral strictures or following posterior urethral trauma (Sankey and Heller 1967; Moulonguet and Jaupitre 1972; Court et al. 1973; Vincent and Anquetil 1976). The results of urethral replacement in man are shown in Table 7.2.

Alternatives to Urethral Replacement or Grafting: The Introduction of Intra-urethral Stenting

Milroy et al. (1989) reported the use of the Wallstent (Medinvent, Lausanne, Switzerland) for the stenting of urethral strictures which had failed to respond to surgery. Patients who had been treated by multiple urethrotomy or by urethroplasties which had failed to cure the stricture were treated by an initial optical urethrotomy and followed by the insertion of the Wallstent – an interwoven tubular mesh of stainless-steel wire. The stent attains its diameter of 14 mm and remains within the urethra to become epithelialised within 6–12 weeks. The results with this device have been shown to be excellent in initial experiments in dogs and in later use in man. Successful stricture treatment is the rule rather than the exception. The Wallstent has been used in patients with a hyperactive urethral sphincter to provide sphincterotomy (Shaw et al. 1990) and also as a permanently implanted stent for the treatment of prostatic outflow obstruction (Williams et al. 1989).

Discussion

The use of prosthetic grafts for the replacement of area of abnormal urethra of whatever cause is an attractive alternative to the use of human tissue grafting.

Although there may be very few circumstances in which urethral reconstruction is not possible or is compromised by absence of suitable local graft tissue, urethral substitution by a prosthetic graft would be a considerable advantage. This would make urethral reconstruction possible in even the least favourable circumstances, particularly in the hypospadias cripple, or the patient with strictures and fistulae.

There are many publications on the subject of replacement of the urethra with prostheses in the animal model but few report experience in man. These anecdotal papers have produced interesting results and encourage further study of this subject.

De Nicola's original paper on the successful outcome of urethral replacement with a silicone-tube graft has been supported by subsequent work both in animals and in man. The results from the studies described above do appear to suggest that silicone-tube grafts are associated with a lower incidence of graft complications than the other techniques considered. Apart from the technical aspects of the surgical procedure it would appear that provided the graft diameter is greater than the urethral diameter and proximal drainage is used, the complication rate should be low. In spite of the interest in silicone replacement for the urethra this technique appears not to have been reported for at least 10 years although it appears the most promising of the prosthetic replacements.

Vein grafts did not produce concurring results in the two papers reviewed. The one benefit of this prosthesis comes from its complete replacement by connective tissue lined by transitional epithelium. This would clearly appear to be an advantage. Lyophilised vein grafts are freely available and their attraction would appear to be their complete histological replacement as described. Prosthetic urethral replacement would be more advantageous if the graft is absorbed leaving an epithelium-lined tube behind. Lyophilised human dura and vein grafts appear to have advantages in this respect over silicone replacements which are more likely to be associated with longterm problems of erosion, infection or calcification. No longterm results of any of these techniques have yet been reported.

Knitted siliconised Dacron produced good short-term results, though graft extrusion would also appear to be a possibility in the longterm. The tissue reaction to all prosthetic replacements would appear to be one of transitional cell proliferation supported by a connective tissue layer.

PTFE-patch substitutes did not produce the same tissue response with very little epithelialisation though the graft patches used did not impede satisfactory voiding.

Replacing only part of the urethra, either by the use of a patch or by leaving a small strip of intact mucosa, was associated with a higher success rate than if the whole urethra was replaced.

The use of an intraurethral spiral or stent has provided an alternative to urethral replacement in patients with prostatic or urethral obstruction.

The initial use of an intra-urethral spiral was reported by Fabian (1980) who cystoscopically implanted a "urological spiral" into the prostatic urethra to relieve retention in 2 patients. In 1983 Fabricius showed that patients with intra-prostatic spirals developed complications. Amongst the complications encountered were urinary incontinence, encrustation and displacement. More recently two different spirals have been produced: the Prostakath – a gold-plated spiral – and the Urospiral. Both of these devices have been recommended for the alternative treatment of prostatic obstruction in patients unfit for transurethral surgery either because of age or contraindications for anaesthesia. Both of these devices are under evaluation and no published results are available. The authors' experience with 3 patients have shown satisfactory voiding after their implantation with no longterm complications at one year.

Milroy et al. (1989) developed the use of the Wallstent for the treatment of urethral strictures that had failed to respond to urethrotomy or urethroplasty. An initial urethrotomy was followed by the placement, under direct vision, of the Wallstent: an implanted self-expanding spiral woven of stainless-steel wire. The stent attains its diameter of 14 mm and remains within the urethra, gradually becoming covered by urethral epithelium in a period of 6–12 weeks. The initial experimental work in dogs has been confirmed by successful use of this stent in man.

The Wallstent has also been used to relieve prostatic outflow obstruction (Williams et al. 1989) by implantation into the prostatic urethra and for the treatment of external sphincter dyssynergia in spinal injured males (Shaw et al. 1990) as an alternative to external striated sphincterotomy.

There are no longterm results of the use of the permanently implanted stent but encouraging early results are reported.

It is likely that new materials for implantable stents will be produced and will offer alternatives to prosthetic urethral substitution.

Summary

Care and attention to detail in the graft substitution of urethral defects with a patient's own tissue should be associated with a high success rate. There are some situations where little of the patient's own tissue is available for urethral replacement and it is here that a prosthetic graft would be ideal. The use of the bladder mucosal graft has recently been rediscovered and has found an important place where salvage urethroplasties are necessary, especially for the complex hypospadias case. In spite of the value of this technique it would be preferable to use a prosthetic graft for urethral reconstruction which would avoid the need for suprapubic bladder surgery with its attendant morbidity.

Further studies need to be performed to look again at different graft materials and to reconsider their place in urethral replacement in man.

References

Anwar H, Dave B, Seebode JJ (1984) Replacement of partially resected canine urethra by polytetrafluoroethylene. Urology 24:583–586

Blandy JP, Singh M, Tressider GC (1968) Urethroplasty by scrotal flap for long urethral strictures. Br J Urol 55:261–267

Brown D (1949) Hypospadias. Post Grad Med J 25:367–372

Campbell CD, Goldfarb D, Roe R (1975) A small arterial substitute: expanded microporous PTFE: patency v porosity. Ann Surg 182:138–143

Court B, Xerri A, Auvert J (1973) Remplacement de l'uretre chez l'homme par un prosthese en elastomere de silicone. J Urol Nephrol 796:643–647

De Nicola RR (1950) Permanent artificial (silicone) urethra. J Urol 63:168–172

Devine PC, Horton CE, Devine CJ Sr, Devine CJ Jr, Crawford HH, Adamson JE (1963) Use of full thickness skin grafts in repair of urethral strictures. J Urol 90:67–71

Dreikorn K, Lobelenz J, Horsch R, Rohl L (1979) Alloplastic replacement of the partially resected canine urethra by expanded polytetrafluoroethylene grafts. Urol Res 7:19–21

Dubernard J-M, Gignoux N, Pin J, Fayol A, Botta J-M, Blanc N (1976) Remplacement de l'urethre perinal chez le chien par des tubes de sparks. J Urol Nephrol 82 (Suppl 2):467–473

Duckett JW (1981) The Island Flap technique for hypospadias repair. Urol Clin North Am 8:503–511

Fabian KM (1980) Der interprostatische "partielle Katheter" (urologische Spirale). Urologe [A] 19:236–238

Fabricius GB, Marz M, Zepnick H (1983). Die Endourethralspirale–eine Alternative zum Dauerkatheter? Z Arztl Fortbild (Jena) 77:482–485

Frang D, Furka I, Koves S (1982) Urethral replacement with autologous venous graft: an experimental study in the dog. Urol Res 10:145–147

Gaur DD (1983) Endourethral urethroplasty – Use of a new catheter. J Urol 130:905–908

Gilbaugh JH, Utz DC, Wakim KG (1969) Partial replacement of the canine urethra with a silicon prosthesis. Invest Urol 7:41–51

Gluck T (1898) Die Moderne Chirugie des Circulations Apparates. Berl Klin 70:1–29

Hakky SI (1976) Urethral replacement by Dacron mesh. Lancet 2:1192

Hakky SI (1977) The use of fine double siliconised Dacron in urethral replacement. Br J Urol 49:167–172

Heller E (1965) Surgical repair of urethral strictures with a silicone rubber patch. J Urol 94: 576–579

Kelami A, Dustman HO, Ludtke-Handjery A, Carcamo V, Herold G (1970) Experimental investigations of bladder regeneration using Teflon-felt as a bladder wall substitute. J Urol 104:693–698

Kelami A, Korb G, Ludtke-Handjery A, Rolle J, Schnell J, Lehnhardt FH (1971) Alloplastic replacement of the partially resected urethra in dogs. Invest Urol 9:55–58

Kelami A, Korb G, Rolle J, Schnell J, Lehnhardt FJ (1972) Replacement of the total resected urethra with alloplastic materials: experimental studies on dogs. J Urol 107:75–77

Kishev S (1962) A new method of urethroplasty for urethral stricture. Br J Urol 34:54–58

Kjaer TB, Nilsson T, Madsen PO (1976) Total replacement of part of the canine urethra with lyophilised vein grafts. Invest Urol 14:159–161

Matsumoto H, Hasegawa T, Fuse K (1973) A new vascular prosthesis for a small calibre artery. Surgery 74:519

Memmelaar J (1947) Use of bladder mucosal graft in a one-stage repair of hypospadias. J Urol 58:68–73

Milroy EJG, Chapple CR, Eldin A, Wallsten H (1989) A new stent for the treatment of urethral strictures. Br J Urol 63:392–396

Moulonguet A, Jaupitre A (1973) Un cas de prosthese de l'uretre posterieur pour retrecissement post-traumatique. J Urol Nephrol 79:292–294

Nedelec M, Auvigne J (1966) Remplacement de l'uretre chez l'homme. Journal d'Urologie 72:18–160

Palleschi JR, Tanagho EA (1978) Urethral tube graft in dogs. Invest Urol 15:408–411

Sankey NE, Heller E (1967) The results of urethroplasty using a silicone rubber patch. J Urol 97:309–313

Shaw PJR, Milroy EJG, Timoney AG, Eldin A, Mitchell N (1990) Permanent external striated sphincter stents in patients with spinal injuries. Br J Urol 66:297–302

Sparks CH (1973) Silicon mandril method for growing reinforced autogenous femoro-popliteal artery grafts in situ. Ann Surg 177:293–300

Thuroff JW, Hutscxhenreiter Rumpelt HJ, Hohenfellner R (1983) Neo-urethra: a new two-stage procedure for reconstruction of the functional urethra. J Urol 130:1228–1233

Turner-Warwick RT (1960) A technique for posterior urethroplasty. J Urol 83:416–419

Turner-Warwick RT (1983) Urethral stricture surgery. In: Glen JF (ed) Urologic surgery, 3rd edn. JB Lippincott, Philadelphia, pp 689–719

Vincent M-A, Anquetil R (1976) Un cas de remplacement de l'uretre par un prosthese en elastomere de silicone. J Urol Nephrol 82:478–484

Willams G, Jager R, McLonghlin J et al. (1989) Prostatic stents: a new treatment for prostatic outflow obstruction in patients unfit for surgery. Br Med J 298:1429

Chapter 8

Urostomy Appliances

R.N.P. Carroll

Introduction

Ever since Bricker popularised supravesical urinary diversion over 30 years ago, urologists, appliance manufacturers, urostomates, stoma care nurses and entero-therapists have been endeavouring to improve stoma appliances. Advances in the biological application of plastics and related substances have, in little over a decade, seen the introduction of the disposable urostomy appliance and with it an ever-increasing consumer choice in the article itself and its accessories. The stage has now been reached where a bewildering choice of appliances faces the consumer and there is no reason to believe that ingenuity, inventiveness and technical advances will do anything but generate further innovations. Our patients can, therefore, expect to be faced with an even wider selection of appliance equipment in the future.

A realisation of the problems involved in stoma patients hastened the acceptance that stoma care required special nursing skills and led to the development of stoma care nurses, greater medical interest in stoma care and the development of self-help organisations for urostomates. These groups have combined with the manufacturers to provide a much greater selection of stoma appliances.

Appliances and Accessories

The Pouch

The basic urinary diversion appliance consists of a pouch or bag which collects the urine and is fitted with an outlet at the bottom for drainage. The material, shape, capacity, colour and transparency or opacity of the pouches vary enormously. Some pouches are of the light, single-use, disposable variety, whilst others are of the heavier, reusable, "permanent" kind. The requirements of the pouch are that it should be light and comfortable to wear, able to keep the patient dry and to give security. By releasing the outlet mechanism, the collected urine can be discarded. However, the outlet tap which is usually of narrow diameter can be attached to extension tubing which is then secured to a drainage leg bag or a night drainage uribag (see chapter on urinary devices for incontinence). In either of these situations the urostomy pouch rarely contains much urine unless the outlet tube becomes blocked. Some pouches incorporate a non-return valve mechanism to prevent back flow of urine when the patient is lying supine. In practice, there is usually a large difference between the stated capacity of a bag and its functional capacity. The functional capacity is usually about 250–350 ml, in other words, the bag is emptied by the patient when it is about half full.

Ideally the disposable pouches should last about a week, but in practice are changed more often. The reusable ones should last 3–6 months. Rubber is considered to be outdated but in parts of the world economic factors determine usage. The problem with rubber bags is that the lining becomes encrusted. This encrustation is thought to be due to an alkaline urine and large doses of ascorbic acid may prevent this although this remedy does not always work. By utilising a combination of a reusable face plate or gasket, together with a disposable pouch, a "semi disposable" appliance can be fashioned. The incorporation of the flange in the pouch or the pouch's independence of it determines whether the appliance is classified as a one- or two-piece variety.

Classification of Pouches

The variety of pouches available on the market is shown in Table 8.1.

1. *Rubber, Reusable or Non-disposable Adhesive – One-Piece*. This black bag is made by Salts of Birmingham, UK. It is oval in shape and has a flange (making it a one-piece pouch) and incorporates a non-return valve mechanism. It comes in three capacity sizes and the aperture for the stoma is variable but not alterable. The adhesive solution (which is also made by Salts) is applied both to the flange or face plate and the skin. This one-piece bag comes fitted with a plastic ring which is incorporated in a rubber flange and the belt hooks into this plastic ring to give support. These pouches, which have been available for many years, have given great service and are frequently preferred by patients who started with them and have not changed to the disposable variety.

Table 8.1. Classification of urostomy pouches

1.	Rubber	Reusable or non-disposable	Adhesive	One-piece
2.	Rubber	Reusable, non-disposable	Non-adhesive	One-piece
3.	Rubber	Reusable, non-disposable	Adhesive	Two-piece
4.	Rubber	Reusable, non-disposabale	Non-adhesive	Two-piece
5.	Plastic	Disposable	Adhesive	One-piece
6.	Plastic	Disposable	Non-adhesive	One-piece
7.	Plastic	Disposable	Adhesive	Two-piece
8.	Plastic	Disposable	Non-adhesive	Two-piece
9.	Plastic	Disposable but durable	Non-adhesive	One-piece

2. *Rubber, Reusable, Non-disposable, Non-adhesive – One-Piece*. This is made by Salts and is similar to that described above except that a foam pad replaces the adhesive solution.

3. *Rubber, Reusable or Non-disposable Adhesive – Two-Piece*. This type of pouch is made by Downs Surgical Ltd. The adult variety is shaped like a hot-water bottle, being oblong rather than oval. There is no non-return valve mechanism and the emptying device is a tap of the stopcock variety. The bag is usually white or honey-coloured and is secured by a separate rubber flange (making it a two-piece appliance) which comes in varying sizes. The rubber flange is secured in place by means of a wire pressure frame which in turn is secured by a web-and-elastic belt. The rubber bag is secured to the rim of the flange by stretching the orifice in the rubber bag over the ring. This bag capacity varies and there are five or six sizes with a corresponding number of flanges. The flange is fixed to the bag by a double-sided adhesive plaster.

Downs Chiron rubber appliances are available for adults and children. The paediatric models are transverse rather than oblong and come in three capacity sizes which are specifically made for either right- or left-sided stomas. The Downs bags are made of white or latex rubber and there is also an odour-proof translet bag of the rubber variety. Downs market a day bag and a night bag which have different capacities, and in addition there is a Chiron double bag which incorporates a valve to prevent back flow of urine where the upper small compartment joins the larger lower compartment of the pouch.

4. *Rubber, Reusable, Non-disposable, Non-adhesive – Two-Piece*. This is made by Downs Brothers and is the same as that described immediately above except that a foam pad replaces the adhesive. The pouch is kept in place by means of a pressure plate and belt.

5. *Plastic, Disposable, Adhesive – One-Piece*. A variety of manufacturers make these bags, including Abbott (Hollister), Coloplast, Downs and Salts. They come in a variety of shapes and sizes from rectangular by Hollister, oval by Downs and shamrock-shaped by Salts. The Coloplast one is rectangular but has a wider base. Coloplast offer a one-size-capacity bag and request the patient to cut out the orifice in the bag to fit his stoma size. The other companies offer bags of varying capacities but with fixed diameter aperture sizes. Some of these are applied with adhesive and a belt facility is optional.

6. *Plastic, Disposable, Non-adhesive – One-Piece*. This is made by Downs Brothers and is similar to the adhesive bag except that a foam pad replaces the adhesive and it requires to be secured by a belt.

7. *Plastic, Disposable, Adhesive – Two-Piece*. These bags are made by Squibb, Coloplast and Downs. The Squibb Systems 2 is very popular and comes with a flange incorporated with Stomahesive and the bag snaps onto the rim of the flange. The belt is optional and a new tap has been incorporated to allow Squibb's aquaseal system to be utilised in the urostomy pouch system. The pouch contains a non-return valve. The Coloplast URO 2002 Urostomy System is similar in principle to the Squibb type.

The Downs variety has a non-disposable flange of rubber or plastic and the plastic bag stretches over the rim (the patient needs good fingers for this). There is also a non-return valve and the flange is attached by adhesive. A belt is optional. The bag has a screw cap for emptying.

8. *Disposable, Non-adhesive – Two-Piece.* This is made by Downs and the foam pad replaces the adhesive. These bags are not commonly used because they are easily dislodged.

9. *Plastic, Disposable But Durable Non-adhesive – One-Piece.* Vance Products Inc (Spencer, Indiana, USA) market a pouch which is effectively only available in the USA. This consists of a transverse-lying plastic pouch which is secured with a web elastic belt. It is worn on the front of the abdomen and the aperture is located on the right, centre or left depending on the siting of the stoma. The pouch size varies from 300 ml to 1100 ml, there being four sizes in all. There is a silicone ring rather like a washer which acts as a seal and this comes in three sizes, small, medium and large. This seal fits into the flange which is incorporated in the pouch itself. There are three stoma sizes. The pouch itself is compartmentalised so that the contents are evenly distributed within the bag. There is a central outlet tap at the bottom of the bag. The effectiveness of this bag is that it is rather easy to disguise and can be worn underneath male underpants or female undergarments and cannot be seen. The manufacturers recommend that patients use two on a "wear-one, wash-one" basis and the pouches can be used for a few weeks at a time. In other words they last longer than the disposable ones described above but not as long as the rubber reusable ones of the permanent variety. Because of their expense, these bags are not available in the United Kingdom or continental Europe.

Pouch Covers

For transparent disposable pouches some patients prefer to use a pouch cover which is made of cotton in either plain colour or floral design. However, Abbott (Hollister) market a paper cover and both of the varieties have the advantage of preventing the pouch from sticking to the patient's skin.

The Flange

The flange is a circular object incorporating a rim to which the pouch is attached when it is secured in place. The flange is usually separate from the pouch (two-piece appliance) but sometimes it is incorporated in the pouch (one-piece) as in the newer disposable appliances. The function of the flange is to support the weight of the bag and to protect the stoma and surrounding skin. The flange is usually made of rubber or plastic and comes in different internal diameters and different depths. The base of the flange can be as much as twice its internal diameter. The flange depth can be critical because if it is too deep in the presence of a low profile stoma, then urine can pool inside the flange and give rise to peristomal skin irritation and leakage. On the other hand some flanges incorporate a canopy to protect the excessively protruding stoma. The base should not be too large as it will affect the adhesion to the body, especially if the stoma is sited near a ridge or fold in the abdominal wall.

Pressure Plates and Belts

Some flanges are secured in place by means of pressure plates which are made of either stainless steel or plastic. These in turn are secured by means of a buckle, tape or Velcro device. Some of the disposable pouches incorporate the pressure plate in the pouch. The belts which basically secure the urinary diversion device are frequently made of web and elastic. Rubber varieties exist and one special type is a sausage-shaped belt which is useful in patients with physical deformity. It is inadvisable for the restraining belt to be applied too tightly because of the risk of herniation of the stoma or peristomal tissue into the flange. Because the stoma itself is insensitive, it can be damaged without the patient realising what has happened.

Adhesives

In those situations where a pressure plate is not incorporated for securing a flange, double-sided adhesive plasters are used instead. These provide a water-tight seal between the skin and the appliance. These adhesive plasters can be made of either zinc or titanium oxide and there are also microporous and acrylic adhesives. There are also specially treated adhesives, such as Clearseal (Downs Surgical Ltd., Mitcham, England) and Stomaseal (3M), which reduce skin sensitivity. The double-sided adhesive plaster can be secured further by painting Tincture Benzoin Co, both on the flange and the skin and then allowing the tincture to dry before applying the plaster. This has the added effect of protecting the skin. Tincture Benzoin Co in aerosol form contains a higher proportion of alcohol, takes longer to dry but is relatively inexpensive. Nobecutane or Octaflex may be used instead of an adhesive plaster to secure the flange. Again, both the flange and the skin are coated and allowed to dry before being applied to each other. These types of adhesives are not easy to remove and various layers can build up over a period of time, but can always be peeled off later. In addition to securing the flange with adhesive, silver-coloured kidney-shaped seals of the same diameter (Downs) may be applied over the flange base for further security. The advantage of using a kidney seal or waterproof tape to overlap the edge of the flange, adhesive and the skin is that it makes the appliance waterproof externally and allows the patient to bath or shower without having to remove the appliance. These seals also prevent residual adhesive from sticking to the pouch or the patient's clothing. Alternatively, if a small arc of adhesive is protruding, talcum powder can be sparingly sprinkled on this adhesive to prevent adhesions but it ought to be remembered that talcum powder can in fact damage the adhesive substance itself.

Skin Protectives

There are a wide variety of barrier creams made by different manufacturers and skin protective pads available such as Stomahesive (Squibb, Convatec, Hounslow, Middlesex), Hollihesive (Abbott, Queenborough, Kent, England),

Comfeel (Coloplast, Peterborough, England) and Seal-a-peel (Eschmann, Lancing, Sussex, England). In addition there are washers made of karaya gum which are incorporated into but easily removable from the flange.

Implements

Scissors, supplied by the manufacturers, are necessary for the application of many pouches. Cutters, like pastry cutters, are useful for cutting out the correct diameter in the appliance to fit over the stoma. Cutters are satisfactory if the stoma is round but less helpful if it is oval.

Solvents

Solvents are frequently necessary to remove the adhesive when the appliance is being changed. The ones in common use are Ethermeth, acetone and Zoff (trichloroethane). Some of these solvents are highly inflammable substances which should be used with great caution in removing skin cement. One must always protect the stoma against splashes from the solvent because a severe reaction can occur on the delicate mucosa if contact is made.

Initial Patient Interview

Once the decision has been made by the urologist that the patient requires a urinary diversion, the opinion should be conveyed to the patient by the consultant in charge even if he himself is not going to perform the surgery. It is a considerable advantage to have a third person present at the discussion who can either be a nurse or a relative of the patient. Either can fulfil the role of supporting and comforting the patient when the bad news is imparted to them.

After the surgical details have been discussed and irrespective of whether a cystectomy is being carried out or not, the conversation inevitably will come around to the stoma and the appliance. It is good practice to enquire early on in the conversation whether the patient has ever seen or spoken to a urostomate. If the answer is in the affirmative, the patient should be encouraged to relate his understanding of urostomy because up to now the conversation may have been dominated very much by the surgeon. Because of disappointment, apprehension or emotion the patient may have played only a passive role in the discussion up to now and giving him an opportunity to speak often has the effect of relaxing him. If the patient has no previous knowledge of stomas or appliances then the surgeon's task is very much more difficult and it can be beneficial to introduce a urostomate. After the stoma has been discussed the conversation will naturally turn to the appliance.

Almost without variation the patient's first expressed concern is whether the urine-filled pouch could be noticed by others. Without avoiding the answer, the question can be circumvented by elaborating on the wide selection of urostomy pouches which are available and explaining that it is not really difficult to find an appliance which will allow the patient to wear his or her normal clothes without too much embarrassment. This brings up the question of body image and in practice the rotund, overweight middle-aged or elderly patients seem much less concerned about body image than younger ones. The patient's next query will concern leakage and odour. Strong reassurance can usually be given about odour and most of today's appliances are odour-proof in respect of urine. In respect of leakage, it is important to tell the patient that while he is in hospital, he will have accidents every day. This needs to be reinforced with the encouragement that by the time he leaves hospital, his skin will have adapted to the appliance and the leakage rate will have fallen considerably. It is important at the initial interview to stress to the patient that a urostomy is not a reason to retire from life. There are only a few manual jobs that remain problematical and most leisure activities can be pursued although contact sports should be avoided. We are, however, aware that many of our young urostomates play football.

Towards the end of the interview one should stress the back-up services and expertise that are available. It is important to explain the expertise of the clinical nurse specialist and stoma care nurse both in the hospital and on a domiciliary basis, and also the role of voluntary organisations who concern themselves with the welfare of the urostomates. It is important to highlight the explosion in high technology which has taken place in respect of appliances and their availability, reinforcing the idea that the patient will not be abandoned once he leaves hospital. Finally the patient must be made to understand clearly that irrespective of how much support and help is available to him he must set out to become the sole expert on his own stoma.

This initial interview has to be followed up with another conversation as soon as possible afterwards. If the patient is in hospital, this can easily be done in a day or so but if the initial interview is conducted on an out-patient basis it is advisable to bring the patient back in a few days to answer his queries, reinforce the things that have been to him and possibly to introduce him to a urostomate or the clinical nurse specialist.

Hospital Admission

Once the patient has been admitted to hospital, the surgeon or ward sister will usually introduce the patient to the stoma care nurse, the appliance consultant or technician and the approved hospital visitor who is somebody who has already undergone urinary diversion himself.

Role of the Stoma Care Nurse

Our practice is to introduce the stoma care nurse to the patient in the ward about 48 hours before surgery. Her role is to discuss the surgery briefly and highlight the support she will be giving to the patient on a daily basis once the immediate post-operative care has been undertaken in the high-dependency part of the hospital. Provided that the patient lives within the locality of the hospital the same stoma care nurse will be able to visit him at home but if this is not the situation she should arrange for the patient's own local stoma care nurse to make domiciliary visits once the patient has been discharged.

The stoma care nurse will usually introduce another ward patient to the one about to undergo surgery in order to reassure him that patients do come through these operations without mishap. The patients under-going urinary diversion surgery need that form of reassurance and are always very grateful for it. The next task is to select a site on the abdominal wall for the stoma to be positioned. This is usually done in the right iliac fossa if an ileal conduit is being fashioned. The chosen site should always be away from depressions such as the umbilicus and away from other surgical scars or swellings on the abdominal wall. If the patient has undergone several surgical procedures in the past, an ideal situation may not present itself and the site chosen may be less than perfect. In those patients with spinal deformities it may be impossible to find a site in the right iliac fossa for the positioning of the stoma and it may have to be put on the left side of the abdomen. The same problem can apply to unilateral amputees whose harness may cross over the preferred stoma site on the right side and consequently the stoma may have to be fashioned on the left side of the abdomen. We have inherited patients who have had the urostomy fashioned at the umbilicus and this usually ends up as a very unsatisfactory urostomy and frequently these have to be resited later, particularly if the patient puts on weight.

The patient's abdomen is examined in the supine position first and then in the standing and sitting positions before the site is chosen. When this is done a pouch half-filled with warm water is placed over the site. Preferably this pouch should be of the disposable type and should be a one-piece bag. It is important to avoid incorporating the accessories when applying the pouch for a trial period. It is psychologically bad for the patient to be encumbered with more than a minimum amount of equipment during his first experience of the appliance. When the pouch has been placed on the abdomen, the patient is encouraged to mobilise himself as much as possible during the first day and to remove the pouch before retiring at night. During that first day, the patient is encouraged to wear his normal street clothes and not his hospital clothes, in order to ascertain if the chosen site is the correct one. The next day the stoma care nurse will equire about the accuracy of the chosen site. Minor adjustments may need to be made to the positioning of the pouch, after which an indelible mark is placed on the skin. If this is not done with such a pen, the chosen site may be lost after the patient has showered or bathed.

Role of the Appliance Consultant or Technician

Most hospitals employ appliance technicians who have knowledge of the availability of appliances, and when the stoma care nurse is not available, these people may be introduced to the patient instead. Appliance consultants are independent contractors with a good deal of experience in the urostomy field and should not be confused with somebody of the same interest who is in fact employed by a manufacturer or supplier (see Role of the Manufacturer's

Agent). The appliance consultant's role is to elaborate on the wide selection of appliances, their availability and their merits or defects. The patient at this stage needs strong reassurance about being able to obtain appliances in a hurry and this the appliance consultant can usually do. Once the patient has left hospital, the hospital does not act as a supplier of appliances, and the responsibility devolves onto the general practitioner. Independent appliance consultants may offer to supply the patient with appliances once the patient has obtained a prescription from his own general practitioner and in practice the arrangement works quite well.

Role of the Manufacturer's Agent

It is bad practice for a manufacturer's agent or supplier to be allowed direct access to the patient in hospital. Inevitably the manufacturer's agents will extol the virtue of their employer's products to the exclusion of their competitors'. These restrictive practices may not be in the patient's best interests. In the United Kingdom, some stoma care nurses are employed by the manufacturers or their suppliers rather than by the hospital or local authority and in this situation, these people lose a measure of independence because of the nature of their employment. In the United States the same sort of system pertains and entero-therapists are often employed solely by one particular manufacturer who is responsible for their salary.

Role of the Hospital Visitor

The patient who has an established urostomy for some years and who is clearly well and active can, if he has the appropriate personality to cope with the task, be trained as a hospital visitor. In the United Kingdom, hospital visitors are usually invited by welfare organisations, such as the Urostomy Association (UA) to undergo a training programme. In the United States, the same programmes are supervised by the Ostomy Association (OA). These programmes are designed to teach the hospital visitor to be tactful and diplomatic, sympathetic and considerate to the patient undergoing surgery. Ideally the hospital visitor should be matched for sex and age with the patients who they are going to visit but matching for occupation and social status can be very difficult. Most hospital visitors, even at the first visit, will usually demonstrate their own stoma and appliance to the potential urostomate. The essence of careful matching of hospital visitor and urostomate is that the patient undergoing surgery is able to identify with the existing urostomate rather than the other way round. The hospital visitor's role is to try to remove by encouragement any inhibition that he may recognise in the potential urostomate. It is axiomatic that the hospital visitor should refrain from relating horror stories about the surgery, the appliances or the stoma that may have come to his attention. It is of enormous encouragement to the patient actually to see somebody with a urostomy leading a normal life and demonstrating confidence and positiveness in their lifestyle. These hospital visitors are also in a good position to advise the patient about the welfare organisations if this has not already been done by the stoma care nurse.

Training programmes are run by some of the welfare organisations to help select and train urostomates for the role of hospital visitor. It can be difficult to persuade chosen urostomates to undergo a training programme in order to become an approved hospital visitor but such reticent people usually make very good hospital visitors and from our experience are willing to visit patients in hospital and in their homes regularly. Unfortunately the urostomates who volunteer freely and brashly for the role of hospital visitor (and in doing so run down the value of the training programme) are almost certainly the very people who should be prevented from visiting hospitals. Some organisations and hospitals require the hospital visitor to have satisfactorily completed a training programme before being allowed access to patients.

Role of Relatives

At the pre-operative stage it is usually not necessary to involve the patient's relatives in the details of the stoma and appliance. This can come in the post-operative period when the patient is coping with his changed body image and is beginning to talk about his appliance and stoma (usually during visiting time). Introducing the relatives to the patient's stoma can, in certain instances, cause more upset and anguish to the relatives than it ever did to the patient. It is good practice to allow the stoma care nurse to introduce the relatives to the patient's stoma. The reaction of the relatives to the stoma depends on the relationship between the patient and his relatives and also the extent to which the relatives are willing to be supportive. There is always apprehension about relatives who openly declare support but decline the invitation to be shown the stoma. Some women prefer that their husbands are not shown the stoma, at least while they are in hospital. This stance can be interpreted in varying ways but it usually means an independent attitude and positive determination on the part of the patient to succeed on her own. Parents of children who are undergoing urinary diversion are introduced to the stoma and appliance very early on because it is initially the parents who will end up by managing the stoma and appliance rather than the child.

Operating Theatre Procedure

Before the start of the operation making a scratch mark with a scalpel over the chosen site which has already been identified with a pen is good practice because inevitably during surgery the indelible skin mark will be erased. From the patient's point of view, the most important aspect of the surgical procedure is the appearance of his urostomy. At the end of a long operation, it may be tempting for the surgeon to delegate the closing of the abdominal wound and the fashioning of a urostomy to one of his assistants but we would strongly counsel against delegating the fashioning of the stoma.

Some surgeons have a preference for actually fashioning the spout when the ileal loop is still wholly within the abdomen and others prefer to site the stoma first and then evert it afterwards. When the everted stoma is sitting proudly in place, there will inevitably be a certain amount of blood oozing between the sutures that have secured the everted mucosa to the skin. If, as is common, the uretero-ileal anastomosis has been fashioned over splinting tubes, these will project from the stoma for about 10 cm. By now the patient should be well hydrated and urine should be emanating from both splinting tubes.

The abdominal wound closure should be completed before the stoma is finally dressed. In those cases where tension sutures have been used (particularly after the patient has received a course of radiotherapy) it may be necessary to apply a gauze dressing to the wound, but in other circumstances a narrow adhesive dressing should be applied over the wound. Abdominal and pelvic drainage tubes should be sited on the contralateral side to the stoma. The peristomal skin should be cleaned and dried with a gauze swab and covered with a swab while the appliance is being prepared for positioning.

It has always been our practice to use the same procedure at the end of the operation for dressing the stoma. Stomahesive is favoured as the skin protective and then a Hollister urostomy bag is applied on top of the Stomahesive. When the stoma care nurse will have used a trial urostomy pouch to assess the site of the stoma, we always request that she uses a Hollister bag because this is the one the patients will see when they recover from their operations. Stomahesive, which no longer comes sterile, needs to have an aperture cut in its centre with curved scissors. In the first instance the aperture should be cut no bigger than about two-thirds the requirement. Because of the effect that the fat in the mesentery has on the shape of the stoma, there is usually nothing symmetrical about a newly fashioned stoma and although one can sometimes cut out quite a reasonable circular aperture, the fit is rarely perfect. When the aperture has been cut, six radial cuts are made into the aperture for a distance of 5–7 mm. The white backing paper is removed from the Stomahesive, exposing the adhesive surface. The gauze swab which has been covering the stoma is then pressed a little into the peristomal tissues to encourage any further oozing in the abdominal stomal site to seep out. Care must be taken in performing this manoeuvre to ensure that the mucocutaneous sutures do not disrupt. The two ureteric splints are then lifted from the abdominal wall and the Stomahesive is placed over the splints and the stoma. By applying circumferential pressure the Stomahesive is secured to the abdominal skin. If the surgeon has been reasonably accurate in the sizing and shaping of the aperture, then those parts of the Stomahesive between the radial cuts will sit up like a collar around the stoma and protect it. This collar of Stomahesive protects the delicate stoma from the flange of the urostomy bag. In placing the Stomahesive it may be necessary to overlap the edge of the wound dressing that has previously been applied.

Our preference is to choose a 30-cm Hollister urostomy bag with a flange diameter of 42 mm. The transparent cellophane and Karaya gum are removed from the back of the face plate (it is unnecessary to use Stomahesive and Karaya gum at the same time). The front surface of the pouch is pinched forward to allow air into the bag and the white backing paper is removed from the adhesive face plate. The face plate of the bag is almost the same size as the Stomahesive sheet and can be made to fit quite easily over the stomahesive sheet. Before this is done, the two ureteric splints are inserted into the bag and pointed towards the outlet tap. The adhesive surface of the face plate adheres to the non-adhesive shiny surface of the Stomahesive. Very often the free top margin of the urostomy bag overlaps the wound dressing and it is advisable to stick down the free edge of the bag to the wound dressing using sleek. In the immediate post-operative period peristomal bleeding can occur and track underneath the Stomahesive, lifting it off and with it the urostomy bag. By using a piece of sleek as described above to secure the urostomy bag, this hazard of displacing the pouch can be reduced but not totally eliminated. The outlet of the urostomy bag usually comes in the shut situation and does not have to be interfered with initially.

At surgery it is our preference to place the long axis of the urostomy pouch (which is V-shaped) at right angles to the long axis of the patient. For the first 48 hours the urinary output is monitored every hour by the nursing staff and it is easier for the nurses to gain access to the urostomy outlet if the bag is at right angles to the patient's body. In this situation, the outlet tap will lie on the bed by the patient's flank and will not be lying in the groin area or between the patient's legs, which might mean disturbing the patient from sleep in order to measure the urine and empty the pouch. If the bag is placed in the long axis of the patient's body, this may have the effect of kinking the bag but it is usually only a problem in the first couple of days. Some surgeons prefer to attach the urostomy pouch to a night extension bag immediately after surgery. There are arguably two good reasons why this should not be done. If the nurses are having to empty the urostomy pouch every hour in the immediate post-operative period, they can also check on the colour of the stoma and report any adverse change. Also, mucus production is very often maximal in the first couple of days and the outlet tube may become blocked, which means that the pouch will fill with urine but not the uribag at the patient's bedside. This renders the night extension tubing and uribag redundant. If Karaya gum has been used when the first pouch is placed around the stoma, it will melt quite quickly and have the effect of adding to the nurses' problems on deciding whether the stoma has changed in colour from a healthy red or pink to foreboding dark brown or black. For this reason it is inadvisable to use Karaya gum in the immediate post-operative period. The nurses' problems in assessing stoma colour are further compounded by bleeding and clot formation around the stoma, added to which any mucus that emanates from the urostomy site will probably tend to lie on top of the stoma, obscuring the nurses' vision of the very mucosa which they wish to inspect.

Immediate Post-operative Care

In the immediate post-operative period numerous factors, excluding accidents, influence the number of times the urostomy appliance is changed by the nursing staff. When the wound dressing is changed of necessity, some nurses feel the need to tidy up the patient's abdomen and are unable to resist the temptation to change the urostomy appliance at the same time. As these patients are frequently in high dependency areas we rely on the indigenous staff to look after the patients and tend not to involve the stoma care nurses or urology-ward nurses at this stage. Probably the main factor that determines why the bags are changed so often is their appearance. If it is blood-stained or tacky that is often a very good reason for changing it. Mucus which the patients produce in great quantity at this stage may easily block the outlet, which cannot be unblocked by a toothpick. We have now reluctantly come to accept that it is almost impossible to enforce our policy of leaving the initial bag on for at least 48 hours.

After 48 hours or so the patient usually returns to the urology ward from the high-dependency ward. By now the patient is usually feeling well enough to sit out of bed and the stoma care nurse takes over the management of the patient's stoma and appliance. It is entirely at the discretion of the stoma care nurse as to which is the best type of appliance for that particular patient.

The stoma care nurse at this stage usually encourages the patient by telling him that his stoma is doing well and that in a few more days the splinting tubes and the mucocutaneous sutures will be removed. If leakage is a major problem, however, it might be best to attach a night extension tube and uribag to the end of the pouch so that any urine emanating from the splinting tubes and urostomy will be drained away immediately thus minimising leaking hazards. Thereby, the peristomal skin may not be subjected to so many pouch changes with the associated trauma which occurs each time the Stomahesive and face plate have to be removed and replaced.

Patient Involvement in Changing Appliances

By the time the splinting tubes have been removed (about the 10th day) the patient is usually identifying with the stoma and at this point we start the training programme under the supervision of the stoma care nurse. At first the patient is introduced to the barrier cream and then the urostomy bag and when he is familiar with these he progresses to apply them himself over his stoma. The experience of the stoma care nurse is very important here because she may recognise that a particular pouch is not to a patient's liking. By now the patient is mobile and so when he is walking around the ward he gets the feel of being happy with his bag. We have never yet had to ask a patient how he is getting on with his instruction. Just as soon as the patient has adequately positioned his first pouch and it has stayed on, he will volunteer the information immediately coupled with the request to be given a discharge date. It is then that we know that the patient has succeeded in accepting the stoma and appliance.

Discharge Home

At the time of discharge from hospital the patient is given at least 2 weeks' supply of the appliance of his preference. In the United Kingdom an exemption certificate can be obtained by the patient which allows him to obtain all his appliances and medicines pertinent to the urostomy free of charge. An application form (number FP91) is issued by the Department of Health in the United Kingdom and can be obtained from any Post Office. Once the form has been completed by the patient or the relative it needs to be countersigned by the general practitioner or the hospital doctor for the patient to obtain the necessary exemption certificate from the local Family Practitioner Committee. Patients are given a list of equipment of their own choice together with the sizes and catalogue numbers. The patient retains one copy, the second copy is sent to the general practitioner and the stoma care nurse frequently keeps the third copy or alternatively it is kept in the patient's hospital records. We prefer not to discharge patients at the weekend but rather at the beginning of the week. This policy has the advantage that the stoma care nurse can usually visit the patient the day following discharge, whereas if the patient is discharged home at the weekend, the particular nurse may not be available to look after him at the weekend. When the patients come from an area outside the hospital's sphere of influence the stoma care nurse usually contacts her counterpart in the patient's home area and asks that nurse to make a domiciliary visit within 24 hours of the discharge home. By now the hospital visitor will have come to see the patient in the post-operative period and will probably make a domiciliary visit in the first few days after the patient's discharge. Provided a relationship has developed between the hospital visitor and the patient, an early home visit is always found to be of great comfort to the patient.

Principle of Appliance Change

In those situations where a surgeon finds himself without a stoma care nurse, an appliance consultant or technician of expertise, he himself or his ward sister will probably have to take on the responsibility of instructing the patient in using the appliance and changing it. He may also have to undertake part of the training programme for the patient before his discharge home. In these circumstances the following principles apply.

1. The appliance should be changed in the early morning before fluids are taken and while the patient is relatively dehydrated
2. Although the patient will at first be instructed in the technique of appliance changing while sitting up in bed, in time the patient will probably change the appliance standing in front of a mirror in his own home
3. The new appliance should be prepared before the old one is removed and in doing so the new pouch, skin-protective barrier cream, paper tissues and cleansing substances should all be set aside on a suitable surface within easy reach of the patient standing in front of the mirror. New appliance preparation may involve cutting out an aperture in the appliance or cutting an aperture in the skin-protective substances or preparing the size of adhesives to fit the orifice of the flange. Scissors to carry out such adjustments are commercially available from the appliance manufacturers for such purposes
4. Before the old pouch is removed it is emptied of urine. The bag together with the skin protective is removed after any restraining devices such as a belt or pressure plate have been removed first. The old pouch should not be discarded down the WC but placed in a receptacle, preparatory to being disposed of according to local health regulations
5. The stoma is wiped with tissue paper or gauze and then wrapped in the same material
6. Any "skin cement" must then be removed with the appropriate cleanser, tissue paper or gauze
7. The peristomal skin is then washed in soapy water and thoroughly dried
8. A non-greasy skin barrier cream such as Chiron Barrier Cream (Downs) is thoroughly rubbed into the peristomal skin and the residue wiped off using

tissue paper or gauze. The adhesive can be then applied over the prepared skin. Alternatively, a skin protective such as Stomahesive, Hollihesive, Comfeel or Seal-a-peel may be applied over the prepared skin instead

9. The pouch is then centred over the stoma and stuck down onto the adhesive by firm pressure. The flange of the disposable appliance is secured using Micropore or some similar tape. Finally the pressure place and belt are secured

Reusable Device – Two-Piece

A reusable device differs in many ways from the disposable device (described above) and frequently the two-piece device is preferred.
   The following considerations then apply.

1. The care of the flange is very important because the flange must be clean, free of adhesive substance and dry
2. The base of the flange is painted with Tincture Benzoin Co using either gauze or a brush until the surface is tacky
3. The double-sided adhesive is then applied to the tacky flange. It is very important that air bubbles and creases are eliminated from the two adhering surfaces as either can be responsible for leakage
4. A commercially available centralising tube is filled with tissue paper and placed over the stoma in order to soak up any moisture and urine during the preparation of the peristomal skin. The skin is prepared with either a barrier cream or a spray such as Tincture Benzoin Co. If the skin is tender, Tincture Benzoin Co should not be used. The flange and adhesive are then picked up. The second side of the adhesive is bared of its paper and the flange is threaded over the centralising tube and secured to the peristomal skin. The flange may need to be further secured to the skin using kidney-shaped seals or tape. The pressure plate and belt are now applied and the centralising tube removed
5. The rubber bag is then applied to the flange and this is done by slipping the bottom half of the opening in the rubber bag underneath the flange and then stretching the rest of the opening around the flange
6. Irrespective of whether a disposable or reusable appliance is being used it may be necessary, particularly in men, to shave the hairs from the peristomal area. Scissors can sometimes be equally effective in removing the hairs but if the skin is shaved it is preferable to use an electric shaver rather than a safety razor which tends to damage the skin and take off some of the top layers of cells. It may be necessary to use solvents to remove "skin cement". Acetone or Zoff are commonly used preparations but they must be used sparingly as they can irritate the skin and must never be allowed to come into contact with the stoma as they can set up a severe reaction in the stoma. Some of these substances are flammable

It is important to point out to the patient that the size of the stoma imme-diately after surgery will not be its final size and therefore the size of the aperture in the pouch will need to be reduced in time. Usually the final size is achieved at 2–3 months after surgery but sometimes there is quite a reduction in the stoma size in the first couple of weeks after surgery and the patient will need to be made aware of this possibility.

Stoma Clinics

These special clinics have been introduced in the last few years and may be for ileostomy, colostomy or urostomy patients or alternatively can be specialised for one of the subgroups. They are usually held in hospital clinics but sometimes, for the patients' convenience, in health centres. They are usually attended by the stoma care nurse, the appliance consultant or technician and, if in a hospital, by the consultant urologist. Attendance should not be delegated to junior staff because most of the junior assistants only have a fleeting acquaintance with urostomy appliances. It is our practice to hold these clinics every 2–3 months but of course in the interim periods the patients can attend the ordinary urology clinics if necessary.

Usually the appliance consultant or technician will have available most of the different manufacturers' products, so that on the advice or recommendation of the consultant urologist, the stoma care nurse or in fact the appliance consultant, a patient may be offered a different appliance to the one that he was using when he came to the clinic. In this situation the decision to alter the patient's appliance is not made from any commercial motive.

Associations and Institutions

Urostomy Association

In 1956 the Ileostomy Association of Great Britain and Ireland (IA) was established in Birmingham and for many years this patient self-help welfare association looked after the interests of people with ileostomies, colostomies and urostomies. In 1971 the Urinary Conduit Association (UCA) was founded in Manchester and this organisation gradually took over responsibility for the urostomy patients who were already members of the IA and for new patients who came to surgery in the 1970s and 1980s. In 1984 the Urinary Conduit Association changed its name to the Urostomy Association (UA). The Colostomy Association was established in 1967 so in the United Kingdom there exist three separate organisations for patients with different types of diversions. The three organisations work closely together, particulary in the field of publicity and fund raising. The Ileostomy Association continues to look after urostomates who live in parts of the country where the UA is not established. By contrast, in the United States there is one organisation, the Ostomy Association, which looks after all three categories of patients. This situation pertains in most other Western countries. The welfare organisations provide tremendous support for their members who must first of all possess a stoma but members of the medical and nursing professions in addition to the manufacturers' representatives can be associate members of the organisations. Over the years the organisations have had a considerable influence in modifying public opinion and bringing to the attention of the public the fact that people with diversions can lead normal lives. In practice most patients are invited to join the pertinent welfare organisation at about the time that they are having surgery and they are usually introduced to the concept of the associations by the hospital visitor or alternatively the stoma care nurse.

International Ostomy Association

In 1975 the first meeting of the International Ostomy Association (IOA) took place in Amsterdam. Very few countries attended the inaugural meeting but there are now 45 registered countries of the IOA. The IOA exists to monitor and advise member nations on how patients with stoma problems ought to be helped. A recent survey by the IOA into the availability of appliances in various countries has shown marked differences in governments' attitudes to appliances. The IOA is contemplating devolving itself into Regional Associations throughout the world because it feels that this new system will become more efficient.

World Congress of Entero-Therapists

The World Congress of Entero-Therapists (WCET) has a wide membership among the nations of the world. The international meetings act as a forum for the dissemination of product information, skills and expertise in the field of stoma care. Unfortunately, there are still many countries in the world where stoma care nurses have not yet been recognised and do not really exist and in these situations it is very much the province of the ordinary trained nurse to look after stoma patients. The contribution of the WCET has probably been greater than that of the IOA in getting the message across that those with stomas, particularly in the Third World, are not freaks, can lead relatively normal lives and be accepted by their societies.

British Standards Institution

A subcommittee of the British Standards Institution (BSI) which is a member of the International Standards Organisation (ISO) is looking into the standardisation and reproducibility of products used in urostomy care. This committee's (SGC/47) work is bedevilled with problems about standardisation and definitions and it will be some time before minimum standards can be agreed within the BSI with a view to making a proposal to the ISO. Attempts by the BSI to standardise urostomy equipment is a welcome step but there remains a large gap between the manufacturers' interests and those of the consumers, represented by the urologists who themselves have no commercial interests in products. Unfortunately, there is little immediate hope of standardisation.

However, when standardisation has been agreed it will be enormously to the patients' benefit and should prevent the flooding of the market place with unacceptable appliances.

Other Surgical Considerations

Patient Selection and Suitability

It is really outside the remit of this chapter to talk about patient selection and suitability but the dexterity of the patient must be taken into account in recommending urinary diversion surgery, particularly if the patient lives alone. Patients suffering from multiple sclerosis, spinal injuries and rheumatoid arthritis may not have the necessary dexterity to change their appliances and in these situations it is particularly important to make sure that their relatives or the people looking after them will be available to change an appliance at fairly short notice should an accident occur.

Different Urostomy Types

Most of the remarks in this chapter apply to ileal loop urostomies. However the principles for colonic loop urostomies are the same. In most patients who have single ureterostomies, the ureterostomy will end up flush with the abdominal wall and a one-piece bag such as a Coloplast bag is usually ideal for these people. One simply fashions an aperture in the face plate and applies the one-piece bag over the urostomy site. There are other people who have both ureters brought out together at the one site in the abdominal wall. This situation usually pertains in older children who because of the effects of spina bifida or a spinal abnormality undergo urinary diversion. Their ureters may be found to be dilated at the time of surgery and this finding obviates the need for an ileal or colonic conduit. The single-stem ureter or the double-barrel ureters are everted and a cuff is fashioned so that the urostomy sits up like a spout. Thus, a urostomy appliance as for an ileal conduit can be used. However, as the children grow, the ureters retract and the urostomy will end up being flush with the abdominal wall and so a single piece appliance will be required in later life.

Some patients are unfortunate and have to have not only a urostomy fashioned but also a colostomy. In these people it is not uncommon to find that they use one manufacturer's products for the urostomy and a different manufacturer's for the colostomy.

Continent Urostomies

The Kock continent urostomy is increasingly being fashioned by urologists throughout the world. This differs from the ileal loop or colonic loop in that the patient catheterises the loop several times a day. There is no need to wear a urostomy pouch unless the operation has not worked. In that situation a one-piece urostomy appliance is usually used until corrective surgery can be performed. Normally the patients catheterise themselves using a catheter inserted through the stoma in the abdominal wall. When they have completed their urine excavation, they merely cover over the urostomy with a piece of micropore or similar material.

Non-surgical Considerations

Pregnancy

A urostomy is not in itself a bar to becoming pregnant and having a normal delivery. Hormonal changes in pregnancy can affect the skin and these changes have the effect of inhibiting appliances sticking to the skin; consequently the appliances need to be changed more frequently and additional skin adhesives may be necessary to help keep the bags in place. As the abdomen enlarges the urostomy will almost certainly change shape and it is probably best for the patient to try a softer more moldable flange. There are not usually any problems with the stoma during delivery either by natural birth or Caesarean section. In the post partum period, as the abdomen subsides, the stoma reduces in size. These alterations mean that the bag changes have to be carried out more frequently. After delivery, hormone changes can affect the greasiness of the skin causing adhesion problems. It is usually advised that the bag should be emptied before feeding, especially breast feeding, because an active baby can easily dislodge a pouch and cause it to leak.

Drugs

There is no doubt that certain drugs affect the adhesiveness of the peristomal skin. These include anticoagulants and the fertility drug Clomid. Individual patients complain that drugs that they are taking affect skin adhesiveness but so far no other identifiable drug group has emerged that can be implicated in causing problems with skin adhesiveness. Teenage girls frequently complain that at the time of menstruation they have great difficulty in keeping their pouches in place but this problem seems to be less noticeable as they grow into adult life.

Religious Considerations

In some parts of the world it is very important to enquire whether the siting of the stoma on the abdominal wall offends religious beliefs. It may be that the stoma has to be sited above the umbilicus and only in this situation will the patient accept a stoma. This pertains not only for urostomies but also for ileostomies and colostomies. In some religions the left hand is considered to be unclean and the right hand may not be used for attending to the stoma. In some religions cleansing of the orifices is carried out before praying can commence and this can cause problems for patients who have a urostomy because if they pray several times a day it may mean that in order to comply with their religious beliefs they have to change the pouch each time. In these situations they are recommended to speak to their religious leaders who are usually very understanding and point out that medical necessity prevails over religious belief. If the patient's religious beliefs are not taken into account and a stoma is fashioned below the level of the umbilicus then this may so offend the patient that he may not want to pray at all because he considers himself unclean.

Seat Belts

In many parts of the world the use of seat belts is compulsory. Following the introduction in the United Kingdom of legislation making seat belts compulsory for people sitting in the front seats of motor cars, the stoma welfare organisation lobbied the Department of Health and Social Security and Members of Parliament about the particular problems stoma patients have. It is now possible for stoma patients to be issued with certificates exempting them from wearing seat belts. If the urostomate is driving a car then the diagonal part of the seat belt may in fact not interfere too much with either the stoma or the appliance but the horizontal strap of the belt may well do so. Arguably it is preferable to have a stoma injury rather than run the risk of a severe head or neck injury. Many patients who obtain an exemption certificate use the certificate for local driving only, but apply the seat belts when travelling on motorways and highways in order to minimise the risk of severe injury to other parts of the body.

Travel

It is advisable when urostomates travel abroad that they keep their supply of appliances with them at all times in their hand luggage. The appliance equipment should not be placed in the main suitcase for fear of the latter being lost in transit. Sufficient appliance equipment should be taken to last throughout the holiday. The hand luggage will be checked at the security baggage check before boarding. It is advisable for the urostomates to carry a list of the equipment that they are carrying in order to show to the security officer or alternatively to obtain a travel certificate from the Central Office of the Urostomy Association. This document, which vouches that the traveller has a urostomy, needs to be signed by a medical practitioner. The urostomate should have a small travel bag with him containing the items necessary to change his appliance en route. However, under no circumstances should a urostomate take inflammable solvents in the cabin with him. When booking he should request an aisle seat close to the toilet.

Road travel is usually less of a problem. It is advisable for urostomates to use any toilets along the motorway or highway in case there are any unexpected and unscheduled stops that might cause embarrassment. Long distance coach journeys in vehicles without toilet facilities may present problems.

In these situations it is probably preferable for urostomates to sit by a window seat and connect the pouch to a night extension drainage bag which can be placed in a holdall on the floor out of sight.

When staying in hotels it is essential to ensure that the urostomate's supplies are secure and to observe the manufacturer's advice about storage. The appliances should be kept in a cool place which is frequently the bathroom and this is particularly so in warm climates. It is important for the urostomate to keep up a high intake of fluid when in a hot climate in order to minimise problems such as renal infection.

Within the European Community there are many health agreements which entitle urostomates to free emergency treatment. To obtain this treatment they must carry with them form E111 which is available from the local DoH office. There is also an accompanying leaflet SA36 entitled "How to get treatment in other European countries", which gives precise details on what treatment is free and what patients have to pay for.

Envoi

The urostomate must be persuaded that it is in his best interests to become the supreme authority on his own stoma and appliance. However, this philosophy should never be allowed to permit the medical and nursing professions to shirk their responsibility for stoma care. Unless the patients are severely handicapped, they must be prevented from allowing their spouses to take on the responsibility for looking after the urostomy excretory function. After all, before the diversion surgery was carried out, the patients were not in the habit of being accompanied by their spouses to the lavatory. However harsh this philosophy may appear from time to time in clinical practice, it should be impressed upon the urostomate to regard it as the norm rather than the exception.

Urostomy Association
Central Office
Buckland
Beaumont Park
Danbury
Essex CM3 4DE

Telephone: 024-541 4294

Chapter 9

Penile Prostheses

J.P. Pryor

The implantation of a paired penile prosthesis into impotent men is a simple procedure, usually without serious complications, and can greatly improve the quality of life for both the patient and his partner. The success of these operations is not disputed but depends upon the correct selection of patients who have a realistic expectation for the procedure. The surgery itself is straight-forward but should be carried out with a minimum of tissue trauma in order to lessen the risk of infection. The overall success rate is 90% but in some groups of patients it will be much higher.

Patient Selection

There is a tendency to replace the term "impotence", or the inability of a man to initiate and sustain penile erection sufficient to allow penetration and orgasm, with the more embracing and less threatening term "erectile dysfunction". The latter term covers a wider spectrum of sexual disorders but should not broaden the indications for a penile prosthesis. Those patients with irreversible organic impotence are the prime candidates for operation and Table 9.1 summarises the indications for operation in a collected series of men who have had a prosthesis.

Diagnosis of Organic Impotence

The diagnosis of organic impotence may be made on the basis of the clinical history and examination and the injection of a vasoactive agent into the corpus cavernosus. A characteristic of organic impotence is that the erectile deficiency is constant with all forms of sexual activity, during sleep and on waking in the morning, and that orgasm and ejaculation may be preserved despite the lack of erection. Variability in the quality of erection is much more likely in

Table 9.1. Indications for penile prosthesis in
collected series of 3884 men

Condition	% of cases
Diabetes	25.6
Vasculogenic causes	19.5
Peyronie's disease	6.2
Post priapism	1.0
Pelvic trauma	7.5
Pelvic surgery	15.9
Spinal injury	5.1
Psychological	7.8
Other causes	11.8

psychogenic impotence, particularly if the erectile failure varies with the sexual
partner or at the time of vaginal penetration.

Enquiries should be made as to the general health of the patient and in
particular as to the use of any medication or drug abuse including alcohol and
tobacco. The harmful effect of smoking has been demonstrated in both animal
experiments and as a high-risk factor in impotent men (Virag et al. 1985). The
presence of marital disharmony or other stress factors may be apparent and the
possibility of depression noted. Most impotent men are convinced that their
problems are organic in nature whereas the doctor knows that there is always a
functional element. It is impossible to give any useful figure for the relative
incidence of the various causes of impotence since those centres which undertake a full diagnostic screening usually have a referral practice. In a study of 86
consecutive patients seen during a 3-month period at St. Peter's Hospital,
approximately 60% of patients were unable to have intercourse for predom-
inantly psychogenic reasons although in some of these the quality of erection
was less than perfect due to vasculogenic factors. It is important to examine the
man thoroughly in order to convince him that there is no underlying disease. A
latent carcinoma of the prostate is detected in about 1% of men by the routine
rectal examination.

The history and examination may provide evidence for the nature of the
impotence and in all patients it is advisable to check the plasma testosterone
level to exclude hypogonadism and also to exclude diabetes, the incidence of
each being about 1%. The diagnosis of vasculogenic or neurogenic impotence
may be suspected from the history and is confirmed by investigation.

Vasculogenic Impotence

A history of incomplete erections under all circumstances is suggestive of
vascular impotence, particularly if the patient is an obese diabetic who smokes
and gives a history of hypertension, ischaemic heart disease or peripheral
vascular disease (Virag et al. 1985). Some variation in the quality of erection
during intercourse may occur in those patients with the gluteal steal syndrome

(Michal et al. 1978) but this is uncommon. Major vessel disease is a rare cause of impotence in urological practice and may be detected by abnormalities of the femoral pulses or abdominal bruits. The detection of penile pulses using a simple Doppler technique and the measurement of penile blood pressure correlate poorly with erectile capacity and have been abandoned and replaced by the intracorporal injection of a vasoactive agent for screening purposes. Virag et al. (1984) demonstrated that the local injection of papaverine into the corpus cavernosus would induce an erection and Brindley (1983) demonstrated that alpha adenoreceptor blocking agents had a similar effect. These agents may be injected for diagnostic purposes and are useful in distinguishing vasculogenic and psychogenic impotence, two categories which often coexist and of which it is difficult to distinguish the relative importance. The initiation of full tumescence following intracavernosal injection of 80-mg papaverine excludes a significant vascular cause for impotence and is a useful screening test (Buvat et al. 1986; Strachan and Pryor 1987; Zentgraf et al. 1988). An impaired response is suggestive of vasculogenic impotence and further investigation is required to distinguish between arteriogenic and venogenic causes. It should be noted that a false-negative response rate of up to 10% may occur in those patients who are anxious (Buvat et al. 1986) and the response should always be correlated with the clinical history. It seems that the incidence of false-negative response is less when prostaglandin E_1 is used and there is also less risk of inducing a prolonged erection with this drug.

A full evaluation of the penile blood supply is necessary in those patients who are candidates for revascularisation (that is less than 40 years of age, non-smokers and not diabetic) or venous surgery. Ultrasound-directed Doppler studies of the penile vessels provide the best methods for studying penile blood flow and the newer apparatus with colour coding is a major advance (Lue et al. 1985) even though expensive.

Venogenic impotence is detected by cavernosometry (Virag et al. 1984; Wespes et al. 1986) and this should be performed following the relaxation of the cavernosus smooth muscle by the injection of vasoactive agents. Five patterns of response have been noted (Dickinson and Pryor 1989). The failure to induce full tumescence despite high flow rates is indicative of veno-occlusive dysfunction. Cavernosography has a small role in such patients as it only opacifies the normal venous drainage and there is now a realisation that the cavernosus smooth muscle is abnormal rather than there being a primary abnormality of the veins.

In the past, abnormalities of the corporal bodies usually occurred following priapism: the early resolution of a priapism – preferably by medical means – is essential if corporal fibrosis is to be prevented. Some impairment of function is common after a priapism and there is always a psychological component. Surgical intervention should not be considered for post-priapism impotence until there has been a return of orgasm and ejaculation. It is worthwhile excluding a patent shunt causing impotence as the closure of this may restore potency. A penile prosthesis is indicated in those patients with extensive fibrosis although the operation may be difficult. Cavernous fibrosis may occur after penile trauma or in some patients with Peyronie's disease.

Patients with irreversible vasculogenic impotence, be it due to arterial insufficiency, corporal fibrosis or veno-occlusive dysfunction are the largest group of patients requiring a penile prosthesis.

Neurogenic Impotence

Neurogenic impotence may be diagnosed from the history and is usually associated with obvious neurological problems such as spinal injury, multiple sclerosis or following radical pelvic surgery. It is more difficult to diagnose neurogenic impotence in patients with a lumbar disc lesion or a peripheral neuropathy especially as impotence may be the first evidence of a peripheral neuropathy in diabetics. Patients with neurogenic impotence often obtain full tumescence with a reduced dose of intracavernous vasoactive agents. This may not occur in diabetic neuropathy as many of these patients also have vasculogenic problems. Tests of autonomic function (Fowler et al. 1988) may be useful and when there is doubt it may be necessary to monitor the erections that occur during sleep.

Nocturnal penile tumescence (NPT) occurs three or four times each night during "rapid eye movement" (REM) sleep and may be monitored by placing two – to eliminate artefacts – strain gauges around the proximal and distal parts of the penis. It is necessary for the patient to sleep undisturbed and this is often difficult in a strange environment such as a hospital or sleep laboratory. Home monitoring machines have been developed to reduce these problems and also to contain costs. Nocturnal penile tumescence was once the gold standard for the diagnosis of organic impotence and our understanding of it owes much to the work of Karacan (Karacan and Moore 1987). The necessity for the test has been reduced by the use of intracorporal papaverine, especially as it is recognised that false-positives may arise due to the penis increasing in size but not being sufficiently rigid to permit intercourse. In an attempt to overcome this problem, it is now possible to monitor the increase in penile size and rigidity (Bradley et al. 1985).

Psychogenic Factors

Most men with an erectile problem become anxious but a full psychological evaluation is not always necessary in those patients with an obvious organic cause for the impotence. In contrast, in those patients where the causation is uncertain, particularly so far as the patient is concerned, psychosexual counselling is advisable.

Men with psychological impotence require psychological advice and this may be given by psychosexual counsellors, psychiatrists or psychologists. Patients with psychogenic impotence should not be implanted until they have been thoroughly treated and assessed by two different therapists, preferably of different background and outlook. The role of a penile prosthesis in psychogenic impotence remains a matter of debate and surgeons should exercise caution as there is an increased risk of patient dissatisfaction. Many patients with psychogenic impotence fail to respond to treatment and may be considered candidates for the operation. The operation is essentially destructive as it destroys the normal corpus cavernosus and in younger patients it may be better to implant a single prosthesis in the hope that potency may improve at a later date. Despite these warnings, many patients with psychological impotence benefit from the procedure.

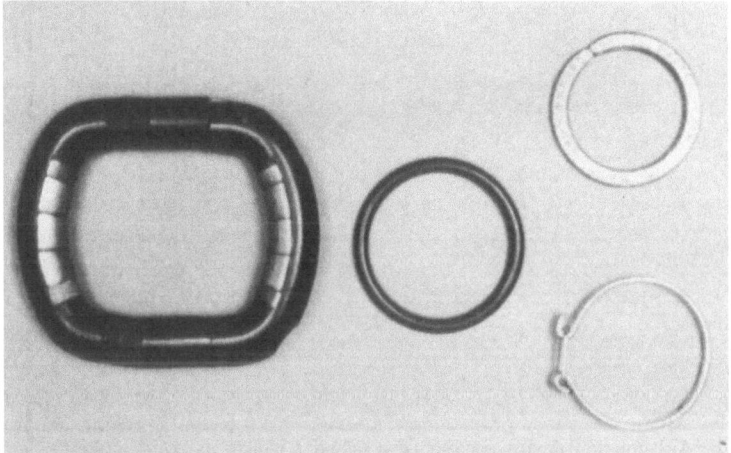

Fig. 9.1.   Constriction rings that have been used around the penis.

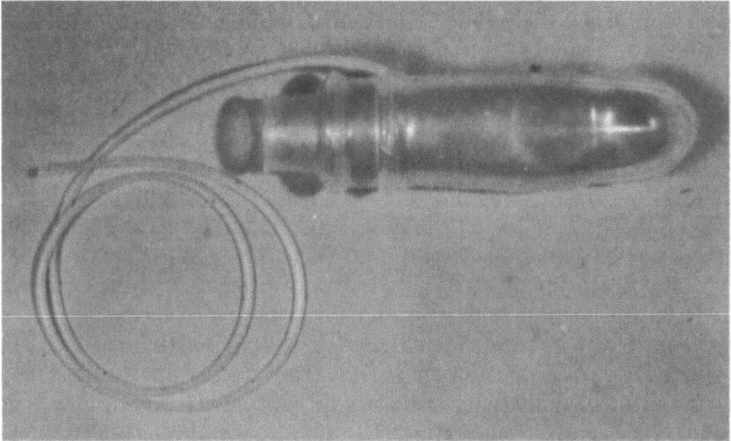

Fig. 9.2.   Correctaid suction device to produce erection. It is worn during intercourse.

Choice of Patient for Operation

Those patients who are judged to have irreversible organic impotence, or who
have failed with psychological treatment, are candidates for the implantation of
a penile prosthesis. It is rarely necessary to exclude patients on the grounds of
fitness to undergo the operation as the procedure may be performed using local
or regional anaesthesia. Severe myocardial insufficiency causes the greatest
difficulty and some men would prefer to proceed with the operation even
though the risks may be increased.

Patients should be informed of alternative methods of management and this
includes external aids to assist erection. For many years a variety of rings (Fig.

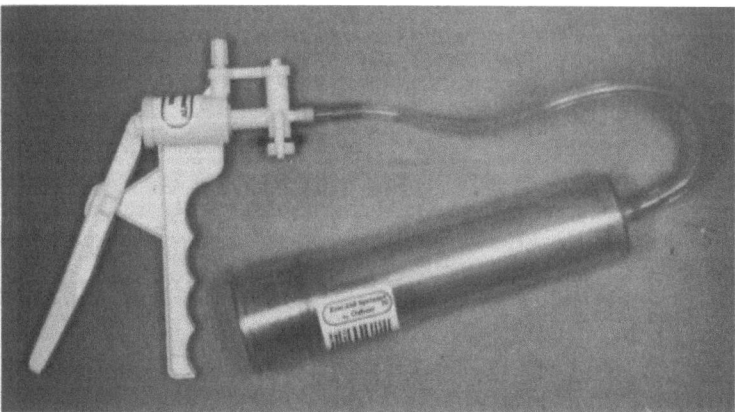

Fig. 9.3. The ErecAid erection device consists of a cylinder which fits over the penis and a mechanical pump to create the vacuum. The erection is maintained by a plastic band which is placed around the penis and the cylinder is then removed.

9.1) have been available by mail order or from sex shops and some men have experimented with home-made constricting devices. Gerow devised a "super condom" suction device with the objective of preventing penile contraction following the removal of an infected penile prosthesis. This device is marketed as the Correctaid (Fig. 9.2).

A vacuum device to create an erection was patented in the United States in 1917 (Nadig et al. 1986) but it was not until 1986 that the use of such devices attracted attention. Many versions (Fig. 9.3) have been produced since that time, with many reports of their successful use (Wiles 1988; Witherington 1989; Korenman et al. 1990; Turner et al. 1990). It would appear that these devices are most effective in the presence of a good arterial inflow of blood.

Many patients elect not to proceed with an operation on the grounds that they are too old or unfit, do not wish to have an operation, or that such techniques are unnatural. These factors vary in different societies and are changing constantly as a result of changes in public opinion – usually due to television. There is no purpose in trying to persuade a patient to proceed with an operation although education and counselling may influence the decision. The patient should usually be seen with his partner before the final decision is made, and it is advisable that there should be an interval between the discussion of an implant and the final decision and operation. In some patients it is desirable to insert a prosthesis at the time of surgery of malignancy (Bennett 1982), e.g., radical cystectomy, whilst in others it is useful to insert the reservoir of an inflatable prosthesis whilst closing the abdominal wound.

It is essential for patients to have a realistic expectation for the operation. The penile prosthesis provides sufficient rigidity to permit vaginal penetration but it is not possible to guarantee sexual satisfaction. The patient should be informed that the penis remains at its flaccid length and only with an inflatable prosthesis is there any increase in girth. Most patients, and their partners, obtain sexual gratification but there are some who find sexual intercourse with a prosthesis unsatisfying. It is important for the patient to realise that an implant does not restore normality and this is particularly important in those men with functional impotence or with vasculogenic problems, particularly if coitus is possible but the erection is incomplete or poorly sustained. In the group of 86 patients referred to earlier who were referred for investigation and possible implantation only 16% of patients proceeded to an operation.

Choice of Prosthesis

The first operations to implant a penile prosthesis were carried out on men undergoing reconstructive procedures following the traumatic amputation of the penis. Bogarus (1936) and Frumkin (1944) used cartilage to give the phalloplasty rigidity and this was also used later in the operations developed by Bergman et al. (1948) and Gillies (1948). Autologous tissue was slowly reabsorbed and in order to overcome this difficulty synthetic materials were implanted into the penis. Goodwin and Scott (1952) reported the use of acrylic to stiffen the penis in two men who underwent penile reconstruction following amputation of the penis in the treatment of a neoplasm. Later Loeffler and Sayegh (1960) reported the use of acrylic implants in men with impotence secondary to the surgical attempt to correct a "congenital short urethra" and in another man who was impotent following a priapism. In 1960 Beheri, working in Cairo, reported the technique of implanting polyethylene implants into each corpus cavernosum and by 1966 he was able to report his results in 700 patients: 95% of these implants were carried out in men with psychogenic impotence and in no other series have penile prostheses been used so readily for this condition. He described the technique of dilating the corpora cavernosa with Hegar's dilators in order to place the prosthesis within the erectile tissue and this has now become a standard technique.

Acrylic and polyethylene implants were not ideal substances for implantation into the body as they were rigid and tended to fracture. Rubin et al. (1971) showed that deeply implanted polyethylene was well tolerated by the tissues (only 10.6% of 244 implants were extruded when they were used as a bony replacement) but its use was abandoned with the discovery of the silicones (Brown et al. 1953). In 1964 Lash et al. reported the use of silicone for implantations into the body and showed a photograph of its use as a penile implant. The early results with this single prosthesis proved satisfactory (Lash 1968; Loeffler and Iveson 1976) but the shape of the implant was modified to a Y-shape in an attempt to stabilise the penis. Pearman (1967) also described the use of silicone for a single penile implant which was originally placed in the penis between Buck's fascia and the tunica albuginea. In 1972 he reported its satisfactory use but had modified the technique to place a single implant within a corpus cavernosum.

The disadvantage of all these prostheses was that the penis remained stiff all the time and it was not until the flexible Small–Carrion prosthesis (Small and Carrion 1975) and the inflatable prosthesis of Scott (Scott et al. 1973) were introduced that penile prosthetic surgery became an acceptable form of treatment. There is now a wide choice of prostheses and the selection depends upon financial considerations as well as the preferences of the patient and surgeon, the availability of each type and the back-up from the distributors. During the period 1975–1990 I have used 370 prostheses as shown in Table 9.2.

Table 9.2. Types of penile prosthesis implanted by the author (1975–1990)

Small Carrion	162
Finney Flexirod	7
Subrini	5
Jonas	8
AMS 600	59
Mentor malleable	79
Flexiflate	2
Hydroflex	21
Dynaflex	6
GFS Resipump	2
AMS 700	18
Mentor inflatable	1
Total	370

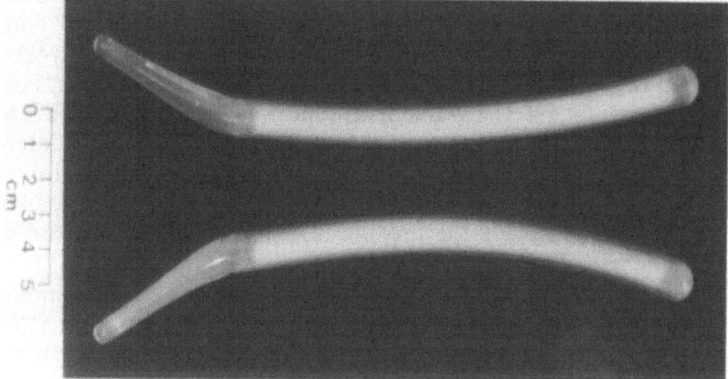

Fig. 9.4. Small–Carrion penile prosthesis.

All prostheses that are implanted at the present time are paired and are made, with the exception of the Mentor inflatable ones, of a silicone polymer. This is inert and is well-tolerated by the body (Habal 1984). The prostheses currently available fall into three main categories: malleable, mechanical and inflatable. The Small–Carrion prosthesis (Fig. 9.4) was for many years a popular choice and good results were obtained with its use (Chaikin et al. 1981; Small 1987). Its use has now been largely abandoned in favour of the malleable prostheses which offer similar functional results but with lower capital costs in providing a complete inventory of sizes, and permit better concealment.

The hinged prostheses of Subrini and Couvelaire (1974) and Finney (1977) consist of a firm penile and a softer crural element. This hinge mechanism permits the penis to be folded down to facilitate unobtrusive dressing. The length of the prosthesis is adjusted at the time of surgery by trimming the crural end with a scalpel. These prostheses are still used by some surgeons. The Subrini prosthesis is manufactured by Dow Corning and was widely used in Europe. Austoni (1988, personal communication) observed that penile tumescence occurred in the presence of the prosthesis and has recommended the use of intracavernous papaverine in order to produce a complementary erection.

The Finney prosthesis is produced by Surgitek and is marketed as the Flexirod. It is important to determine the correct length of the more rigid penile part prior to implantation in order that the hinged area is correctly sited. The prosthesis is available in a range of diameters and lengths and the conical tip of the distal end was designed to fit snugly into the distal part of the corpus cavernosus. The prosthesis gives good concealment, is extremely durable and gave good results in the first 763 patients (Finney 1984). The manufacturers state that over a 10-year period 20 000 pairs were sold and only 4 were returned for mechanical failure.

Malleable Prostheses

Malleable prostheses have an inner metal core that allows the penis to be bent into different positions. This allows the penis to be folded downwards when not required for coitus although in reality many men continue to dress with the penis against the abdominal wall.

Jonas Prosthesis

The Jonas prosthesis (Jonas and Jacobi 1980) was the first of the malleable prostheses and was introduced in 1978. It consists of a pair of silicone prostheses with an inner core of 10 silver wires, 0.6 mm in diameter which are surrounded by a PTFE coat (Fig. 9.5). It is available in three diameters and in varying lengths from 16 to 25 cm. It is also available as a "trimming tip" version in an attempt to reduce the inventory of sizes. The prosthesis was tested in a laboratory prior to its introduction, but after some years failure of the silver wire was reported by some patients (Tawil et al. 1984; Tawil and Gregory 1986). The authors noted that laboratory testing had shown that when the prosthesis was bent to 115° with a bend radius of 30 mm the first break in the silver wire was observed at greater than 6000 double bends and up to 7000 double bends were required to break all 10 strands. The manufacturers' report stated that of 15 000 prostheses implanted into patients in the United States prior to 1984 only 18 breaks were confirmed and a further 19 assumed. Some of the patients remained satisfied with the prosthesis despite the broken wires and did not consider reoperation necessary. The manufacturers believe that the problem has been diminished by modification of the prosthesis.

Jonas (1983) summarised the experience of 309 physicians implanting 1890 prostheses and other favourable reports are quoted by Krane et al. (1981), Benson et al. (1983) and Rowe and Royle (1983). In conclusion it is worth while noting that cheaper "lookalike" implants are manufactured in some countries but these are less reliable.

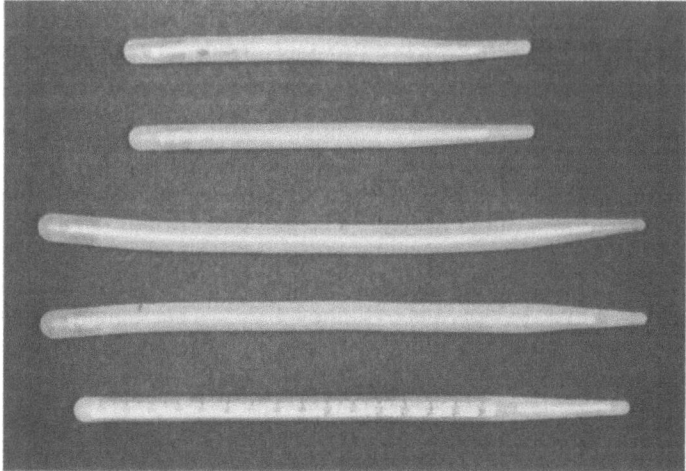

Fig. 9.5. Jonas penile prosthesis.

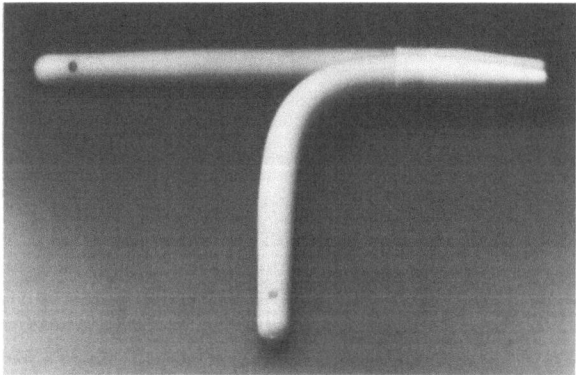

Fig. 9.6. AMS 600 malleable penile prosthesis. (Courtesy of American Medical Systems.)

American Medical Systems Malleable Prosthesis (AMS 600)

The AMS 600 prosthesis (Fig. 9.6) was introduced by American Medical Systems in 1983 and a report of its use in 56 patients was published in 1986 (Moul and McLoed 1986). It has a core of steel wires which are surrounded by an outer cloth sheath in order to minimise the risk of a fractured wire perforating the surrounding silicone. The prosthesis is manufactured in three lengths (12, 16 and 20 cm) and has rear tip extenders (1-, 2- and 3-cm long) which are fitted to the prosthesis at the time of surgery in order to obtain the correct length. The prosthesis is 13 mm in diameter but the outer silicone

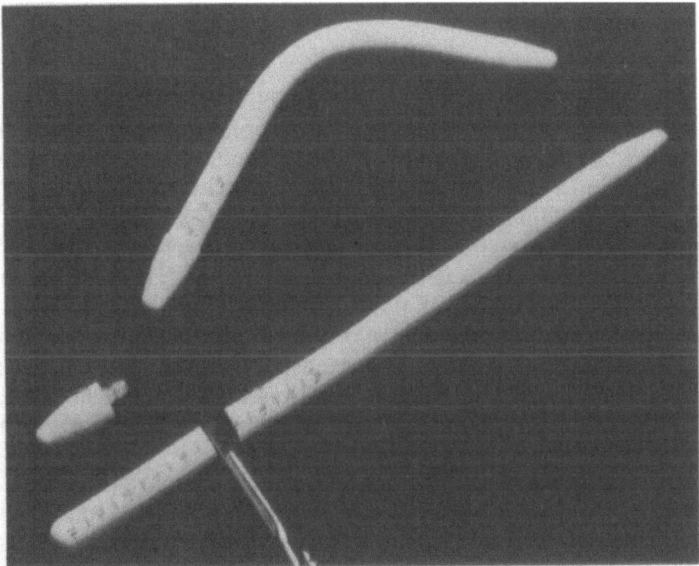

Fig. 9.7. Mentor malleable prosthesis.

jacket may be removed at operation to reduce the diameter to 11 mm. This is easily accomplished by carefully sliding the tip of a blunt scissors under the rear portion of the jacket and sliding the scissors along the entire length of the rod. Care is taken not to damage the surface of the white silicone. The outer jacket is then peeled away and discarded.

The manufacturers report that of the first 500 prostheses implanted (1983–1986) there was only one revision for mechanical considerations and there were no mechanical failures in the first 12 000 to 15 000 implanted (Nielsen and Bruskewitz 1989). In 1987 we reviewed the results obtained in 19 patients and found that 7 prostheses had been removed, usually for erosion. The prosthesis has been modified to become more flexible and in the period 1988–1989 only two prostheses have been removed and these were for infection. Dorflinger and Bruskewitz (1986) also found a high incidence of complications.

Mentor Malleable Prosthesis

The Mentor malleable prosthesis (Fig. 9.7) consists of a moulded silicone elastomer incorporating a trimmable tail section of softer silicone. The shaft part of the prosthesis contains a silver wire to give additional rigidity and also limit flexibility. The prosthesis is trimmed to the correct length at the time of operation and the rear cap fitted. Minor adjustment of length may be made by further trimming or adding caps which are 0.5 or 1 cm in length. The prosthesis is available in three diameters (9.5, 11 and 13 mm). Results obtained with this prosthesis have been very satisfactory with no mechanical failures.

Mechanical Prostheses

The OmniPhase (Dacomed Corporation, Minneapolis, Minnesota, USA) is a paired prosthesis and each element consists of three main components. The proximal and distal tips are made of medical grade silicone, a flexible body that is encased in polytetrafluoroethylene (PTFE) and a sheath of silicone. The prosthesis is available in two diameters (10 or 12 mm) and by varying the length of the proximal and/or distal tips the overall length of the prosthesis may vary from 16 to 29 cm. The correct length is selected at operation. The body of the prosthesis is composed of a column of plastic segments held together by a tension cable which passes through the centre of the column. When the cable is tightened the prosthesis becomes rigid and on releasing the cable the prosthesis lengthens by 4 mm and the prosthesis may be positioned like a malleable one. A further description of the prosthesis and the results are to be found in the initial report of Krane (1986).

A modification of this prosthesis – the DuraPhase (Dacomed) (Fig. 9.8) – does not have an activator mechanism. Unlike the OmniPhase, it may be implanted through a penoscrotal incision (Krane 1988). Mulcahy (1989a) described his early experience with the OmniPhase and found that the manufacturers had observed a 7% incidence of mechanical failure in the first 1400 prostheses implanted. Despite this he concluded that these prostheses have a role because of the ease of the manipulation of the implant by the patient, and more recent reports remain optimistic (Mulcahy et al. 1990).

Inflatable Prostheses

The advantage of these prostheses is that they permit the flaccid penis to become rigid enough to permit intercourse. The original prosthesis designed by Brantley Scott has undergone many modifications since its introduction but it remains the standard against which all others are compared. The past 5 years have seen the introduction of self-contained and two-part (cylinders and combined pump and reservoir) prostheses and the role of these has yet to be fully evaluated.

The advantage of all the inflatable prostheses has to be offest by the increased risk of mechanical failure and the increased cost of the prosthesis. It should also be remembered that the prosthesis may give an increasing girth of the penis but as yet it does not permit an increase in the length of the penis on inflation although the recently introduced Ultrex attempts to remedy this problem.

Self-contained Inflatable Prostheses

Hydroflex and Dynaflex

The hydroflex prosthesis was introduced by American Medical Systems in 1985. Each cylinder consisted of a pump situated in the distal portion of the

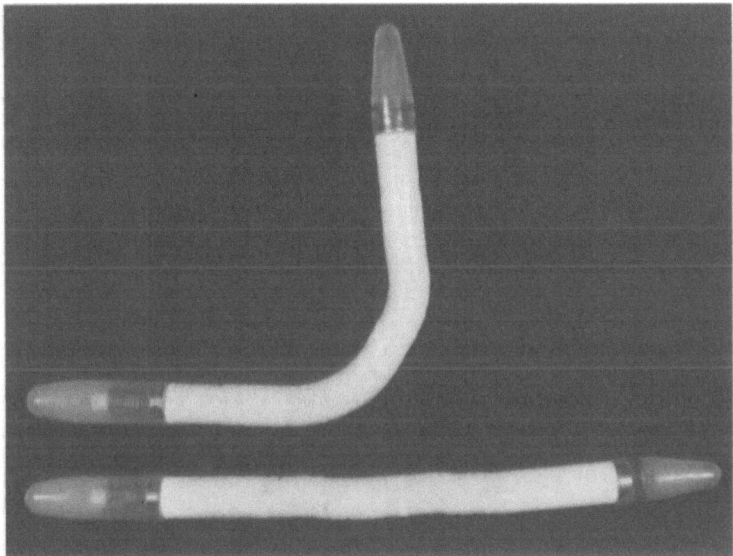

Fig. 9.8. Duraphase prosthesis.

prosthesis, an inflation cylinder in the central zone and a reservoir in the rear. The prosthesis was filled with isotonic solution as silicone rubbers are all semi-permeable. The prosthesis was activated by pumping the distal tip between the thumb and forefinger in order to transfer the fluid from the reservoir to the inflation chamber. Deflation occurred when steady pressure was applied to the deflation valve situated just behind the glans penis. Patients usually found it easy to activate the prosthesis but deactivation was more difficult. It was for this reason that the prosthesis was withdrawn in 1990 and replaced by the Dynaflex (Fig. 9.9). Flaccidity is obtained with this prosthesis by bending the penis over the forefingers and holding it in that position for 10 seconds (Fig. 9.10a,b). The Dynaflex is prefilled by the manufacturers and has two diameters (11 and 13 mm) and is supplied in four lengths (13, 16, 19 and 22 cm). The correct size is obtained at the time of surgery by using rear tip extenders. These prostheses have relatively little change in fluid volume between flaccidity and erection and there tends to be little variation between flaccidity and erection when first implanted. This begins to improve after 3 months. The variation in the quality of erection is less satisfactory in patients with a short or long penis due to the relative imbalance between the size of the reservoir and the inflation chamber. The development of the Hydroflex is a fascinating story and has been described by Porter (1989). Early experience with the Hydroflex was reported by Fishman (1986) and a larger experience by Mulcahy (1989b). In the first 12 patients operated upon at St. Peter's hospitals there was a high incidence of post-operative pain (7) or infection (4). This was ascribed to an excessive amount of tissue handling at the time of surgery. The contrast in rigidity of the penis when the prosthesis is inflated or deflated is not impressive at the time of surgery but improves during the subsequent 2–3 months. The incidence of post-operative pain and infection was reduced when the prosthesis was implanted in the same manner as a malleable one and not subjected to repeated

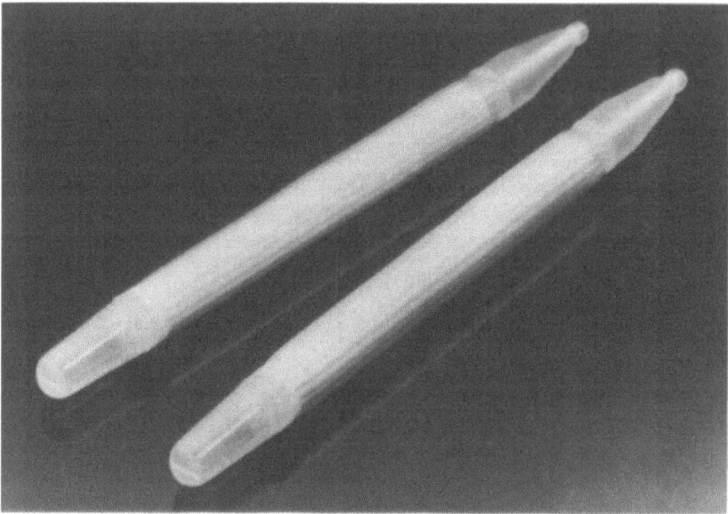

Fig. 9.9. Dynaflex penile prosthesis (courtesy of American Medical Systems).

inflation/deflation cycles at operation. Fracture of a Hydroflex prosthesis was reported by Goulding (1987).

The Hydroflex has been discontinued due to the difficulty some patients found with the deflation mechanism and has been replaced by the Dynaflex. The deflation mechanism has been simplified and occurs when the patient bends the prosthesis for 10 seconds and then releases it. This delayed release mechanism reduces the risk of inadvertent deflation during coitus. The degree of flaccidity has been enhanced by increasing the number of channels connecting the reservoir and inflation pump and the volume of the reservoir has been increased and matches the size of the cylinders.

Flexiflate

The flexiflate is a self-contained inflatable prosthesis, developed by Surgitek (Racine, Wisconsin, USA) in an attempt to provide a simple inflatable prosthesis. The prosthesis is activated by squeezing the distal part and deflation occurs by flexing the prosthesis within the penis. The initial prosthesis (Flexiflate I) was filled during the operation but Flexiflate II is prefilled. There was a tendency for the initial prosthesis to deflate spontaneously during intercourse (Finney 1986) but this problem has been reduced in the current model (Flexiflate II) from 73% to 58% (Stanisic and Dean 1989).

The Flexiflate II is available in two diameters (11 and 13 mm) and in penile shaft lengths of 10–15 cm. The trimmable rear tips of the Flexirod are retained and permit accurate sizing during operation. The initial experience with this prosthesis is found in the report of its designer (Finney 1986) and by Stanisic and Dean (1989). The latter report a mechanical failure rate of 11.6% due to leakage of fluid.

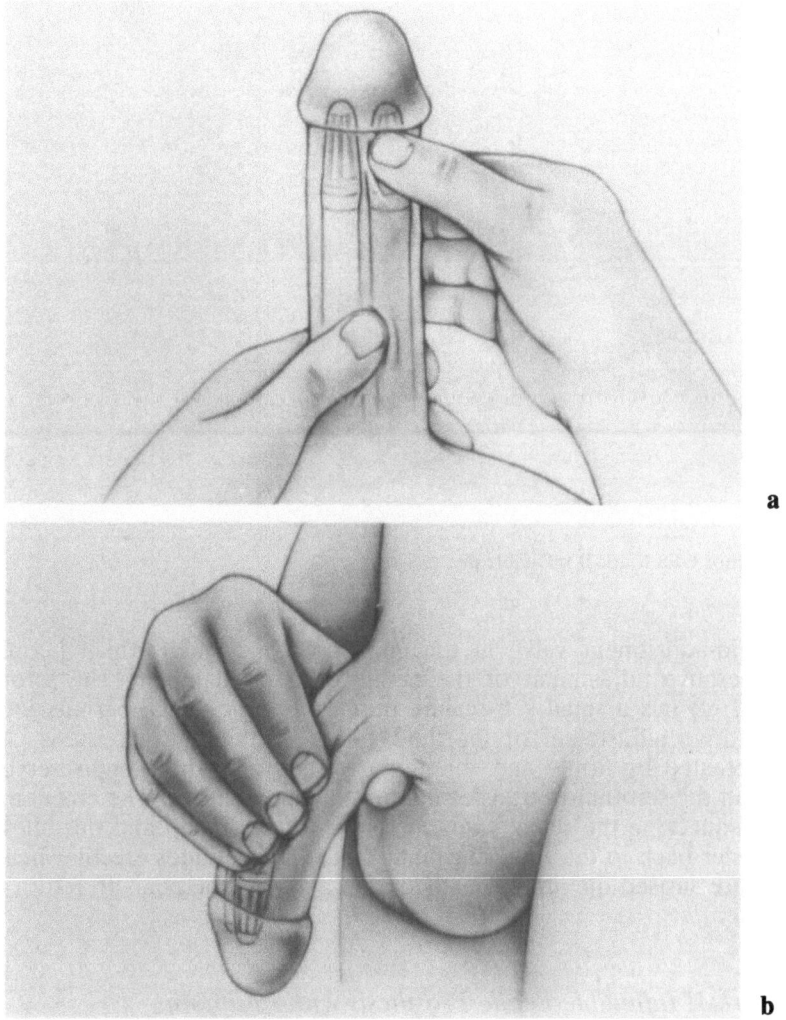

Fig. 9.10. **a** Inflation and, **b**, deflation technique for the Dynaflex prosthesis. (Courtesy of American Medical Systems.)

Two-Part Inflatable Prostheses

Uniflate 100

The Uniflate 100 is the latest prosthesis available from Surgitek and consists of a pair of inflatable penile cylinders which are attached to a combined scrotal pump and reservoir with kink-resistant tubing. The prosthesis is prefilled but the final fluid volume may be adjusted at the time of operation. The prosthesis is available in 11 and 13 mm diameters and five cylinder lengths (pubis to mid glans lengths of 8, 10, 12, 14 and 16 cm) and with connecting tubes 10 or 13 cm long. The penile cylinders are made of Dacron-reinforced silicone and there

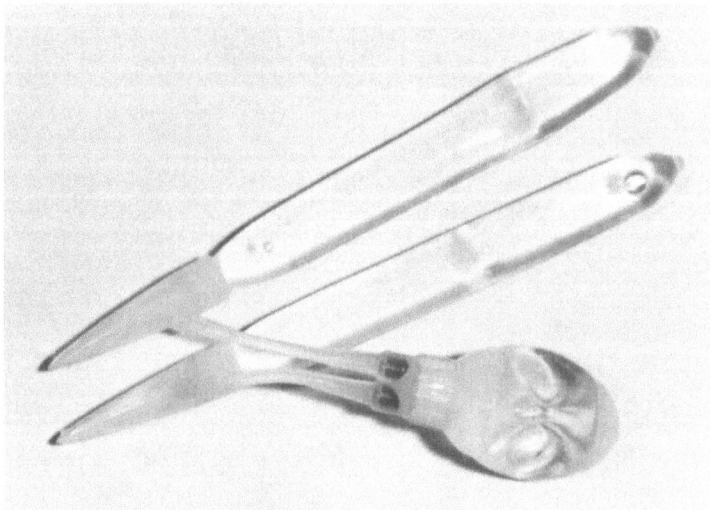

Fig. 9.11. Mentor GFS Mark II inflatable prosthesis.

is a fine fluid-adjustment valve at the end of each cylinder which permits the intra-operative adjustment of the penile cylinder diameter. The scrotal reservoir (20 ml) has a small self-sealing port at its base which permits intra or post-operative adjustment of the fluid volume within the prosthesis. An erection is created by firmly and continuously squeezing the pump/reservoir located within the scrotum to transfer fluid to the inner sheath. The erection is released by squeezing the release ring at the tip of the pump and this allows fluid to transfer back to the reservoir/pump bulb. As the inner erectile sheath becomes depressurised the inner sheath softens allowing the penis to return to a flaccid state.

Mentor Mark II Inflatable Penile Prosthesis with Resipump

The Mentor inflatable penile prostheses differs from all others by being constructed of bioflex polyurethane elastomer. This is considered to be more durable than silicone polymers, does not have crease-fold failures and allows

Table 9.3. Modifications of the AMS 700 penile prosthesis

Year	Modification
1974	Single inflate/deflate pump introduced
1978	Seamless spherical reservoir
1980	Rear tip extenders
1983	Kink-resistant tubing
	Non distensible cylinders
	EPTFE tubing sleeves
1985	"Quick connect" mechanism for joining tubes
1987	AMS 700CX cylinders

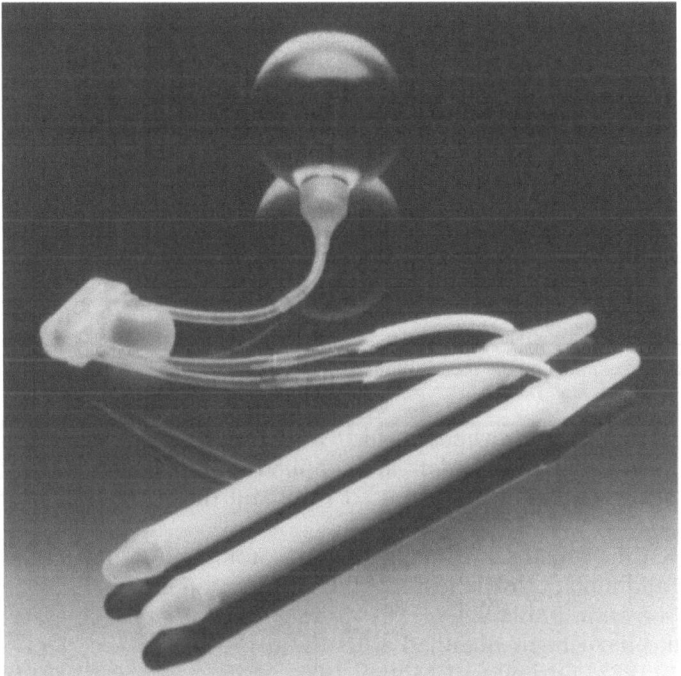

Fig. 9.12. AMS inflatable 700 CX penile prostheses. (Courtesy of American Medical Systems.)

the manufacturers to give a 10-year warranty. In the small number of these prostheses that I have implanted there appears to be more post-operative pain and fibrosis.

The Mark II prosthesis (Fig. 9.11) consists of two inflatable penile cylinders (12 to 22 cm in length at 1-cm intervals) connected to a GFS Resipump of 20 or 25 ml capacity. The system is filled peroperatively and the tubing connected with special Snap-Lock connectors.

Multipart Inflatable Prostheses

American Medical Systems AMS 700

The AMS 700 is a development of the original Scott inflatable prosthesis. The original model consisted of two penile cylinders and two pumps and reservoirs but was soon simplified by the elimination of one pump. The prosthesis has undergone many modifications since its introduction (Table 9.3) in an attempt to improve its mechanical reliability. The current model is shown in Fig. 9.12. Each penile cylinder consists of outer and inner silicone layers with an expandable woven fabric between that prevents aneurysm formation. Each 700 CX cylinder expands from a flaccid diameter of 12 mm to an erect diameter of 18 mm ensuring that the flaccid penis appears and feels more natural. The small 700 CXM cylinder expands from 9.5 mm flaccid to 14.2 mm when inflated. A

Table 9.4. Filling solutions for inflatable prostheses

Contrast medium[a]	(ml)	Sterile water (ml)	Total Volume (ml)
Hypaque 25%	50	60	110
Conray 280	20	60	80
Cysto-Conray II	60	15	75
Isopaque-Cysto	60	27	87
Iopamiro 300	47	53	100
Hexabrix	53	47	100
Urografin 30%	49	51	100
Solutrast 300	53	47	100
Conray FL	58	42	100
Telebrix 12	53	47	100

[a] If the patient is sensitive to contrast media then isotonic saline solution should be used.

recent innovation is the Ultrex cylinder which increases in length as well as girth on inflation. The standard cylinders are supplied in four lengths (12, 15, 18 and 21 cm) and rear tip extenders are used to obtain the correct length at the time of operation.

It is important that the prosthesis is filled with an isotonic solution as silicone is semi-permeable and fluid is slowly lost from demonstration models. A list of filling solutions is shown in Table 9.4.

Impressive results have been obtained with these prostheses (Scott et al. 1983; Malloy et al. 1987; Furlow and Motley 1988; Scarzella et al. 1988) but their longterm mechanical reliability is uncertain. Fluid loss can occur from any part of the multiple-component inflatable prostheses and require reoperation. The improvements that have been introduced are designed to overcome leaks which were usually from the penile cylinders. CX cylinders have not only reduced the rate of leakage but largely prevented aneurysm formation. The latter may occur due to inherent weakness of the tunica albuginea or as a consequence of weakness where the corporotomy was closed (Diokno 1983).

The site of a leak may be detected by a simple radiograph or at operation by testing each component in turn. Silicone is non-conductive and there should be no loss of current from the system when fluid is injected and an ohmmeter is attached to the tubing.

Self inflation may occur due to raised intra-abdominal pressure or when the space for the reservoir is too small to prevent its expansion. This is avoided at operation by filling it and checking that there is no tendency of the reservoir to empty. It is for this reason that the reservoir is kept filled during the early post-operative period. The penile cylinders may expand by having the fluid forced into them by the pump mechanism but the filling of the reservoir is on a more passive basis.

Mentor Multipart Inflatable Prosthesis

The Mentor multipart inflatable prosthesis is similar in appearance to the AMS 700 prosthesis but is manufactured from bioflex for added durability. The manufacturers are sufficiently confident of its reliability that they offer a 10-year replacement policy. The rounded pump has a collar which allows easy release without the need to orientate the scrotal pump. The kink-free tubing is readily joined by the use of Snap-Lock connectors.

The overall satisfactory results with this prosthesis have been summarised by Merrill (1989) but whereas he had a reoperative rate of 2% some authors had a reoperative rate as high as 39%.

Which Prosthesis?

The ideal prosthesis does not exist. It should allow the penis to be dependent in the flaccid state and with the prosthesis difficult to feel. Inflation of the prosthesis should make the penis expand in both length and girth and be sufficiently rigid to make for easy vaginal penetration during intercourse and with no tendency for buckling. There should be little risk of mechanical failure and it should be inert when placed in the tissues. The implantation procedure should be simple and the prosthesis cheap.

The final choice of prosthesis is far from easy and depends upon reliability, cost, personal preference of both surgeon and patient and availability. In general terms, it is likely that a malleable prosthesis will be cheaper and more reliable especially as inflatable prostheses are likely to require reoperation in 5–10 years on account of wear. The benefits of the inflatable prosthesis are the flaccidity for those groups who require it (those who take communal baths at work or sport) and that the tumescence is associated with an increased girth of the penis. Beutler et al. (1986) found that patients' and their partners' satisfaction was greater with the inflatable prosthesis but this issue is far from resolved.

The manufacturers have invested much time and money into the current prostheses in an attempt to improve them. They all try to provide an excellent service but the limited number of suppliers makes for difficulties in providing a satisfactory world-wide network of agents. The choice is varied and there is no single "best buy".

Preoperative Considerations

Proper informed consent is essential and, although the meaning of this may vary in different countries, the basic requirements are common to all. The need for operation should have been assessed and the patient advised as to the alternative methods of treatment, his expectations and the risk of complications. It is the latter that most frequently give rise to litigation. Any focus of infection must be eliminated prior to operation and it is also advisable to correct any urinary outflow obstruction. Prophylactic antibiotics are essential and these and other techniques to reduce infection will be discussed under complications.

The Operation

Surgery is best learnt in the operating theatre and it is not intended to give more than a broad outline. Fuller descriptions may be found in textbooks of operative surgery (Montague 1986; Hinman 1989). In addition the prosthesis manufacturers have useful videos of operative technique and also educational programmes for prospective implant surgeons.

Anaesthesia

This may be general, regional or local and the choice depends on the preferences of the patient, surgeon and anaesthetist. Inhalation anaesthetics are best avoided in patients with respiratory problems but are to be preferred in those with cardiac disease. Some surgeons, and patients, prefer out-patient day surgery under local anaesthesia but this preference is often made on financial grounds. Surgeons wishing to implant on a day-case basis could benefit from reading the articles on technique by Scott (1987) and Small (1987).

Incision

The original perineal incision has been abandoned and a penoscrotal incision (Barry and Seifert 1979) is the most practical. A small dorsal sub coronal incision (Jonas and Jacobi 1980) is convenient for a simple malleable prosthesis but should be avoided in the uncircumcised. The transverse infrapubic incision popularised by Kelâmi (1980) is useful but not recommended in the obese as corporal dilatation may be difficult. It is a safe incision for the beginner to use when implanting an inflatable prosthesis with an intra-abdominal reservoir. Once the surgeon has acquired more experience, he may elect to implant the prosthesis through the inguinal canal and this may be facilitated by a transverse penoscrotal incision (Scarzella 1989).

Implantation Technique

Surgery

The prevention of infection is of prime importance and the patient should receive prophylactic antibiotics. Movement within the operating theatre should be kept to a minimum and it is preferable to shave the lower abdomen and scrotum once the patient arrives in the operating theatre. The skin should be thoroughly cleansed with povidone-iodine.

The following description is for the implantation of semi-rigid or malleable prostheses. The most versatile incision is a longitudinal one, approximately 5 cm long at the penoscrotal junction. The skin and underlying subcutaneous tissue are incised down to the facia overlying the corpus spongiosus; if there is any doubt about the anatomical landmarks it is easy to insert a urethral catheter. The tunica albuginea is exposed on either side of the urethra and stay sutures inserted. Longitudinal corporotomies are performed using a scalpel. Whilst obtaining experience it is helpful to insert stay stitches through the cut edge of the tunica albuginea as this facilitates measuring the correct size for the prosthesis to be inserted. The corporotomy should be approximately three times as long as the diameter of the prosthesis (3–4 cm). A space is created within the corpora by gentle dilatation with a measuring tool or Hegar's dilator. The dilatation is kept to the minimum that is required to receive the prosthesis, and it is important to ensure that the prosthesis will fit to the end of the corpus cavernosum and can be felt beneath the glans penis.

It is important to obtain an accurate measurement of the internal lengths of the corpora, and the marker suture provides a fixed point for all measurements. The diameter of the prosthesis is of less importance, but it is advisable to implant the widest prosthesis that will fit the corpus. This is particularly important in those patients with a long penis as the pencil-like appearance of a very long penis is unsatisfactory. It is most uncommon for the length of prosthesis inserted into each corpus to differ by more than 1 cm.

The second prosthesis is fitted into the opposite corpus cavernosum in the same manner as the first and the corporotomies are closed with interrupted 00 synthetic absorbable sutures. The operation to insert the penile cylinders of an inflatable prosthesis is very similar to the above description. An additional aid is found in the Hydroflex and AMS 700 prostheses, which have a suture placed through the tip which facilitates traction of the prosthesis down to the sub-glandular region. The traction sutures are conveniently placed using a Keith needle mounted in a Furlow (Furlow 1978) introducer. Once the traction sutures have been inserted it is convenient to preplace sutures in the edges of the corporotomies to avoid the risk of puncturing an inflatable cylinder at the time of closure. Should it be necessary to place an additional suture a closure tool is another useful accessory. The length of the corporotomy is adjusted so that the connecting tube from the penile cylinder exits from the corpus at the proximal margin of the corporotomy. With an inflatable prosthesis it is convenient to inflate the cylinder and place it proximal and then to deflate the prosthesis and use the stay suture to pull the prosthesis down the penile shaft to the subglandular region.

Before inserting the reservoir it is sensible to ensure that the bladder is empty. Once the reservoir is inserted in the extraperitoneal space, it is important to test it to make sure that there is sufficient room for expansion. The pump mechanism is placed as low as possible in the scrotum and a Babcock used to secure it at the base of the scrotum. The skin incisions are closed with 30 polydioxanone and the patient receives antibiotics for at least 3 days. An indwelling urethral catheter may be left overnight if there is any possibility of retention, and wound drainage is not used routinely unless there has been a considerable amount of oozing at the time of operation. It is removed when there is less than 10 ml of drainage each day. The penis is left deflated with the reservoir full but the penile cylinders may be inflated as soon as is comfortable for the patient.

Care should be taken to avoid perforating the tunica albuginea or urethra. The former is of little importance provided that the perforation is recognised and the prosthesis is correctly positioned. An exception to this is when the distal end of the corpus cavernosum is perforated and the dilator appears through the glans or distal meatus. In these circumstances the attempt to implant the prosthesis should be abandoned on that side and a further attempt made in three months' time. Urethral perforation should also lead to the attempt at implantation being abandoned on that side and a urethral or supra-pubic catheter should be left in place for 1 week. When the corporal perforation is proximally, then provided it is not at the end of the corpus it is of little significance.

Post-operative Care

The penis is left lying on the anterior abdominal wall and inflatable prostheses are left deflated. The use of bupivacaine reduces the need for post-operative analgesics and oral medication is often all that is required. Some discomfort may persist for up to 4 weeks. Patients may be discharged as soon as comfortable and usually on the second post-operative day. Showering is permitted after 48 hours and bathing after 5 days. Coitus is prohibited until the patient is pain-free and the wounds have healed (usually 4–6 weeks). No attempt is made to inflate the hydraulic prosthesis until 3–4 weeks after surgery in order to allow healing and the pain-free operation of the prosthesis. This may be initiated at the post-operative visit and the patient given further instruction as to its operation. A water-soluble lubricant facilitates intercourse and both partners should be warned that there is a learning period in order to adjust to the new prosthesis. A further appointment is made for 3 months after the operation to check that all is well and the couple advised to seek further help should they have difficulties either with the mechanics of the prosthesis or with intercourse.

Complications

The overall incidence of complications varies widely and depends upon the cause of the impotence, the type of prosthesis used and the experience of the surgeon. The true incidence of complications is unknown but may be as high as 36% in some series reviewed by Kabalin and Kessler (1989a). Most of the complications were minor and 265 of the 290 patients (91%) were left with a functioning penile prosthesis although reoperation was necessary on 152 occasions in 96 patients. Many patients are able to have intercourse satisfactorily following the loss of a single prosthesis and Krauss (1985) obtained satisfactory results when he chose to implant a single prosthesis in selected patients.

Operative

Perforation of the tunica albuginea may occur during dilatation – usually if there is an element of fibrosis. This is not important unless the perforation is through the glans or into the urethra and under these circumstances a prosthesis should not be inserted into that corpus. The safest course of events with a urethral perforation is to insert a suprapubic catheter for 7 days. Should the perforation of the tunica not be at the end of the corpus, be it proximal or distal, and not into the urethra, then it is safe to implant the prosthesis provided that the two ends of the prosthesis are safely seated. Failure to recognise a proximal perforation may result in the migration of the prosthesis into the perineum. This situation may be rectified by a perineal approach to repair the tunica.

Mechanical Failures

Mechanical failures have been discussed with the individual prostheses and the manufacturers have worked with surgeons to improve the quality and design of all prostheses.

Technical Failures

Technical failures occur through failure of operative technique. The implantation of a prosthesis that is too short leads to the ST or Concord deformity whereas too long a prosthesis may produce post-operative pain and subsequent erosion with extrusion of the prosthesis. When a prosthesis protrudes through the glans or urethral meatus it may be easily removed and the capsule around the prosthesis prevents any bleeding. Urethral catheterisation is unnecessary.

It is a simple matter to exchange a short prosthesis for a larger one and it may be necessary to strengthen the distal part of the tunica albuginea with a Goretex or Dacron patch.

Needle stick injuries of an inflatable prosthesis should be recognised at the time of surgery but partial injury may cause a weak area which will subsequently cause leakage.

Post-operative Urinary Retention

Catheterisation is avoided whenever possible and any outflow obstruction should have been corrected before the operation. Urethral catheterisation may be kind if the operation is performed in the late afternoon, and the catheter is removed the next morning. Should a patient develop post-operative retention then a stab suprapubic cystostomy is the method of choice for managing this complication.

Haematoma Formation or Penile Oedema

Some bruising may occur but it is rarely severe enough to warrant any specific measures. Penile oedema is not uncommon following the insertion of the self-contained inflatable prostheses and is more likely if there have been repeated attempts at inflation and deflation of the prosthesis. Care should be taken to avoid a constricting dressing around the penis as this may lead to gangrene. This is particularly likely to occur if the dressing has become soaked in blood and hardened and the tissues are compressed between the dressing and the prosthesis. The presence of a urethral catheter is an additional hazard as it permits the passage of urine without inspection of the penis. The glans penis should always be visible and the use of constricting tape should be avoided.

Infection

Infection is the major complication and results in the loss of up to 10% of prostheses. The overall incidence of infection is difficult to assess and is

Table 9.5.   Incidence of penile prosthesis infection (after Carson 1989)

Type of prosthesis	Number of centres	Number of patients	Number (%) of infections
Rod	9	2806	50 (1.8)
Inflatable	9	2278	60 (2.6)
Inflatable rod	2	66	4 (6)

Table 9.6.   Complications of penile prosthetic surgery related to aetiology of impotence

Aetiology	Number	Infection	Removal or extrusion of prosthesis
Diabetes	30	7	9
Priapism	9	2	3
Peyronie's disease	20	4	4
Vasculogenic	17	2	3
Pelvic surgery/fracture	18	2	1
Neurogenic	21	4	1

Table 9.7.   Complications of penile prosthetic surgery related to type of prosthesis implanted (1983–87)

Prosthesis	Number	Infection	Removal or extrusion of prosthesis
Small Carrion	56	4	4
AMS 600	15	1	7
Mentor malleable	12	0	1
Hydroflex	11	4	3
Others	21	2	6

very low in some series. Blum (1989) and Carson (1989) have reviewed the incidence and the results are summarised in Table 9.5. Scott et al. (1983) reported an incidence of 2.4% in 1300 operations to implant an inflatable prosthesis whereas, in a personal series of 115 operations, the overall incidence of infection was 10% and the removal or extrusion of the prosthesis occurred in 18% of patients. Thanalla and Thompson (1987) found a similar incidence. The incidence of infection and removal rates was related to the original cause of the impotence and the type of prosthesis (Tables 9.6 and 9.7).

The infecting organism is usually a *Staphylococcus epidermiditis (albus)* (Thanalla and Thompson 1987; Montague 1987; Carson 1989) although other organisms may be responsible.

The importance of preventing infection is shown by the number of prophylactic measures that may be taken and are briefly described. No patient should be operated upon until all septic foci have been eliminated and the urine is sterile.

Urinary outflow obstruction should be relieved before operation and the patient be free of catheters and urinary collection apparatus.

The patient should have a bath, possibly containing antiseptic, before surgery and the pubic shave should be deferred until the patient is in the operating suite.

Prophylactic antibiotics are commenced 1–24 hours preoperatively and continued for 2–10 days. The antibiotics should be active against staphylococci, gram-negative organisms and anaerobes. Cephalosporins, aminoglycosides and metronidazole are popular choices. The surgeon should scrub for 10 minutes and the patient's skin preparation should also be thorough.

Theatre traffic should be kept to a minimum and gloves should be changed at the moment of handling the prosthesis. Peroperative antibiotics may be used topically and also to wash the prosthesis. Meticulous haemostasis should be obtained and although bleeding from the corporotomy may occur during the operation this ceases when the corporotomy is closed with a continuous suture. A closed suction drainage apparatus may be used if there is any continued oozing.

A superficial wound infection may occur without the loss of the prosthesis but post-operative infection of the periprosthetic tissues is accompanied by pain, fever, local tenderness and swelling. Most infections are apparent within the first month but some infections do not appear for weeks or months (Montague 1987). The prosthesis usually has to be removed when infection occurs but there have been reports of successfully irrigating the cavity with antibiotic solution and reimplanting a new prosthesis (Montague 1987; Maatman and Montague 1987). A safer alternative is to wait for the tissues to heal and to implant a new prosthesis after an interval of 3 months although it should be remembered that many patients are able to have satisfactory intercourse with a single prosthesis. Infection of one prosthesis does not inevitably lead to the loss of both prostheses.

Tissue necrosis and gangrene may occur (Shelling and Maxted 1980; Bour and Steinhardt 1984; McClellan and Masih 1985) in rare circumstances and usually in diabetics. Underlying ischaemia is an additional factor and this may be related to the original impotence or be due to a constricting dressing around the penis. The latter is more likely to occur if there is an indwelling catheter in addition to the prosthesis. Necrosis of the cavernous tissue may occur and it may be necessary not only to remove the prosthesis, but also the necrotic tissue, by curettage. A large drainage tube is inserted and the cavity allowed to heal rather like an empyema cavity. Necrosis of the superficial tissues may lead to the loss of part of the penis and debridement and the addition of a temporary urinary diversion is advisable.

Gerow (1990 personal communication) designed a vacuum device to fit around the penis after explantation of a prosthesis in an attempt to maintain penile size prior to reoperation. Moul and McLoed (1989) tried this in 14 patients, 10 of whom were able to have intercourse with such a device. Its efficacy in maintaining penile size was not stated.

Post-operative Pain and Erosion

Some pain is to be expected following the operation and this may be minimised by avoiding excessive handling of the tissues and the intra-operative use of bupivacaine and post-operative analgesia. The worst of the pain is usually over within one week and most patients are pain-free in 4–6 weeks by which time the wound is healed and the polydioxanone sutures have fallen out.

Persistent pain is usually due to infection, particularly if there was a postoperative fever. The antibiotics may damp down the infection, which may not be apparent for many weeks. If the prosthesis is too long this may be a source of pain and the prosthesis may erode through the tunica albuginea and become subcutaneous in the penis or ulcerate through the skin. This may account for the loss of a prosthesis after many years but in some instances this will be due to a haematogenous infection.

In some patients the pain may persist for many months and sometimes for as long as a year and then cease without apparent reason. Some patients with persistent pain are diabetics and it may be that there is a neuropathic element to the pain. On rare occasions it is necessary to explant the prosthesis on the basis of pain alone and the earliest that this was necessary was after 8 days. Before proceeding to remove the prosthesis for persistent pain, it is worthwhile injecting local anaesthesia into the corpora (Krauss 1986) before changing to a smaller prosthesis or removing an existing one.

Special Circumstances

Peyronie's Disease

Raz et al. (1977) recommended the implantation of a prosthesis in all patients with Peyronie's disease who required surgery. This is unnecessary and a prosthesis should be reserved for those men with an impaired quality of erection.

Dilatation is seldom difficult in Peyronie's disease except in those uncommon instances when the condition is primarily a cavernous fibrosis rather than fibrosis of the tunica albuginea. A malleable prosthesis is usually sufficiently rigid to overcome the deformity associated with Peyronie's disease but this may not be the case with an inflatable prosthesis. Simple plaque incision – carried out with cutting diathermy if the prosthesis is in situ – may be sufficient to correct this (Malloy et al. 1981) although there will be a tendency for the cylinders to herniate through the defect. The stronger cylinder of the AMS 700 or the Mentor inflatable device should be used. Alternative strategies are to combine the incision with a patch of dermis, Dacron or Goretex or to correct the deformity with the Nesbit (1965) procedure at the time of implantation (Mulcahy and Rowland 1987).

Priapism

Post-priapism impotence is often the result of the erectile tissue being replaced with fibrous tissue. The extent of the fibrosis is variable and may be assessed by clinical examination, ultrasound examination or cavernosography (Herzberg et al. 1981). The crura may be spared from the fibrotic process but dilatation of the penile part of the corpora cavernosa may be difficult or impossible. The procedure resembles the secondary placement of a penile prosthesis

(O'Donnell 1986) and is best carried out through a penoscrotal incision. This allows access to the whole length of the corpora cavernosa and the penis may be invaginated to allow removal of the fibrous tissue under direct invagination. A urethral catheter facilitates orientation during the procedure and minimises the risk of damaging the urethra. Douglas (1987) described a technique which utilised a dorsal penile incision and only incises the tissue in the penile part of the corpora. Kelâmi (1985) was able to implant 12 patients successfully using an infrapubic incision and Bertram et al. (1985) were successful in 5 of 6 patients.

Dilatation is sometimes possible and an Otis urethrotome may be inserted to cut a suitable space for the prosthesis. Even when the corpora are replaced by fibrous tissue it is sometimes possible to dissect in a plane beneath the tunica albuginea and excise a core of fibrous tissue. A corporal corer – a cross between an apple corer and an endarterectomy knife – is sometimes useful but even with this instrument care should be taken to avoid injury to the urethra.

On some occasions it is not possible to create a space in which to place the prosthesis and on these occasions it is sufficient to implant a single prosthesis. On other occasions it is not possible to close the tunica around the prosthesis and a patch of Dacron may be used to fill the gap. An alternative procedure would be to place the prosthesis within a tubed Dacron vascular graft which is anchored to both ends of the crura (Fritzler et al. 1986; Fishman 1989; Mulcahy 1987). These circumstances are uncommon. This technique of implanting into a Dacron tube has also been used in "hypospadias cripples" in whom the penile erectile tissue thrombosed during one of the considerable procedures that these unfortunate men underwent in childhood or adolescence. The difficulties encountered post-priapism were shown when 6 of the first 10 patients (Pryor and Hehir 1982) had minor or no difficulties but in the remaining 4 patients extreme difficulty was encountered although 3 of them ended up with a satisfactory result in that they were able to have intercourse. In one of these patients success was only obtained after the fifth operation.

Traumatic Paraplegia

Golgi (1979) inserted Small–Carrion prostheses in 30 patients with paraplegia. In two of them the operation was carried out primarily to stabilise the penis in order to make the application of a condom incontinence appliance easier and this was an additional consideration in 6 of the other men. It is important to evaluate bladder emptying before operating to implant the prosthesis and many of the patients will require external sphincterotomy or a bladder neck procedure prior to the implantation. Some patients have found it easier to manage their bladders following the insertion of the penile prosthesis and gain continence as a result of the increased urethral resistance. Paraplegics have an increased risk of prosthesis failure due to erosion and infection.

Immunosuppressed Organ Transplant Recipients

Impotence occurs commonly in patients requiring organ transplantation and is usually vasculogenic in origin. It is possible to implant these patients despite immunosuppression (Sidi et al. 1987; Kabalin and Kessler 1989b) although there might be an increased risk of infection (Walther et al. 1987).

Phalloplasty

Bogarus (1936) described the first penile implants when he utilised rib cartilage to stiffen a phalloplasty. Cartilage, or rib, is slowly reabsorbed and nowadays a silicone-based prosthesis is used. In male patients the base of the prosthesis fits securely into the crura of the corpus cavernosum. It has been suggested (Bogarus 1936) that a prosthesis may be inserted in an early stage of the Gillies phalloplasty. The blood supply of the pedicle is at risk at this stage and it would seem better to wait until a later stage in the operation (Pryor et al. 1981). It is also unnecessary to implant two prostheses and the technique is now modified to insert only a single implant.

The implantation of a prosthesis into the phalloplasty in transsexual patients is more difficult. The corpora cavernosa cannot accept an implant although an attempt can be made to anchor a 7-mm Flexirod prosthesis into the crura. The dilatation of the phallus is also difficult and may compromise the blood supply as a whole. An Amplatz tube may be used to facilitate placement of the prosthesis into the phallus. Pressure necrosis over the edge of the prosthesis is not uncommon and the phallus may have to be carefully positioned in order to avoid such a risk. Despite these difficulties it is possible to insert a prosthesis satisfactorily into the neophallus and enable the patient to have sexual intercourse and even father children.

Results

The results of a penile prosthesis are usually satisfactory and most dissatisfaction arises when there are complications even though these may be rectified by a further operation. Preoperative counselling of the patient, which includes information about the complications, is most important in order to obtain satisfactory results. Provided that the prosthesis is functioning and in the correct position this avoids dissatisfaction stemming from false expectations. It is most important for the patient to realise that the penis will not increase in length during intercourse.

Patients rarely complain of difficulties concealing the prosthesis and when they do it is important to check that the prosthesis is functioning satisfactorily. Some patients prefer to keep the penis against the abdominal wall whilst others prefer to keep it against the thigh. These measures are not necessary with the inflatable prostheses but occasionally patients complain of self inflation of a multipart inflatable prosthesis. This occurs when the intra-abdominal pressure is raised by standing or when a capsule forms around the collapsed reservoir. It is for this reason that the prosthesis is kept deflated for the first 3–4 weeks after operation. The pump mechanism is sufficient to transfer fluid into the penile cylinders and stretch the capsule around the prosthesis but the return mechanism is a passive one and pressure is barely sufficient to distend the reservoir.

Dissatisfaction in the presence of a normal prosthesis usually stems from psychological reasons and further counselling is required (Schovar 1989). Dissatisfaction from a non-functioning prosthesis requires further operation and some of the patients resort to litigation. The legal aspects in the United States were reviewed by Irwin (1989). A satisfactory outcome should occur in 90% – 95% of patients despite the complications that may occur, and sexual satisfaction is usual for both the patient and the partner – in fact many partners consider sexual performance to be enhanced as the erection may be maintained as long as they wish.

References

Barry JM, Seifert A (1979) Penoscrotal approach for placement of paired penile implants for impotence. J Urol 122:321–326

Beheri GE (1966) Surgical treatment of impotence. J Plast Reconstr Surg 38:92–97

Bennett AH (1982) Placement of penile prosthesis during surgery for malignancy. Urology 20: 276–277

Benson RC, Barrett DM, Patterson DE (1983) The Jonas prosthesis: technical considerations and results. J Urol 130:920–922

Bergman RT, Howard AH, Barnes RW (1948) Plastic reconstruction of the penis. J Urol 59: 1174–1182

Bertram RA, Carson LC, Webster GD (1985) Implantation of penile prostheses in patients impotent after priapism. Urology 26:325–327

Beutler LE, Scott FB, Rogers RR, Karacan I, Baer PE, Gaines JA (1986) Inflatable and non inflatable penile prostheses: comparative follow up evaluation. Urology 27:136–143

Blum MD (1989) Infections of genitourinary prostheses. Infect Dis Clin North Am 3:259–274

Bogarus N (1936) Über die volle plastische wiederherstellung eines zum koitus fahigen Penis (peni plastica totalis). Zentralbl Chir 63:1271–1276

Bour J, Steinhardt G (1984) Penile necrosis in patients with diabetes mellitus and end stage renal disease. J Urol 132:560–561

Bradley WE, Timm GW, Gallagher JM, Johnson BK (1985) New method for continuous measurement of nocturnal penile tumescence and rigidity. Urology 26:4–9

Brindley GS (1983) Cavernosal alpha blockade: a new technique for investigation and treatment of erectile impotence. Br J Psychiatry 143:132–37

Brown JB, Fryer MP, Randall P, Lu MP (1953) Silicones in plastic surgery. Plast Reconstr Surg 12:374–376

Buvat J, Buvat-Herbaut M, Dehaene JC, Lemaire A (1986) Is intracavernous injection of papaverine a reliable screening test for vascular impotence? J Urol 135:476–478

Carson CL (1989) Infections in genitourinary prostheses. Urol Clin North Am 16:139–147

Chaikin L, Carrion H, Plitano V (1981) Complications of the Small–Carrion prosthesis: long term follow up. J Urol 126:44–45

Dickinson IK, Pryor JP (1989) Pharmacocavernometry: a modified papaverine test. Br J Urol 63:539–545

Diokno AC (1983) Asymmetric inflation of the penile cylinders: etiology and management. J Urol 129:1127–1130

Dorflinger T, Bruskewitz R (1986) AMS malleable prosthesis. Urology 18:480–485

Douglas LL (1987) Technique for placement of Small–Carrion prosthesis post priapism. Urology 30:273–274

Finney RP (1977) New hinged silicone penile implant. J Urol 118:585–587

Finney RP (1984) Finney Flexirod prosthesis. Urology 23:79–82

Finney RP (1986) Flexiflate penile prosthesis. Semin Urol 4:244–246

Fishman IJ (1986) Experience with the Hydroflex penile prosthesis. Semin Urol 4:239–243

Fishman IJ (1989) Corporal reconstruction procedure for complicated penile implants. Urol Clin North Am 16:73–90

Fowler CJ, Ali Z, Kirby RS, Pryor JP (1988) The value of testing for unmyelinated fibre, sensory neuropathy in diabetic impotence. Br J Urol 61:63–67

Fritzler M, Flores-Sandoral FN, Light TK (1986) Dacron "sock" repair for proximal corporeal perforation. Urology 28:524–526

Frumkin AP (1944) Reconstruction of the male genitalia. Rev Soviet Med 2:14–21

Furlow WL (1978) Inflatable penile prosthesis: new device for cylinder insertion. Urology 12: 447–449

Furlow WL, Motley RC (1988) The inflatable penile prosthesis: clinical experience with a new controlled expansion device. J Urol 139:945–946

Gillies H (1948) Congenital absence of penis. Br J Plast Surg 1:8–28

Goodwin WE, Scott WW (1952) Phalloplasty. J Urol 68:903–908

Golgi H (1979) Experience with penile prosthesis in spinal cord injury patients. J Urol 121: 288–289

Goulding FJ (1987) Function of Hydroflex penile implant. Urology 30:490–491

Habal MB (1984) The biological basis for the clinical application of the silicones. Arch Surg 119:843–848

Herzberg Z, Kellett MJ, Morgan RJ, Pryor JP (1981) Method, indications and results of corpus cavernosography. Br J Urol 53:641–644

Hinman F (1989) Atlas of urologic surgery. WB Saunders, Philadelphia

Irwin JR (1989) Legal aspects of urologic prosthetic devices. Urol Clin North Am 16:165–174

Jonas U (1983) Five years' experience with the silicone-silver penile prosthesis: improvements and new developments. World J Urol 1:251–256

Jonas U, Jacobi GH (1980) Silicone-silver penile prosthesis: description, operative approach and results. J Urol 123:865–867

Kabalin JN, Kessler R (1989a) Penile prosthesis surgery: review of 10 year experience and examination of reoperations. Urology 23:17–19

Kabalin JN, Kessler R (1989b) Successful implantation of penile prostheses in organ transplanted patients. Urology 33:282–284

Karacan I, Moore CA (1987) Diagnosis of impotence. In: Pryor JP, Lipshultz LI (eds) Andrology. Butterworths, London, pp 133–147

Kelâmi A (1980) Atlas of operative andrology. De Gruyter, Berlin

Kelâmi A (1985) Implantation of Small-Carrion prosthesis in the treatment of erectile impotence after priapism. Difficulties and effects. Urol Int 40:343–346

Korenman SG, Viosca SP, Kaiser FE, Mooradian AD, Morley JE (1990) Use of a vacuum tumescence device in the treatment of impotence. J Am Geriatr Soc 38:217–220

Krane RJ (1986) OmniPhase penile prosthesis. Semin Urol 4:247–251

Krane RJ (1988) Penile prostheses. Urol Clin North Am 15:103–109

Krane RJ, Freedberg PS, Siroky MB (1981) Jonas silicone-silver prosthesis: initial experience in America. J Urol 126:475–476

Krauss DJ (1985) Single cylinder penile prosthesis. Urology 26:466–467

Krauss DJ (1986) Elimination of pain caused by Small-Carrion penile prosthesis. Urology 28:22–23

Lash H (1968) Silicone implant for impotence. J Urol 100:709–710

Lash H, Zimmerman DC, Loeffler RA (1964) Silicon implantation, inlay method. Plast Reconstr Surg 34:75–79

Loeffler RA, Iveson RE (1976) Surgical treatment of impotence in the male. Plast Reconstr Surg 58:292–297

Loeffler RA, Sayegh ES (1960) Perforated acrylic implant in management of organic impotence. J Urol 84:559–561

Lue TF, Hricak H, Marich KW, Tanagho EA (1985) Vasculogenic impotence evaluated by high-resolution ultrasonography and pulsed Doppler spectrum analysis. Radiology 155:777–781

Maatman TJ, Montague DK (1987) Intracorporal drainage after removal of infected penile prostheses. Urology 30 (suppl):42–43

Malloy T, Wein A, Carpiniello VL (1981) Advanced Peyronie's disease treated with the inflatable penile prosthesis. J Urol 125:327–328

Malloy T, Wein A, Carpiniello VL (1987) Reliability of AMS 700 inflatable penile prosthesis. Urology 28:385–387

McClellan DS, Masih BK (1985) Gangrene of the penis as a complication of penile prosthesis. J Urol 133:862

Merrill DC (1989) Mentor inflatable penile prostheses. Urol Clin North Am 16:51–66

Michal V, Kramer J, Pospichal J (1978) External iliac steal syndrome. J Cardiovasc Surg 19: 355–357

Montague DK (1986) Penile prosthesis. In: McDougal WS (ed) Rob and Smiths' operative surgery: urology. Butterworths, London, pp 599–610

Montague DK (1987) Periprosthetic infections. J Urol 138:68–69

Moul JW, McLoed DG (1986) Experience with the AMS 600 malleable prosthesis. J Urol 135: 929–931

Moul JW, McLoed DG (1989) Negative pressure devices in the explanted penile prosthesis population. J Urol 142:729–931

Mulcahy JJ (1987) A technique of maintaining penile prosthesis position to prevent proximal migration. J Urol 137:294–296

Mulcahy JJ (1989a) The OmniPhase and DuraPhase penile prostheses. Urol Clin North Am 16:25–31

Mulcahy JJ (1989b) The Hydroflex penile prosthesis. Urol Clin North Am 16:33–38

Mulcahy JJ, Rowland RG (1987) Tunica wedge excision to correct penile curvature associated with the inflatable prosthesis. J Urol 138:63–64

Mulcahy JJ, Krane RJ, Lloyd K, Edson M, Siroky MB (1990) DuraPhase penile prosthesis – results of clinical trials in 63 patients. J Urol 143:518–519

Nadig PW, Ware JC, Blumoff R (1986) Noninvasive device to produce and maintain an erection-like state. Urology 37:126–131

Nesbit RM (1965) Congenital curvature of the phallus: Report of three cases with description of corrective operation. J Urol 93:230–232

Nielsen KT, Bruskewitz RC (1989) Semirigid and malleable rod penile prosthesis. Urol Clin North Am 16:13–23

O'Donnell PD (1986) Operative approach for secondary placement of penile prosthesis. Urology 28:108–110

Pearman RO (1967) Treatment of organic impotence by implantation of penile prosthesis. J Urol 97:716–719

Pearman RO (1972) Insertion of a silastic penile prosthesis for the treatment of organic sexual impotence. J Urol 107:802–806

Porter LH (1989) Development of a penile prosthesis: the Hydroflex. Urol Clin North Am 16:149–164

Pryor JP, Hehir M (1982) The management of priapism. Br J Urol 54:751–754

Pryor JP, Hill JT, Packham DA, Yates Bell AJ (1981) Penile injuries with particular reference to the erectile tissue. Br J Urol 53:42–46

Raz S, de Kernion JB, Kaufman JJ (1977) Surgical treatment of Peyronie's disease: a new approach. J Urol 117:598–601

Rowe PH, Royle MJ (1983) Use of Jonas silicon-silver prosthesis in erectile impotence. J R Soc Med 76:1019–1022

Rubin L, Brombery BE, Walden RH (1971) Long term human reaction to synthetic plastics. Surg Gynecol Obstet 132:622–623

Scarzella GI (1988) Cylinder reliability of inflatable penile prosthesis. Urology 33:486–489

Scarzella GI (1989) Improved technique for implanting AMS 700 CX inflatable penile prostheses using transverse scrotal approach. Urology 34:388–389

Schovar LR (1989) Sex therapy for the penile prosthesis recipient. Urol Clin North Am 16: 91–98

Scott FB (1987) Outpatient implantation of penile prostheses under local anaesthesia. Urol Clin North Am 14:177–186

Scott FB, Bradley WE, Timm GW (1973) Managment of erectile impotence; use of an implantable inflatable prosthesis. Urology 2:80–82

Scott FB, Fishman IJ, Light JK (1983) A decade of experience with the inflatable penile prosthesis. World J Urol 1:244–250

Shelling RH, Maxted WC (1980) Major complications of silicone penile prosthesis. Urology 15:131–133

Sidi AA, Peng W, Sanseau C, Lange PH (1987) Penile prosthesis surgery in the treatment of impotence in the immuno suppressed man. J Urol 137:681

Small MP (1987) Semirigid and malleable penile implants. Urol Clin North Am 14:187–201

Small MP, Carrion H (1975) A new penile prosthesis for treating impotence. Contemporary Urology 7:29–33

Stanisic TH, Dean JC (1989) The FlexiFlate and FlexiFlate II penile prostheses. Urol Clin North Am 16:39–49

Strachan JR and Pryor JP (1987) Diagnostic intracorporeal papaverine and erectile dysfunction. Br J Urol 59:264–266

Subrini L, Couvelaire R (1974) Le traitement chirurgual de l'impuissance virile par intabation prothétique intra cavernseuse. J Urol Nephrol 80:269–276

Tawil EA, Gregory JG (1986) Failure of the Jonas prosthesis. J Urol 135:702–703

Tawil EA, Hawatmeh IS, Apte S, Gregory JG (1984) Multiple fractures of the silver wire strands as a complication of the silicone-silver wire prosthesis. J Urol 132:762–763

Thanalla JV, Thompson ST (1987) Infectious complications of penile prosthetic implants. J Urol 138:65–67

Turner LA, Althof SE, Levine SB, Tobias TR, Kursh ED, Bodner D, Resnick MI (1990) Treating erectile dysfunction with external vacuum devices: impact upon sexual, psychological and marital functioning. J Urol 144:79–82

Virag R, Spencer PP, Frydman D (1984) Artificial erection in diagnosis and treatment of impotence. Urology 24:157–161

Virag R, Brouilly, P, Frydman D (1985) Is impotence an arterial disorder? Lancet 1:181–184

Walther PJ, Andriani RG, Maggio MI, Carson CC (1987) Fourniers gangrene: a complication of penile prosthesis implantation in a renal transplant patient. J Urol 137:299–300

Wespes E, Delcour C, Stragven J, Schulman CC (1986) Pharmacocavernometry-cavernography in impotence. Br J Urol 58:429–433

Wiles PG (1988) Successful non-invasive management of erectile impotence in diabetic men. Br Med J 296:161–162

Witherington R (1989) Vacuum constriction device for management of erectile impotence. J Urol 141:320–322

Zentgraf M, Baccouche M, Jünemann KP (1988) Diagnosis and therapy of erectile dysfunction using papaverine and phentolamine. Urol Int 43:65–75

Chapter 10

Vas Deferens Prostheses

S.S. Schmidt

A variety of vas deferens prostheses have been developed in the past 40 years to allow temporary obstruction of the vas and to provide easier and more successful reanastomosis. Most were experimental and current practice finds none in clinical use.

The indications for vas deferens prostheses are:

1. As solid stents in vasovasostomy. These stents usually are removable, but some are absorbable
2. As internal cannulae in vasovasostomy (endosplints), either loose in the anastomosis or brought out of the vas and fixed to the skin
3. As tubing with external surfaces that permit the body to invade them and form a mechanical bond to the tissues. Such prostheses have been proposed as a means of: (a) bridging an interruption in the vas; (b) replacing a missing segment of the vas; (c) draining spermatic fluid to the outside either for study or for use in artificial insemination
4. As an obstructing device later to be removed, thus permitting subsequent patency of the vas
5. As permanently placed valves, which would permit the vas to be obstructed or not as desired

In the past, surgeons failed to recognise that the vas is a structure with its own specific characteristics (different from the ureter, for example), and also that it is a living structure and not an inert conduit. Many prostheses failed because these factors were not considered. A delineation of the principles of vas surgery shows the problems presented by any such prosthesis and compares them to current vasovasostomy technique. The following factors hold true for both.

1. The procedure can be done under local anaesthesia
2. The procedure is suited to outpatient surgery
3. All sutures should be monofilament and non-reactive
4. Although the procedure can be done as a macroscopic technique, microsurgery permits more precision

5. Contact between sperm and raw tissue should be avoided as much as possible

6. Sperm antibodies are common after either obstruction of the vas or extravasation of sperm

7. A puncture of the vas (for example, a suture into the lumen) heals at once without significant leakage, whereas a device left in the wall of the vas for several days and later removed may leak at the point of emergence and cause the vas to be obstructed there

The following factors are relevant to any permanent prosthesis:

1. It should be made of nonreactive material

2. It should be of a consistency similar to that of the vas

3. It must be bonded to the vas lest it migrate

4. The vas will dilate around an internal prosthesis permitting sperm to pass around it

And finally, certain factors are peculiar to each:

1. A prosthesis might be used to bridge a large defect in the vas, one wherein the ends of the vas could not be approximated

2. A vasovasostomy can be performed in the convoluted vas, while it might be impossible to place a prosthesis there

3. A vasovasostomy should be performed by approximating the mucosa of the vas without intervening raw tissue lest a contracture occur later, while a prosthesis may not require this

4. A vasovasostomy must join ends of the vas having different luminal diameters. This may or may not be a factor in the prosthesis, depending upon when it is placed in reference to a vasectomy

The above factors will be discussed below, as the indications for prostheses are presented along with the advantage and disadvantages.

Stents in Vasovasotomy

The early descriptions of this operation called for the vas to be aligned over a stent that was first silkworm gut, next wire and later monofilament nylon (O'Conor 1948; Dorsey 1957). These stents were removed 7–14 days postoperatively. They were brought out of the vas above or below the anastomosis, or sometimes both, and held to the skin. Wire could be driven through the wall of the vas and through the skin but had the disadvantage of being rigid and, occasionally, of having a hook on its cut end. Nylon was flexible and was either swagged on to a straight milliner's needle or passed through the shaft of a hypodermic needle out of the vas and through the skin (Fig. 10.1). This technique allowed impregnation to occur (average 25%).

The use of these stents derived from comparing vas anastomosis with anastomosis of the thin walled ureter (which could kink and get obstructed). However, in contrast to the ureter, the vas is thick-walled and cannot be kinked

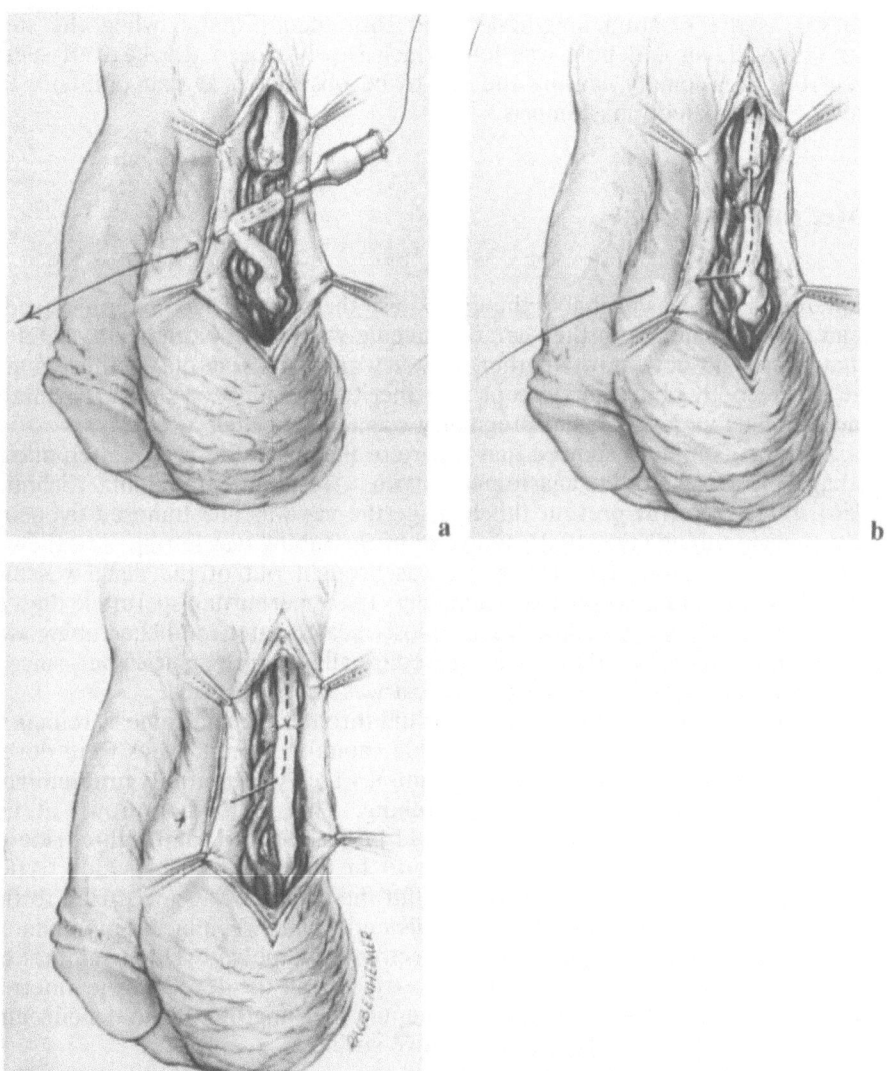

Fig. 10.1a–c. Placement of nylon stent in anastomosis of the vas (Schmidt 1956).

upon itself or at a properly constructed anastomosis. The stent also was said to provide a scaffold for mucosal and muscular regeneration, a possibility perhaps if gross suturing were used, but our present technique of precise tissue approximation leaves no defect at the anastomosis and thus no need for such a scaffold. (Furthermore, in a technique of gross suturing, raw tissue was sometimes exposed to the irritative effects of spermatozoa, a condition peculiar to the spermatic ducts.)

Positioning these stents created an additional problem. If they were brought out of the vas on both sides of the anastomosis, they did not move, but if they were brought out at one point only, the other end was free to move in the vas as the scrotum lengthened and shortened. Finally, when the stent was removed, an exit hole was left, which slowly closed. Leakage of sperm occurred, occasionally causing the vas to be obstructed at that point, in the presence of a patent anastomosis.

Internal Cannula

Cameron (1945) was probably the first to use the shaft of a hypodermic needle as an internal cannula in the vas. This needle was left in permanently. Unfortunately, we do not know whether it later worked its way out of the vas and out of the body, but the concept had merit. Spermatozoa appeared in the ejaculate postoperatively, but pregnancy was not reported.

Experiments in dogs showed that failure of the anastomosis was often due to leakage of sperm at the anastomosis, with a resultant granuloma (Schmidt 1956). In an effort to prevent this leakage the vas was anastomosed over fine polyethylene tubing (Fig. 10.2). One end of the tubing was left open in the vas to receive spermatic fluid; the other was brought out of the distal vas and through the skin of the upper scrotum (Fig. 10.3), permitting spermatic fluid to drain into the bandages as the anastomosis healed, and until the tubing was later removed (Schmidt 1961). This procedure allowed pregnancies but, since it could not be used in the convoluted vas, it was later discarded.

The idea of conducting the spermatic fluid through the anastomosis remained attractive, but the concept of a removable cannula did not. Thus were developed tapered internal cannules (endosplints), which were entirely intraluminal. The first was made of polyethylene tubing. This was drawn down at the operating table until its smaller end could be passed into the urethral side of the vas, the tubing being large enough to fit into the testicular side. After placement, the vas was sutured over it, but the cannula was not affixed to the vas (Fig. 10.4). One patient in whom this endosplint was placed impregnated his wife. Later, when he requested a vasectomy, the polyethylene could not be found on one side and the vas was obstructed at the level of the internal inguinal ring, apparently because the cannula had migrated to that point and had perforated the vas owing to its relative stiffness.

The next development was a factory tapered tubing of Silastic rubber (Schmidt 1972). It was somewhat difficult to insert as it was so soft. It also appeared to migrate up the vas since there was nothing to bond it in place. Other cannulae made of absorbable materials such as gelatin were also tried. Although they seemed to prevent leakage at the anastomosis (at that time we were not employing the careful approximation of layers that is in use today), other problems occurred such as delayed occlusion of the anastomosis.

Microporous Tubing

A further development, the use of tubing that would bond itself to the vas, was never fully explored. Many years ago segments of polyurethane tubing that had

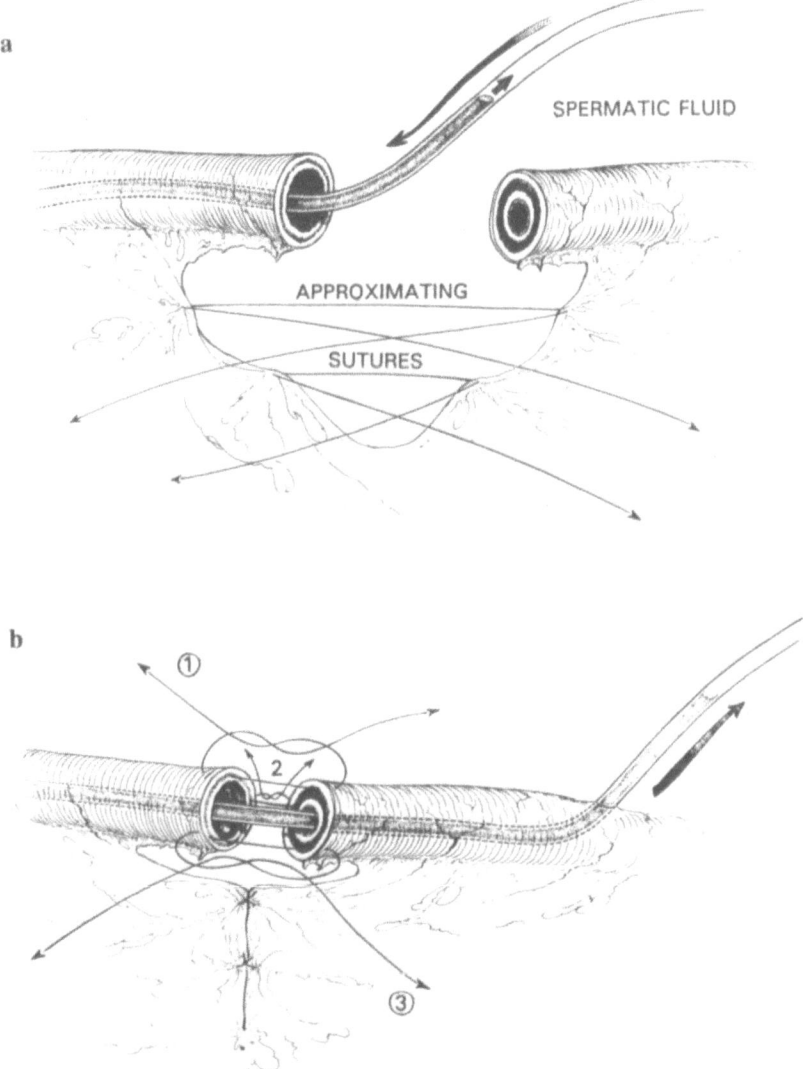

Fig. 10.2a,b. Polyethylene tubing placed in the vas as a cannula (Schmidt 1961).

a microporous outer surface seemed satisfactory when they were used in animal experiments (Schmidt 1976). Similar types of tubing were used by other investigators. All had a shaggy outer coating into which the body would send fibrous tissue to from a firm mechanical bond. These tubes were soft, elastic and non-reactive. They were placed either by (1) reaming out the mucosa of the cut ends of the vas and placing the tubing into these ends; or (2) constructing the device with a shaggy surface at right angles to the tubing so that the bond would occur between the device and the muscular face of the vas end; or (3) stabbing diagonally through the walls of the obstructed vasa into their

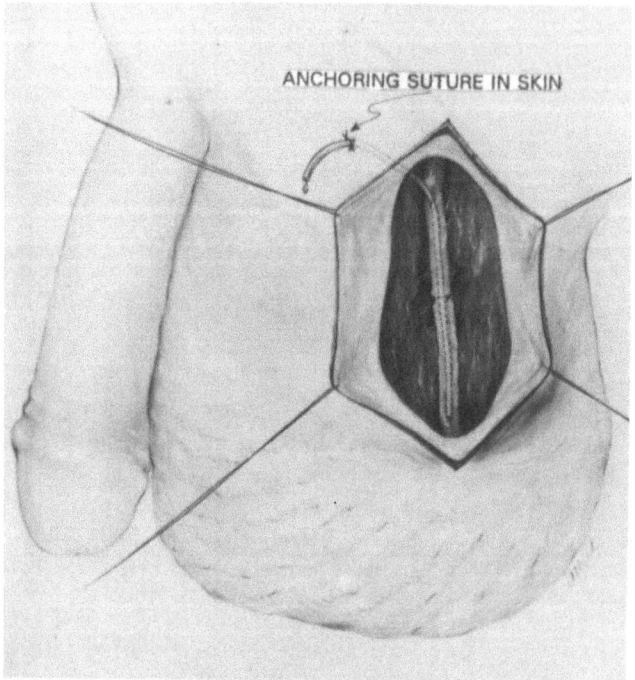

Fig. 10.3. Polyethylene tubing draining spermatic fluid (Schmidt 1961).

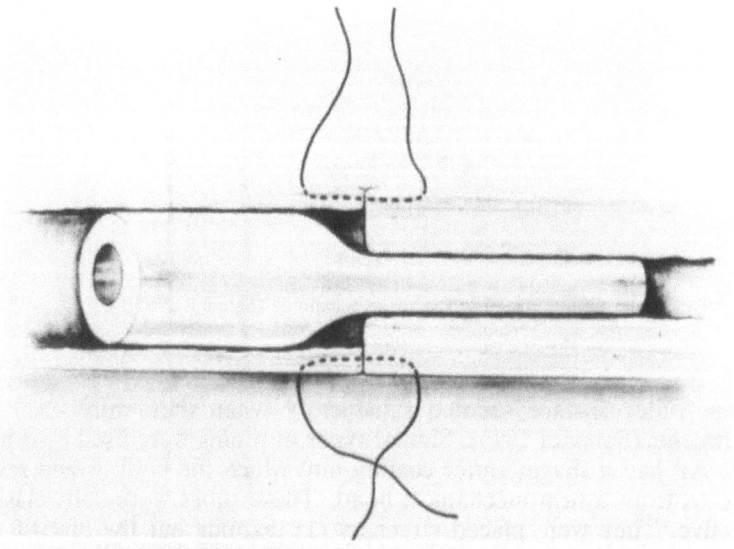

Fig. 10.4. Diagram of endosplint in anastomosis of the vas (Schmidt 1972).

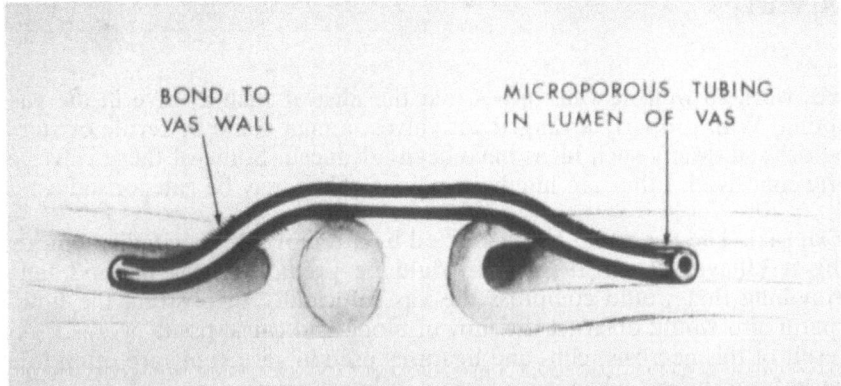

Fig. 10.5.   Diagram of microporous tubing bridging end of the vas (Schmidt et al. 1976).

lumens, placing the tubing through this stab wound so that it formed a bridge between the vas ends, the ends of the tubing being open in the vas lumen to carry spermatic fluid between these ends (Fig. 10.5). Of all vas prostheses, this one seemed to offer the greatest promise, although its softness could cause it to kink if it were used to bridge any significant distance. However, its elasticity would permit it to be compressed shut once it was bonded.

Materials to Obstruct the Vas Temporarily

Many surgeons, although they have studied the properties of tissue and of sound healing, seem to forget these principles and thus treat the vas as if it were a segment of steel water-pipe. Many devices or materials have been proposed (Silastic, cyanoacrylate) to fill the lumen of the vas completely by hardening and thereby obstructing it (Hrdlicka et al. 1967). The understanding was that, since the devices were inert, they could later be removed upon request and fertility thereby restored. This is a tempting idea, until the following points are considered:

1. The lumen of the vas dilates after obstruction, so that a device initially tight enough to obstruct the lumen may become loose, permitting sperm to pass around it
2. Regardless of how the vas is obstructed, blowouts will occur in the epididymis, creating obstructions
3. The value of some of these devices appears to be interference with sperm transport. Such interference may cause the sperm to stay in the vas past their period of viability
4. If the device is to be held in place by constricting ligatures, the ligatures will constrict the flow of blood in the wall of the vas

None of these ideas seem to have stood the test of time and all appear to have been abandoned.

Vas Valves

Valves work so well in water-pipes that the idea of such a valve in the vas is tempting. With properly arranged vas valves, a man could be fertile or sterile, as he desired. Many such ideas have been advanced. Some of these valves are poorly conceived, other are highly ingenious. They may be categorised as:

1. External: The vas could be obstructed by a removable metal clip compressing it (Jhaver et al. 1971). As could be predicted, this method failed. Anything that would compress the vas sufficiently to obstruct the flow of sperm also would obstruct the flow of blood and cause tissue necrosis. As a result of this necrosis, clips and ligatures used in vasectomy are often found away from the vas when it is exposed at later vasovasostomy

2. Internal: The vas would be cut or obstructed and the valve would be placed between the cut ends (Free 1975; Brueschke 1976). A water-tight (sperm-tight) bond would be necessary between the vas and the valve. For that reason, it would probably be necessary to place the valve in the open position, so that the pressure of spermatic fluid in the testicular end of the vas would not disrupt the forming bond. Two types of valves have been proposed.

    a)   Plastic tubing, such as microporous polyurethane. This could be compressed to obstruct the vas. Those types that have been devised would require an operation to expose the valve and change the setting, and the compressing mechanism was usually of metal

    b) Metal valves. The first of these copied a conventional water valve, being entirely of metal and with a stem that could be turned to change the setting. It was modified by adding plastic tubing to the ends of the valve (after the first completely metal valves eroded out of the vas). The most recent innovation employs magnetism of an uncommon wavelength. The polarity of the valve can be changed from outside the body so that the valve can be opened or closed without operation (Politanova (1987) personal communication). The use of this valve remains experimental

Although the idea of easily reversible male sterilisation has vast appeal, it proves of limited practicality when faced with physiological reality. The following problems present themselves:

1. Any operation upon the vas creates the risk that a spermatic granuloma might form at that point. This could lead to a recanalisation, with sperm bypassing the valve

2. The longer the vas is obstructed, the greater is the chance that an epididymal blowout and obstruction will occur, so that sperm would not reach the valve

3. As after conventional vasectomy, sperm antibodies would arise in half of the patients, a small number of whom would have non-motile or agglutinated sperm as a result of these antibodies, just as is seen after vasovasostomy

4. Any such valve would need soft, flexible ends within the vas lest its ends erode out of the vas when the scrotum moves

5. Owing to sperm storage in the ampulla of the vas, there would be a significant delay, as after vasectomy, in achieving sterility after the valve was turned to the off position

6. Finally, the spermatic nerve runs next to the vas. This creates the possibility that it might be pinched against a metal valve, causing severe pain. Although this has not been reported by the experimenters, I would not like to have a metal device in my scrotum and then go horseback riding.

Many different devices have been placed in the vas in past years. Improved understanding of the principles of vasovasostomy have made stents and internal cannulae obsolete. Devices to obstruct the vas reversibly either by external pressure or by plugging its lumen have failed and have been abandoned. Experiments continue, using devices either partly or fully made of soft inert plastic tubing, with an outer surface that can be invaded by fibrous tissue, thus bonding the device to the vas in a leak-proof manner. The future of any device designed to obstruct the vas reversibly seems very limited.

References

Brueschke EE (1976) Reversible occlusive devices. J Reprod Med 17:103–115

Cameron CS (1945) Anastomosis of the vas deferens. JAMA 127:1119–1120

Dorsey JW (1957) Surgical correction of postvasectomy sterility. J Int Coll Surg 27:453–456

Free MJ (1975) Development of a reversible intravasal occlusive device. In: Sciarra JJ, Markland C, Speidel JJ (eds) Control of male infertility. Harper and Row, Hagerstown, pp 124–139

Hrdlicka JG, Schwartzman WA, Hasel K, Zinsser HH (1967) New approaches to reversible seminal diversion. Fertil Steril 18:289–296

Jhaver PS, Davis JE, Lee H, Hulka JF, Leight G (1971) Reversibility of sterilization produced by vas occlusion clip. Fertil Steril 22:263–269

O'Conor VJ (1948) Anastomosis of the vas deferens after purposeful division for sterility. J Urol 59:229–233

Schmidt SS (1956) Anastomosis of the vas deferens: an experimental study I. J Urol 75:300–303

Schmidt SS (1961) Anastomosis of the vas deferens: an experimental study IV. The use of fine polyethylene tubing as a splint. J Urol 85:838–841

Schmidt SS (1972) Vas reanastomosis procedures. In: Richart RM, Prager DJ (eds) Human sterilization. Charles C Thomas, Springfield, pp 76–85

Schmidt SS, Schoysman R, Stewart BH (1976) Surgical approaches to male infertility. In: Hafez ESE (ed) Human semen and fertility regulation in men. CV Mosby, St Louis, pp 476–493

Chapter 11

Alloplastic Spermatocele (Sperm Reservoirs)

A. Kelâmi

The development of sperm reservoirs commenced in 1968 when Schoysman used the saphenous vein. In 1973 Kelâmi and Wagenknecht, independently of one another, began experimental work to construct an alloplastic reservoir of silicone and Dacron (Kelâmi et al. 1976; Wagenknecht 1977). Pregnancies and live births occurred in the laboratory work (Kelâmi et al. 1977a,b; Wagenknecht 1977) and the technique was applied to man. Kelâmi (1981) reported the first successful delivery following the use of such a technique.

Jimenez-Cruz (1980) used a Goretex prosthesis and was able to obtain pregnancies with live births. Colpi et al. (1983) also used a vascular prosthesis but attached it on to the vas deferens instead of on to the epididymis whilst Puppo et al. (1984) sutured the prosthesis from one epididymis to the other. In 1986 Brindley et al. described a new sperm reservoir which was sutured to the vas deferens and contained an intraluminal tube. Successful pregnancies were reported by using this device.

What Is an Alloplastic Spermatocele?

An alloplastic spermatocele is a receptacle for sperms, that can be punctured, the contents aspirated and the aspirate inseminated into the female partner. The alloplastic spermatocele is indicated in the following circumstances:

1. Aplasia of the vas deferens
2. Long-distance stenosis of the vas deferens
3. Obstruction of the ejaculatory ducts
4. Loss of ejaculation after retroperitoneal lymph node dissection
5. Spinal cord injuries

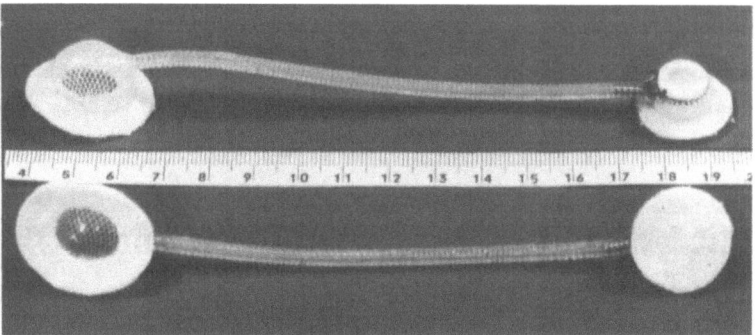

Fig. 11.1. The Kelâmi–Affeld prosthesis is made up of one piece and consists of three different parts, all made from silicone elastomer: (1) the reservoir with a volume of 1.5 ml has a flange which is covered with Dacron velour on one side to allow the ingrowth of granulation tissue which holds the prosthesis in place; (2) a non-kinking connecting tube, and (3) a puncture port (polypropylene) with a self-sealing silicone membrane (Kelâmi 1978).

The Implantation and Aspiration Technique

A scrotal or infrapubic (Kelâmi 1980) approach is used for the implantation. The latter has the following advantages:

1. It is in a hygienic, clean area
2. Wound healing is excellent
3. Scrotal contents can be explored up to the inguinal ring on both sides through one incision
4. If a Kelâmi–Affeld alloplastic spermatocele is used, the puncture port is easily placed through the same incision, also for both sides

After the eventration of both scrotal contents, the epididymis is incised first in the cauda region and checked for sperms. If there are none, this procedure is repeated in the corpus and the caput areas until sperms are found. Only one (proximal) tubule needs to be cut open. As a motility-increasing agent, the operative area is steadily irrigated with Baker's solution. The Kelâmi–Affeld prosthesis (Fig. 11.1–4) is then sutured with 3/0 non-absorbable monofilament material on to the tunica albuginea of testis without handling the tubules, especially the proximal one. After the termination of the anastomosis, the tunical vaginalis is closed with continuous 3/0 synthetic absorbable sutures and the scrotal contents replaced. Then, using Roux retractors, the inguinal region is explored and a subcutaneous tunnel made for the puncture port which is placed without fixing. As the scrotum and its contents are very tender during the first few postoperative days, the subcutaneously placed punctureport button in the inguinal region makes for easy puncturing. By not puncturing the reservoir itself, possible injuries to the epididymis and the reservoir are avoided. The puncture-port contains a base plate which stops the puncturing needle from going through.

The aspiration is done under sterile conditions with an 18 gauge needle and an empty 2 ml syringe. The aspirated amount of about 1.5 ml is called aspirate

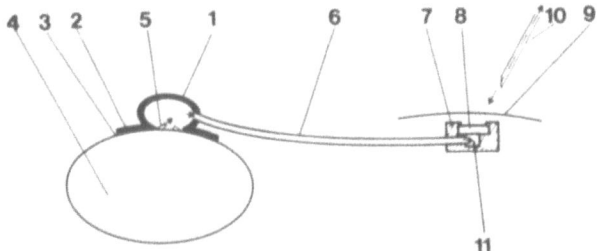

Fig. 11.2. Cross-section of the Kelâmi–Affeld prosthesis: (1) alloplastic spermatocele; (2) the margin of the silicone prosthesis; (3) Dacron velour; (4) epididymis; (5) opened proximal tubule; (6) non-kinking tube between the reservoir and the puncture port; (7) polypropylene case; (8) silicone membrane; (9) skin surface; (10) needle for irrigation and aspiration and (11) the pool of the puncture port (Kelâmi 1978).

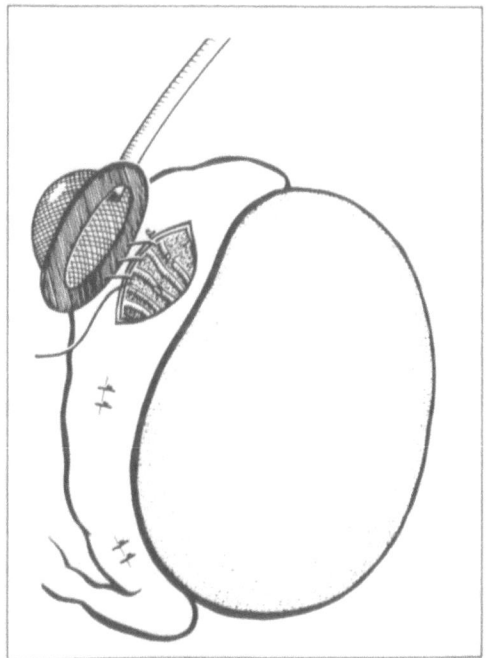

Fig. 11.3. The Kelâmi–Affeld prosthesis is being sutured on to the tunica of the epididymis in the caput region (Kelâmi 1980).

No. 1. The reservoir is then irrigated with 1.5 ml Baker's solution and aspirated again (aspirate No. 2). Another 1.5 ml Baker's solution is then given back into the reservoir and the needle removed. Spermatological examination of the aspirates is essential. For insemination, aspirate No. 1 is mixed with the ejaculate of the patient and 0.2 ml of it inseminated high cervically by the gynaecologist. The rest of aspirate No. 1 and aspirate No. 2 is then applied with a cervical cap. If necessary, motility-increasing agents like caffeine, kallikrein and carnitine may be added (Kelâmi 1981)

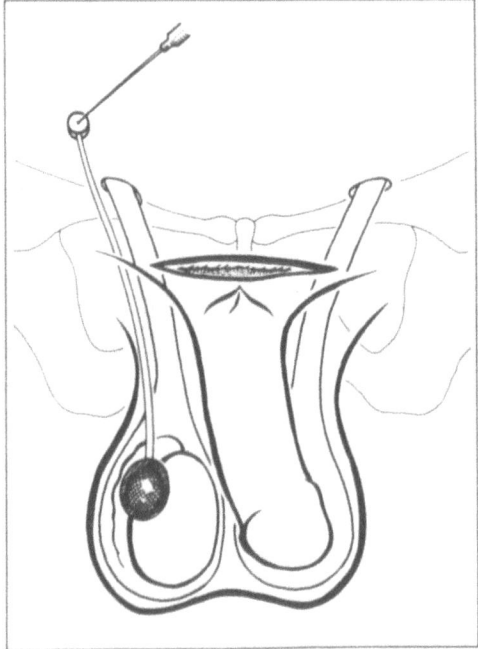

Fig. 11.4. The infrapubic (Kelâmi) incision eases the entire implantation procedure, including the puncture port in the lower abdominal wall (Kelâmi 1980).

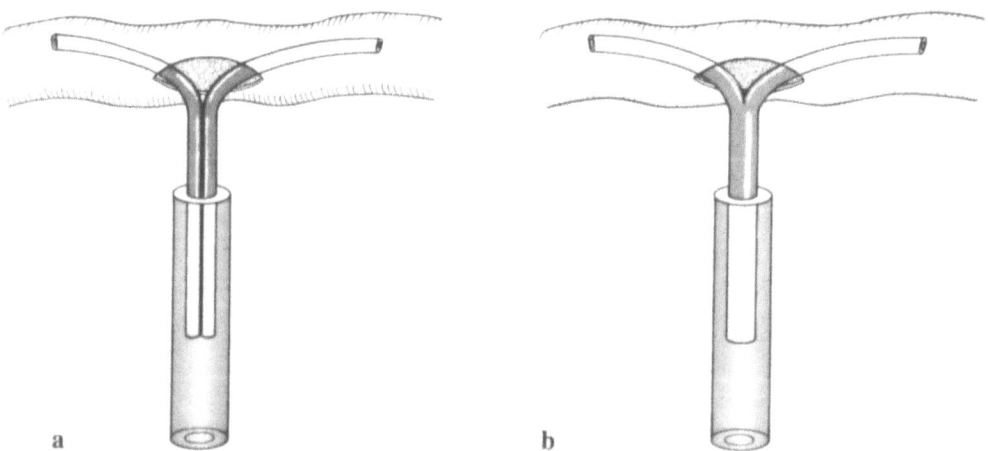

a   b

Fig. 11.5a,b. Intubation of the epididymal tubule in both directions with a microtube (Kelâmi 1978).

The implantation is only performed after thorough investigation of the female partner which should include the following data:

1. At least three cycles of basal temperature
2. Hormonal status
3. Proof of tubal patency

Results

I have implanted 42 prostheses in 27 patients and there has been one abortion and one delivery of a healthy baby who is now nearly 10 years old.

In 1986, Belker et al. reported the implantation of 130 alloplastic spermatoceles in 91 patients in three different centres. Seven pregnancies have occurred, three of which ended with abortion, and four progressed to full-term delivery. The study of these cases showed that the presence of non-motile sperm contraindicates the implantation of an alloplastic spermatocele, because these sperm always remain non-motile.

Brindley et al. (1986) reported that motile sperm were obtained from 8 of the 12 patients and the partners of 2 patients successfully conceived with artificial insemination. Two of the reservoirs became infected and had to be removed.

A very recent publication by Micic et al. (1990) reports the implantation of 12 alloplastic spermatoceles. In 10 of them, forward moving sperm were discovered. The wives of 3 patients became pregnant delivering two sets of twins and one single child.

What Happens to the Alloplastic Spermatocele?

The problem seems to be with the epididymal tubules and not with the prosthesis. The present different types of prosthesis all serve well as a reservoir. The main difference is the puncturing procedure, and there the Kelâmi–Affeld prosthesis shows clear advantages.

The prosthesis remains intact and is undisturbed by the irrigation procedure. Only four of the 42 prostheses had to be removed at the patients' request. In no instance was this due to infection. The open surface of epididymis and the tubule or tubules were covered with a fibrinous layer which caused obstruction and a failure of sperms to enter the prosthesis. Prostheses on the cauda epididymis contain sperm for longer than those in the caput region.

Experience shows that motile spermatozoa could be observed in the epididymal fluid of half of the cases. Only 10% of those with motile sperms at operation still showed motile sperm when first aspirated. In one case motile sperms could be observed even after 6 months, but in no case showing non-motile spermatozoa could motile sperm be seen in the aspirate. This leads to the conclusion that in cases of non-motile spermatozoa in the epididymal fluid, spermatoceles should not be implanted.

A disadvantage of the development by Puppo is that it is limited to cauda-cauda cases and in case of infection on one side, the other side is endangered as well.

How Can the Proximal Tubule be Kept Open?

Jimenez-Cruz sutured the walls of the open tubules outward without success (personal communication). Another possibility would be to develop microtubes to be inserted into the epididymal tubuli as permanent splints (Kelâmi 1978). These microtubes could be inserted, under the microscope, into both sides of the tubule and fixed, leaving the single end free, or be inserted into the vas deferens as in epididymovasostomies (Özdiler and Kelâmi 1980) (Fig. 11.5a,b).

In 1990, Thomas reported his results with such a technique at the 9th International Symposium of Operative Andrology in Berlin, but unfortunately he was unable to improve the results.

The collection of sperms from the epididymes remains problematical. Since the introduction of in vitro fertilisation, gamete intrafallopian transfer (GIFT), zygote intrafallopian transfer (ZIFT), intrauterine insemination (IUI) and microsurgical epididymal sperm aspiration and insemination (MESAI), our way of thinking has changed. In all cases of azoospermia, it is warranted to try MESAI in order to use the very first, and maybe the very last, possibility of insemination. Thereafter, any kind of bypass surgery (vasovasostomy, epididy-movasostomy, tubulovasostomy, alloplastic spermatocele) can be tried. This means, naturally, a high degree of cooperation between the infertile couple, andrologist and gynaecologist.

References

Belker AM, Jimenez-Cruz DJF, Kêlami A, Wagenknecht LV (1986) Alloplastic spermatocele: poor sperm motility in intraoperative epididymal fluid contraindicates prosthesis implantation. J Urol 136:408–409

Brindley GS, Scott GI, Hendry WF (1986) Vas cannulation with implanted sperm reservoirs for obstructive azoospermia or ejaculatory failure. Br J Urol 58:721–723

Colpi GM, Zanollo A, Lange A, Farina U, Baretta G (1983) Artificial spermatocele inserted onto the vas deferens: a clinical report. Acta Eur Fertil 14:203

Jimenez-Cruz JF (1980) Artificial spermatocele. J Urol 123:885–886

Kelâmi A (1978) Alloplastische Spermatocele. Eine kritische Betrachtung und Verbes-serungsvorschläge. Extr Urol 1:245–251

Kelâmi A (1980) Atlas of operative andrology. De Gruyter, Berlin

Kelâmi A (1981) Kelâmi-Affeld alloplastic spermatocele and successful human delivery. Urol Int 36:368–372

Kelâmi A, Rohloff D, Affeld K (1976) Alloplastische Spermatocele – vorläufige Mitteilung. Akt Urol 7:167–169

Kelâmi A, Rohloff D, Affeld K, Schröter A, Blohm B (1977a) Alloplastic spermatocele, insemina-tion from epididymal reservoir. Urology 10:317–319

Kelâmi A, Rohloff D, Affeld K (1977b) Alloplastische Spermatocele – tierexpermimentelle Untersuchungen und die ersten klinischen Versuche. Therapiewoche 27:7538–7542

Micic S, Papic N, Mladenovic I, Prorocic M, Genbacev O (1990) Intrauterine insemination with spermatozoa recovered from the aspirate of artificial spermatocele. Human Reproduction 5: 582–585

Özdiler E, Kelâmi A (1980) Microscopical splint epididymovasostomy. Eur Urol 7:81–84

Puppo P, Belgrano E, Gaboardi F, Trombetta C (1984) Alloplastic bridge spermatocele: an experimental study in the rat. J Androl 5:155–158

Schoysman R (1968) La création d'une spermatocèle artificielle dans les agenesis du canal dèfèrent. Bull Soc Belge Gynec Obstet 38:307–317

Wagenknecht LV (1977) Further experiences with an alloplastic spermatocele: experiments in bulls. Andrologia 9:179–181

Chapter 12

Testicular Prostheses

J.P. Pryor

The implantation of a testicular prosthesis to replace an absent testis is a cosmetic operation carried out at the request of the patient or his parents. Some men or boys with the absence of one or both testes do not feel the necessity to have a prosthesis whilst others suffer severe psychological disturbances. It is these who derive great benefit from this simple yet effective procedure.

Historical Aspects

Since the first Vitallium testicular prosthesis was implanted by Bowers in 1939 (Girdansky and Newman 1941) many other substances have been tried (Table 12.1). Prentiss et al. (1963) tried many materials and concluded that silicone rubber was the most satisfactory. Silicone polymers go a long way towards fulfilling the criteria for an ideal prosthesis and most of the current models are constructed of silicone. Rea (1943) emphasised the need for different sizes; in addition, the manufacturers attempt to give the prostheses a consistency which makes them feel natural on palpation.

Indications

Any male with an absent testis is a candidate for a testicular prosthesis and the only absolute contra-indication is the presence of infection. For this reason a testicular prosthesis should not be inserted at the time of exploration for torsion or trauma. Some surgeons believe that implantation is contra-indicated at the time of orchidectomy for testicular cancer (Rosen and Benson 1984) but whilst implantation may be undesirable in these circumstances, they do not constitute a definite contra-indication.

Young children do not feel anxiety about the absence of testes but by the age of 10 years the absence may give rise to teasing by other children. It is for this

Table 12.1. Development of testicular prostheses

Author	Material
Girdansky and Newman (1941)	Vitallium
Rea (1943)	Lucite
Hazzard (1953)	Glass marbles
	Methacrylate
Baumrucker (1957)	Gelfoam
Prentiss (1963)	Dacron
	Rubber
	Polyethylene
	Plexiglass
	Silicone rubber
Furka and Molnar (1967)	Plastic
	Polymethylmethacrylate
	Polyurethane foam
Puranik et al. (1973)	Ivalon sponge
	Silastic gel
Lattimer et al. (1973)	Foam-filled silicone

reason that it is reasonable to discuss with the parents the desirability of inserting a prosthesis at the time of surgery for cryptorchidism. They should be warned that it might be necessary to exchange the prosthesis for a larger one at adolescence but this is not always necessary.

Adolescents are often acutely aware of the absent testis and may be inhibited in their sexual activities. Team games and communal changing rooms are a source of embarrassment and discomfiture and relationships with the opposite sex may be inhibited. This is more often due to the fear of embarrassment than the result of teasing. It is rare for married men to request a testicular prosthesis following orchidectomy and even rarer for the request to arise before or after a subcapsular orchidectomy for prostatic cancer.

Weissbach et al. (1981) reported two psychological studies on men following orchidectomy and prosthetic replacement of the testis. He found that although there were psychological changes these could not be separated from the effect of orchidectomy. In general terms, the time of greatest effect of testicular loss on a patient's awareness of body image is during and immediately after puberty. The authors also drew attention to the fact that amongst adults, university graduates and civil servants were more likely to opt for a cosmetic replacement than men from lower income groups.

Choice of Prosthesis

The current range of prostheses is shown in Table 12.2. The Dow Corning prostheses are based upon the original design of Lattimer and consist of a Silastic gel-filled implant featuring a unique suture loop made of Dow Corning high-performance elastomer (Fig. 12.1). The suture loop secures the implant in the proper anatomical position and a removable insert in the loop helps to prevent accidental puncturing of the silicone envelope whilst inserting the

Table 12.2. Testicular prostheses that are currently available

Manufacturer	Size	Length (mm)	Diameter (mm)	Volume (ml)
Dow Corning	Child	25	20	5.3
	Youth	34	24	9.4
	Adult (average)	42	28	16.2
	Adult (large)	47	30	22.2
Mentor	Small	33	26	
	Medium	37	31	
	Large	42	37	
Surgitek	Infant	25	17	
	Petite	30	21	
	Small	30	44	
	Medium	33	47	
	Large	40	55	

suture (Fig. 12.2). The prosthesis is supplied sterile but should resterilisation be required, this is easily accomplished by either high-speed instrument (flash) sterilisation (at least 15 min at 270°F (132.2°C) and 30 psi (2 kg/cm^2)) or in a standard gravity steriliser (30 min at 250°F (121°C) and 15 psi (1 kg/cm^2)). The Dow Corning prosthesis is available in four sizes and it is also possible to obtain custom-built prostheses.

The Mentor prostheses (previously Heyer–Schulte) are available in three sizes of reinforced, moulded silicone elastomer (RME) and have an optional Dacron reinforced silicone elastomer pad through which a suture may be placed to anchor the testicular prosthesis in the scrotum.

The Surgitek testicular prostheses are supplied in five different sizes and manufactured in two consistencies – gel-filled, which are extra soft and elastic,

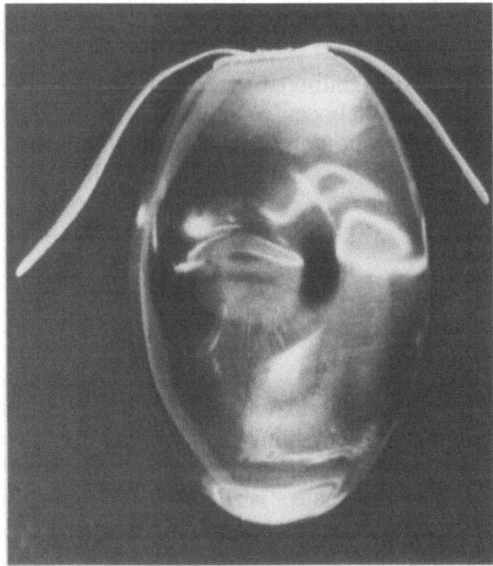

Fig. 12.1. Dow Corning testicular prosthesis prior to implantation.

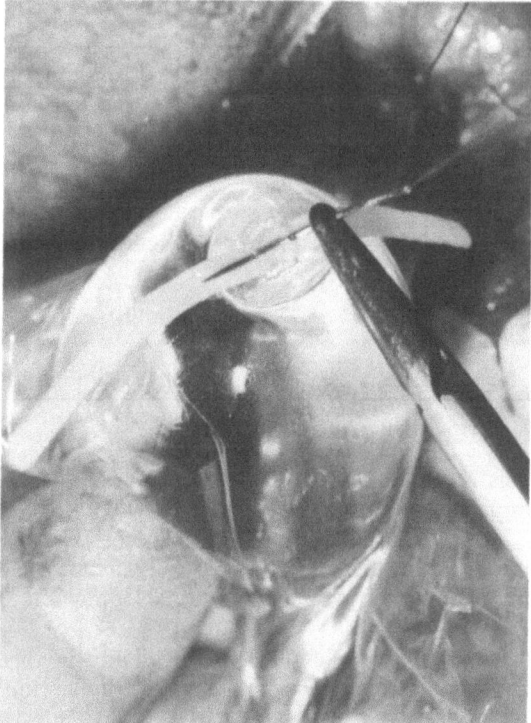

Fig. 12.2. Dow Corning testicular prosthesis showing the protective function of the insert in the suture loop.

and Plastigel, which are firmer but still pliable. The prostheses are supplied plain or may be fixed in the scrotum with a suture through the attached Dacron felt or through the suture loop.

In adults the size of the prosthesis is determined by comparison with the remaining testis. In children the prosthesis is chosen to be a little larger than the remaining testis in the hope that any inequalities in size will not cause embarrassment. It is always possible to replace a small prosthesis with a larger one at a later date.

Surgical Considerations

The operation is usually carried out under general anaesthesia and with an umbrella of prophylactic antibiotics. Prevention of infection is essential and skin preparation and other antiseptic techniques should be meticulously enforced.

In general, the skin incision (Fig. 12.3) should not overlie the prosthesis and although Solomon (1972) advocated a midline incision through the scrotal raphe, this was in patients undergoing bilateral orchidectomy for carcinoma of the prostate. The newer forms of chemical castration or the technique of sub-

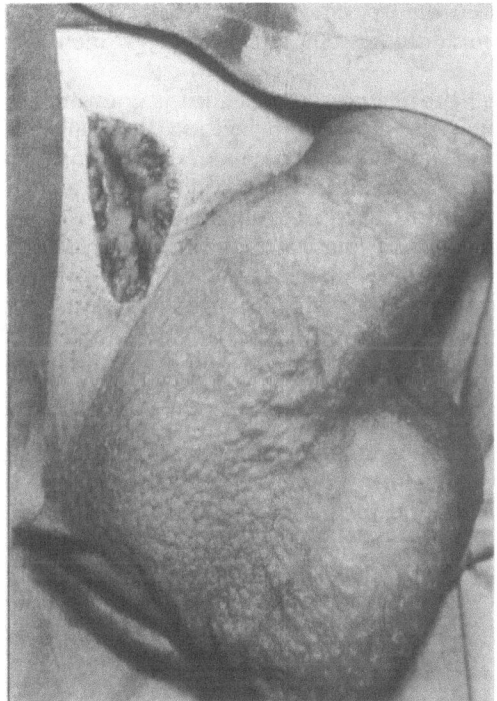

Fig. 12.3. Skin incision may be inguinal or inguino-scrotal but should not be situated so that it will overlie the prosthesis.

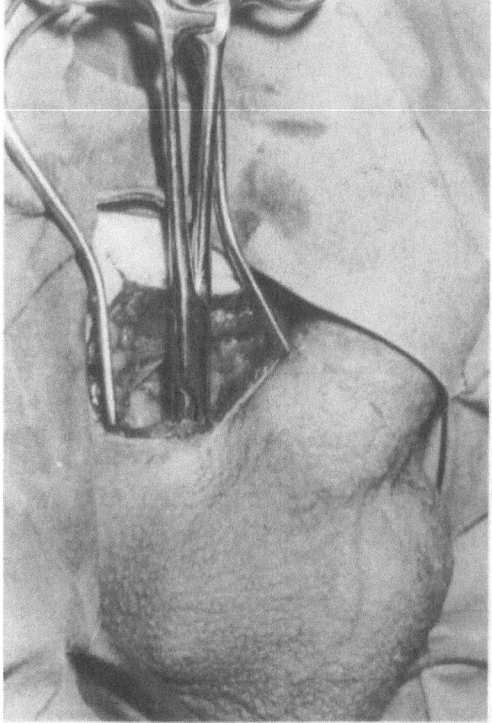

Fig. 12.4. Blunt resection with a swab to create the necessary space for the prosthesis in the scrotum.

capsular orchidectomy have rendered the operation of bilateral orchidectomy obsolete for prostate cancer and, in addition, it is rare for elderly men to be interested in testicular prostheses.

The skin incision may be inguinal or inguino-scrotal and it is convenient to implant bilateral prostheses through the infrapubic incision that has been popularised by Kelâmi (1980). Abassian (1972) recommended a transverse contralateral scrotal incision and the placement of the prosthesis into a dartos pouch. A more satisfactory method is to use the Lattimer et al. (1973) technique and place the prosthesis in a space created in the scrotum by blunt dissection. The space may be prepared by opening the scissors and then enlarged by finger dissection or tucking a swab into the wound to ensure that the cavity is large enough to accommodate the prosthesis (Figs 12.4 and 12.5). This may be difficult but the use of tissue expansion techniques (Lattimer and Stalnecker 1989) is necessary on but rare occasions. A Babcock or Alliss forceps is used to grasp the lower part of the scrotal sac which is then hitched up into the wound (Fig. 12.6). A non-absorbable (000 monofilament nylon) suture is placed through the loop of the prosthesis – the protecting strip of plastic preventing the needle damaging the prosthesis – and through the sub-cutaneous tissues near the forceps, taking care not to puncture the skin (Fig. 12.7). The suture is tied, the protective wrapping is removed (Fig. 12.8), and the testis placed into the scrotal sac. The testis is secured in position by closing the neck of the scrotal cavity with a purse string suture of 000 Dexon. The

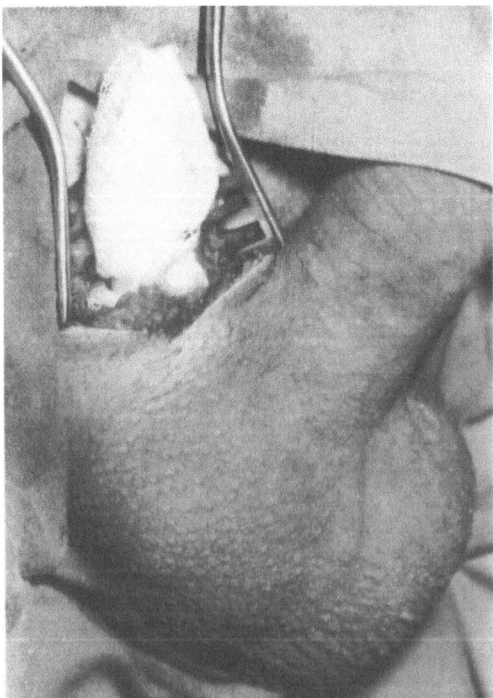

Fig. 12.5. Swab tucked into the scrotum to ensure adequate space for the prosthesis.

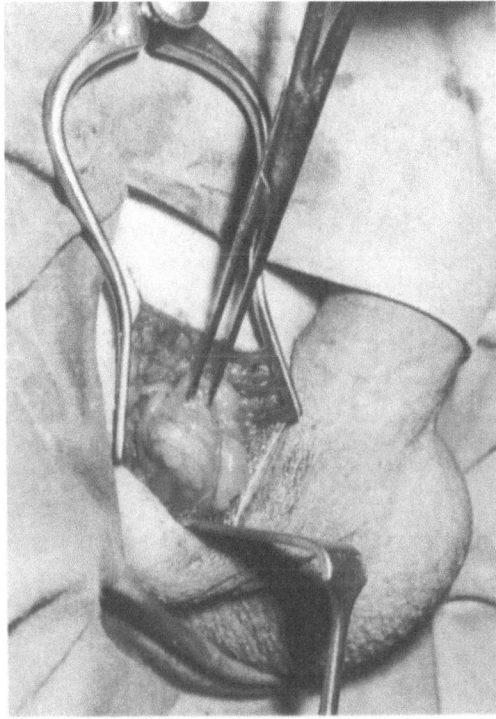

Fig. 12.6. The lowest part of the scrotal pouch is hitched up into the wound in order to place the anchoring suture.

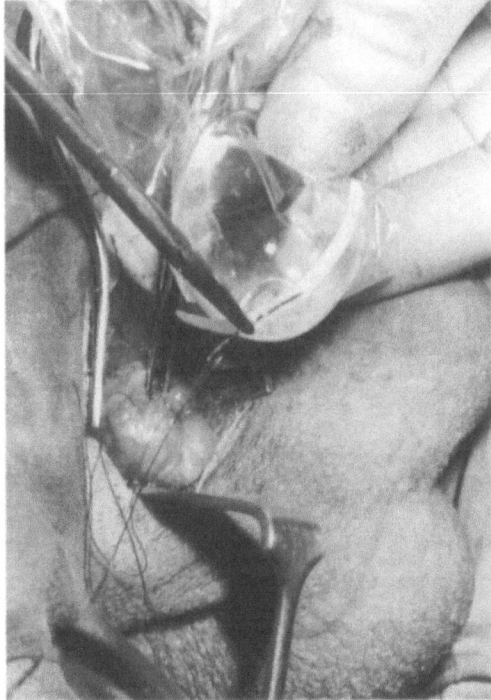

Fig. 12.7. The prosthesis is sutured to the subcutaneous tissues to anchor the prosthesis to the lowest part of the scrotum. Note that the protective wrapping still surrounds most of the prosthesis in an attempt to lessen the risk of skin contamination.

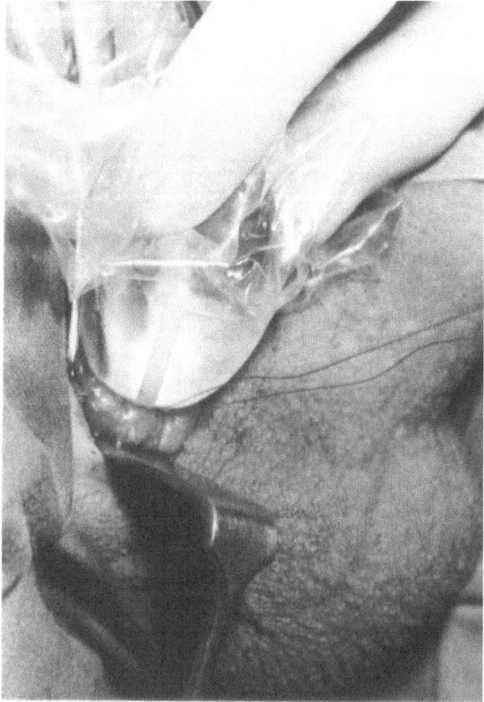

Fig. 12.8. Placing the prosthesis in the scrotum.

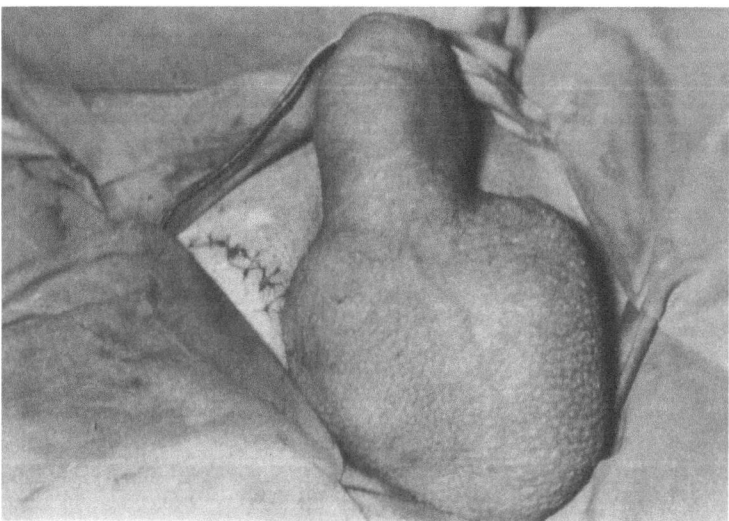

Fig. 12.9. Appearance at the conclusion of the operation.

subcutaneous layers of skin are closed with synthetic absorbable sutures (Fig. 12.9). Throughout the procedure it is desirable to handle the prosthesis as little as possible and to avoid contact between the skin and the prosthesis.

Complications

The incidence of complications is difficult to assess but Marshall (1986) in a survey of members of the Western Section of the American Urological Association found that complications occurred more frequently after previous scrotal surgery for infection or torsion. The incidence of complications in that study is shown in Table 12.3. In addition to the complications shown in the table, transient or persistent contraction of the scrotum was seen in 4% and 3% of the 2533 patients.

Haematoma Formation. Meticulous haemostasis is essential and it is unnecessary to use any scrotal drainage. The risk of haematoma formation can be minimised by using blunt dissection.

Infection. The risk of this should be minimised by using an antiseptic technique and short-term prophylactic antibiotics. Should the prosthesis become infected it is necessary to remove it and wait 3 months before trying to insert another one. Minor skin infection does not necessitate the removal of the prosthesis, particularly if the wound has been closed in layers.

Skin Necrosis. This may occur when too large a prosthesis is inserted and the skin overstretched. It is also more likely to occur if there have been previous scrotal incisions.

Implant Rupture. This may occur if the device was accidentally damaged at the time of insertion or it may follow blunt trauma to the testis.

Malposition and Replacement. This should not occur but at the time of operation it is important to check the lie of the prosthesis to ensure a good cosmetic

Table 12.3. Complications of testicular prosthesis insertion in 2533 patients (Marshall 1986). Complications arising from prosthesis placement in patients with testicular trauma or orchidectomy for carcinoma of the prostate are not included

Indication for prosthesis	Number	Complications (number (%))			
		Wound dehiscence or prosthesis extrusion	Infection	Haematuria	Pain
Epididymitis/orchitis	231	18 (7.8)	5 (2.2)	6 (2.6)	7 (3.0)
Torsion	527	27 (5.1)	7 (1.3)	9 (1.7)	6 (1.1)
Undescended/absent testis	1079	42 (3.9)	7 (0.7)	3 (0.3)	11 (1.1)
Testicular tumour	696	18 (2.6)	4 (0.6)	2 (0.3)	10 (1.4)
Total	2533	105 (4.2)	23 (0.9)	20 (0.8)	34 (1.3)

result. During any subsequent surgery to correct the position of the prosthesis, cutting diathermy is used once the skin has been incised (diathermy does not damage silicone) but care should be taken not to damage the prosthesis with the diathermy point.

Miscellaneous. Scrotal and penile lymphoedema occurred in a 50-year-old man operated upon by Elsahy (1972) and required excision of the affected tissues.

Conclusion

It is difficult to better the conclusion of Rosen and Benson except to add that the patient makes the choice to have the operation rather than the surgeon. They stated that "surgeons should avoid value judgments about sexuality and a particular patient's body image. All patients, young or old, unfortunate enough to have an absent testicle should be offered the operation of a testicular prosthesis. The prostheses currently available all result in a satisfactory cosmetic result, and surgical complications are very low."

References

Abassian A (1971) A new surgical technique for testicular implantation. J Urol 107:618

Baumrucker GO (1957) Testicular prosthesis for an intracapsular orchidectomy. J Urol 77:756–758

Elsahy NI (1972) Scrotal and penile lymphoedema as a complication of testicular prosthesis. J Urol 108:595–598

Furka I, Molnar J (1967) Palliativer Hodenerstatz mit Kunstoff. Acta Chir Acad Sci Hung 8:25

Girdansky J, Newman HF (1941) Use of a Vitallium testicular implant. Am J Surg 53:514

Hazzard CT (1953) The development of a new testicular prosthesis. J Urol 70:959–960

Kelâmi A (1980) Atlas of operative andrology. De Gruyter, Berlin, pp 11–13

Lattimer JK, Stalnecker MC (1989) Tissue expansion of underdeveloped scrotum to accommodate large testicular prosthesis. Urology 33:6–9

Lattimer JK, Vakili BF, Smith AM, Morishima A (1973) A natural-feeling testicular prosthesis. J Urol 110:81–83

Marshall S (1986) Potential problems with testicular prostheses. Urology 28:388–390

Prentiss RJ, Boatwright DC, Pennington RD, Hohn WF, Schwartz MH (1963) Testicular prosthesis: materials, methods and results. J Urol 90:208–210

Puranik SR, Mencia LF, Gilbert MG (1973) Artificial testicles in children: a new silastic gel testicular prosthesis. J Urol 109:735–736

Rea CE (1943) The use of a testicular prosthesis made of lucite: with a note concerning the size of the testis at different ages. J Urol 49:727–731

Rosen JS, Benson RC (1984) Testicular prostheses. Semin Urol 2:176–179

Solomon AA (1972) Testicular prosthesis: a new insertion operation. J Urol 108:436–438

Weissbach L, Bach D, Wagenknecht LV (1981) Clinical applications of testicular substitutes. In: Wagenknecht LV, Furlow WL, Auvert J (eds) Genitourinary reconstruction with prosthesis. George Thieme Verlag, Stuttgart New York, pp 177–187

Chapter 13

Vascular Access

C.J. Rudge

Introduction

The principal conditions for which vascular access are indicated, and in the management of which a urological surgeon may be involved, are acute and chronic renal failure. This chapter concentrates primarily on this topic but will also mention briefly other circumstances in which more prolonged intravenous access is required for longterm intravenous nutritional support and the administration of cytotoxic drugs into large central veins.

Strategies for Dialysis Access

Many of the operations required to provide access for haemodialysis, haemo-filtration or any of the other forms of renal support are intrinsically "minor" operations in the surgical sense – they do not involve major dissection of deep structures, they do not take very long to perform, and they require few specialised instruments or surgical skills. Many of them can be performed under local or regional anaesthesia. However, the single most important error in the surgical provision of vascular access is to consider these "minor" procedures relegated to the most junior surgeon at the end of an operating session. To provide access for a critically ill patient with acute renal failure may be extremely difficult and demanding. To provide good access for a patient with chronic renal failure is to establish their life-line for dialysis which, in the absence of a successful renal transplant, will be required for the rest of their life. Potential sites for access are limited and must be cherished and preserved for as long as is possible. Inappropriate use of a site, or the failure for technical reasons to use each site to its maximum potential is potentially a disaster for the individual patient. Whilst the possibilities today are greater than was the case in the early days of dialysis the nightmare situation of a patient "running out" of dialysis access sites is very real both to medical staff and to the patients themselves. It is essential to have a *very* longterm perspective when the various options and alternatives are considered.

In general terms access procedures fall into one of two groups: those that provide immediate access for a limited time (weeks or occasionally months) and those that potentially provide longterm access (years) but which cannot be used for several weeks following the procedure. It is convenient to describe these two groups of operations separately and then to consider their use in the most appropriate manner in various clinical settings. Before doing so it is useful to describe in general terms the requirements for successful access. Ideally a vascular access procedure would:

a. Provide a blood flow through the dialyser in excess of 300 ml/min
b. Function without the use of a blood pump in the dialysis circuit (i.e., be "driven" by the patient's systolic blood pressure)
c. Be as independent as possible of the patient's blood pressure, and be non-thrombogenic
d. Be safe
e. Be free of the risks of sepsis
f. Be cosmetically acceptable

In practice only one procedure, the arteriovenous fistula, comes close to fulfilling all these criteria. Every other procedure falls short of the ideal in one or more ways and the drawbacks as well as the advantages of each procedure are described below.

Acute Access for Haemodialysis

Percutaneous Dialysis Catheters

Using a pumped dialysis system, if necessary with a "single-needle" system in which the direction of blood flow is alternately reversed through a single-lumen catheter, it is possible to obtain adequate dialysis through a percutaneously-placed central venous dialysis catheter. A number of such catheters are available commercially. They are inserted, usually at the bedside under local anaesthesia, into a central vein. Standard sites of insertion are the internal jugular vein and the subclavian vein although it is also possible to cannulate the femoral vein. Well-described techniques for puncture of these veins are available. Complications of central venous puncture are also well described and apply equally to dialysis catheter insertion. Patients with chronic renal failure have abnormal haemostasis and bleeding is, therefore, a particularly significant complication in such patients, especially following inadvertent arterial puncture during catheter insertion. The use of DDAVP (Desmopressin; Lerring, Leltham, Middlesex) or cryoprecipitated plasma may be advisable.

The Arterio-Venous (AV) Shunt

Described by Scribner and Quinton thirty years ago (Quinton et al. 1960) the AV shunt was the first attempt to provide prolonged vascular access for

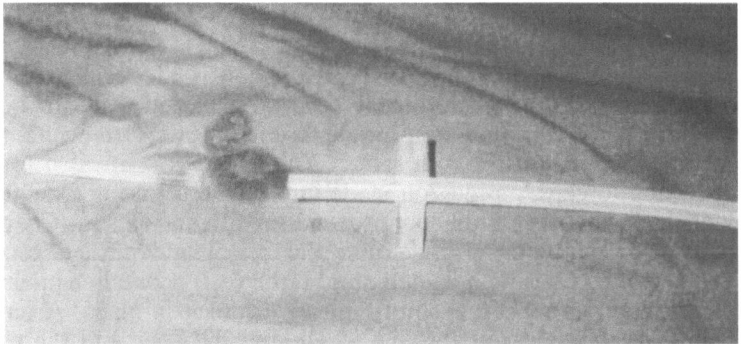

Fig. 13.1. Ramirez winged AV shunt and vessel tip.

haemodialysis and is still a valuable technique. An AV shunt consists of two limbs, each made up of a silastic shunt limb and a Teflon tip (Fig. 13.1). The shunt limbs are standard and, whilst a number of configurations are available, the author prefers to use a straight "Ramirez winged" shunt, as illustrated. Into the shunt limb is inserted a Teflon (PTFE) tip the size of which depends on the vessel into which the shunt is to be inserted. One limb is positioned in an artery, the other in a vein, and when the shunt is not in use blood flow is preserved by connecting together the arterial and venous limbs.

Shunt Sites and Surgical Exposure

Whilst in theory, or in desperation, a shunt can be inserted into any artery or vein there are three standard sites for shunt insertion:

1. The ankle, using the posterior tibial artery and long saphenous vein. An incision is made on the medial side of the leg, 4 cm proximal to the medial malleolus and parallel to, but 1 cm posterior to, the tibia. The posterior tibial artery lies below the deep fascia in the neurovascular bundle between flexor digitorum longus anteriorly and flexor hallucis longus posteriorly. The long saphenous vein lies in the fat under the anterior edge of the incision.

2. The wrist, using the radial artery and forearm cephalic vein. It is possible, though less satisfactory, to use the ulnar artery, and of course, any superficial vein. The incision should be longitudinal and midway between the radial arterial pulse and forearm cephalic vein. The artery is below the deep fascia, the vein lies in the superficial fat.

3. The upper arm, using the brachial artery and one of its venae commitantes. The incision should be directly over the brachial aertery where it can be palpated medial to biceps, 4–5 cm proximal to the elbow. The artery lies below the deep fascia. Care must be taken to avoid the median nerve which lies close to the artery, its exact position depending on the level in the upper arm at which the artery is exposed. There are usually two or three venae commitantes lying close to the artery and joining into a single, larger vein more proximally.

Surgical Technique

Regardless of the site of shunt insertion the technique is identical for both artery and vein. The vessel is ligated distally and a tie placed (but not tied) proximally around the vessel. The appropriate shunt tip is inserted into the shunt limb and the system primed with saline. The vessel is controlled proximally with dissecting forceps, an incision made into the vessel using a number II scalpel blade, and the vessel dilated proximally with a Watson–Cheyne probe. The tip of the shunt is inserted into the vessel and pushed gently proximally. The proximal tie is then ligated around the vessel containing the tip and the distal tie ligated around the shunt limb to secure it in place. Arterial and venous limbs are brought out through small stab incisions and the skin closed with nylon.

Choice of Shunt Site

As always with vascular access there is likely to be a conflict of interests between immediate and successful function and other considerations. In general a shunt should not be used in the arm of a patient with chronic renal failure for whom the arm veins should be preserved for future arteriovenous fistulae (vide infra). However, there are likely to be problems with a leg shunt in older patients with peripheral vascular disease (it is not worth attempting shunt insertion if the posterior tibial pulse is not palpable) and ill, hypotensive patients. In the arm, the forearm site is infinitely preferable to the upper arm because of the risk of distal ischaemia following ligation of the brachial artery. However, in patients who are severely ill and in intensive care with acute renal failure it is not uncommon to find that all superficial veins (including the forearm cephalic) are thrombosed following multiple intravenous cannulations and therefore a brachial shunt may be the only practical site.

Shunt Complications

Shunt complications include infection, clotting, distal ischaemia and disconnection (leading to haemorrhage).

The Permcath

There is now available a semi-permanent, dual-lumen central venous catheter (Permcath, Quinton) that is inserted surgically, provides immediate access but which may function for considerably longer than the percutaneously-placed catheters. The essential component of the catheter is that it has a Dacron cuff at its mid-point (Fig. 13.2). The Dacron cuff on the catheter encourages fibrous ingrowth thus both anchoring the catheter and reducing the likelihood of systemic sepsis.

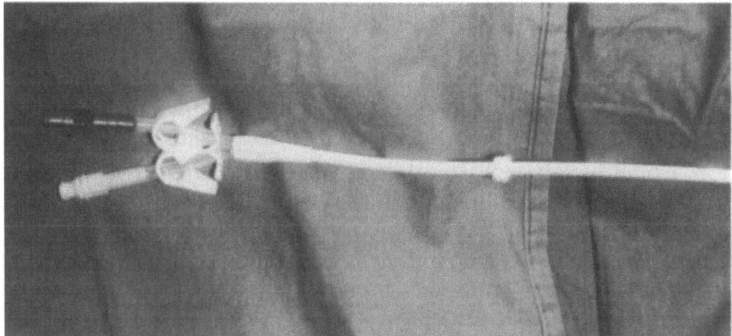

Fig. 13.2. Permcath.

Surgical Technique

The catheter is inserted into the internal jugular vein (preferably on the right) such that there is an 8–10-cm-long subcutaneous tunnel.

The incision lies 2 cm above the medial 2–3 cm of the clavicle. Division of sternomastoid muscle, or (in thin patients) separation of the two heads of the muscle exposes the internal jugular vein. The exit site for the catheter is chosen on the anterior chest wall and the catheter drawn through the subcutaneous tunnel. The catheter is inserted into the vein using a 5/0 Prolene purse-string suture and the position of the catheter confirmed by X-ray or screening (the tip should lie in the superior vena cava). The incision is closed.

Complications of the Permcath are clotting and sepsis, which may be local or systemic.

Chronic Access for Haemodialysis

AV Fistula

Following the description by Brescia and Cimino (Brescia et al. 1966) of the surgically-created arteriovenous fistula this has become the standard first-choice access for maintenance haemodialysis. Following creation of the fistula, blood flow and pressure in the superficial vein increase and as a result the vein dilates and the wall thickens. The vein may be cannulated 6–8 weeks post-operatively with special dialysis needles and provides adequate blood flow for dialysis. A successful fistula may provide good access for many years of dialysis.

Fistula Sites

1. The preferred site for a fistula is in the forearm, with an anastamosis between the radial artery and forearm cephalic vein. The incision may be

over the anatomical snuff-box or more commonly in the forearm immediately proximal to the radial styloid. It is essential to ensure pre-operatively by physical examination that the forearm cephalic vein is patent. Unfortunately it is a favourite vein for use by anaesthetists and others for intravenous cannulae and if as a consequence it is thrombosed a valuable access site is lost.

2. The only reasonably satisfactory alternative to the forearm fistula is the antecubital or brachial fistula, between the brachial artery and the upper-arm cephalic vein. This vein is not always present or patent and there is a temptation to use the median basilic vein. Whilst it is usually possible to perform the operation in this way it rarely provides a useful fistula as the vein passes medially and then deep into the upper arm where it is not accessible for a dialysis needle.

3. It may be possible to construct a fistula between the ulnar artery and a vein on the ulnar aspect of the forearm, but this is rarely as good a fistula as those described above.

Surgical Technique

1. *Forearm fistula*. The incision is similar to that used for a forearm shunt (vide supra). It is necessary to mobilise both artery and vein for 4–5 cm such that they can lie side-to-side without tension. Branches of the vein are ligated if necessary. The two vessels are clamped proximally and distally and opened on their anterior surfaces for about 2 cm. A continuous suture with 6/0 Prolene is performed and it is extremely useful immediately before tying the suture to pass a Watson–Cheyne probe up all four limbs of the fistula whilst releasing the vascular clamps in order to dilate the vessels. A thrill should be palpable over the anastamosis and the proximal vein demonstrating flow through the anastamosis. A pulse but no thrill indicates venous obstruction, whereas no pulse and no thrill indicates an arterial inflow problem.

If the forearm cephalic vein lies too far on to the dorsum of the forearm for a side-to-side anastamosis to be performed without tension the vein may be divided distally and swung across to create an end-to-side anastamosis. In this case the vein should be spatulated to create a 1.0–1.5-cm anastamosis.

2. *Antecubital fossa fistula*. An end-to-side anastamosis is created between the upper arm cephalic vein and the brachial artery. Through a transverse skin-crease incision in the antecubital fossa the brachial artery (medially) and the cephalic vein (laterally) are exposed. It is not necessary to mobilise more than 2.0 cm of the brachial artery – this occasionally involves partial division of the bicipital aponeurosis. The vein is mobilised both proximal and distal to the skin incision as far as is necessary to allow distal ligation and division. The proximal end is then swung medially to reach the artery, spatulated, and a 1-cm anastamosis performed using 6/0 Prolene.

Fistula Complications

1. *High output cardiac failure*. This rarely occurs unless the vein dilates abnormally to produce a particularly large fistula – almost invariably an antecubital fistula.

2. *Venous hypertension*. The thumb and index finger may become swollen and engorged with possible skin changes if there is excessive distal flow following a side-to-side forearm fistula. Ligation of the vein immediately distal to the anastamosis is curative.

3. *A "steal" syndrome*. Occasionally, usually in diabetic patients or those with severe peripheral vascular disease, flow through the fistula may reduce distal arterial flow and produce ischaemic signs or symptoms. If the fistula is large it may be banded to reduce flow through it, but more commonly ligation of the fistula is necessary to restore distal blood flow.

4. *Aneurysm formation*. This usually follows repeated needling over many months of the same site, associated with sepsis.

Grafts

When attempts to create fistulae using native veins as described above have failed it becomes necessary to use synthetic or biological vascular grafts. The advantage of this approach is that the graft may be positioned subcutaneously (and thus accessible for "needling") whilst anastamosed to a deeper artery and vein that themselves cannot be used for a fistula. Whilst in some dialysis centres graft fistulae are used as first or second choice access procedures, the longterm patency of such grafts is less than that of "native" fistulae, and the likelihood of complications is greater. It is, therefore, common practice to restrict their use for those patients in whom all possible sites for a native fistula have failed.

Types of Grafts

Biological Grafts. It is possible to remove a length of long saphenous vein from the patient's own thigh for use as a graft in either the arm or leg. There is available commercially human long saphenous vein, sterilised and preserved, for use. Also available commercially are grafts prepared from human umbilical vein and bovine carotid artery.

Synthetic Grafts. A number of products are available, the majority being produced from expanded polytetrafluoroethylene (PTFE). One interesting option, based on a slightly different principle, is the biocarbon access device. This consists of a length of standard PTFE on to the side of which has been fused a biocarbon access port. The graft is positioned subcutaneously with appropriate arterial and venous anastamosis, whilst the access port is brought through the skin to provide easy access by using specifically designed connectors. This has the theoretical advantage of using deep vessels to produce the blood flow through the graft whilst avoiding the problems of needle insertion into the synthetic graft.

Sites for Grafts

Because the graft uses vessels not themselves used for fistula construction the possible sites are not the same as for a fistula. Wherever an artery and vein are accessible a graft can be interposed, but the three most common sites are (a) the forearm, running from the radial artery to an ante-cubital vein; (b) the upper arm, running from the brachial artery either in the antecubital fossa or higher in the arm to any convenient deep vein; (c) the leg, running most commonly from the superficial femoral artery to femoral or long saphenous vein.

In most sites there is also a choice of configuration – the graft may be straight, running from artery to vein exposed through separate incisions; or looped/curved, running from artery to vein exposed through a single incision.

Choice of Graft Material and Site

Despite a large number of publications (Haimov et al. 1974; Owens et al. 1979; Tellis et al. 1979; Palder et al. 1985; Butler et al. 1977) regarding the use of graft fistulae for dialysis there are very few good comparative studies allowing conclusions to be drawn between the different types of graft available. Consequently there is no clear-cut "best buy" and the surgeon will need to balance cost, availability, ease of handling and the preferences of the dialysis nursing staff. The author's preference is for the Vitagraft (Johnson and Johnson, Anatreim, California), a PTFE graft which is freely available, less expensive than some, and which can be positioned freely in a loop or curve without kinking. The Vitagraft is available with 6 mm or 8 mm diameter – the smaller is normally used. Similarly there is no concensus on the optimal site or configuration for grafts – the thigh has the advantages that during dialysis the patient has both arms free, and also of a greater blood flow because of the larger vessels used.

Surgical Technique

Incisions and exposure clearly depend on the chosen site and configuration of the graft. The author's current preference is to position a 6-mm PTFE graft (Vitagraft) in a loop on the anterior aspect of the thigh. However similar principles apply to implantation of the graft in other sites.

Through a longitudinal incision in the upper thigh, starting 2–3 cm below the inguinal ligament the superficial femoral artery and vein are exposed lying medial to sartorius muscle. Mobilisation for 3–4 cm is usually adequate. The graft is positioned in a subcutaneous tunnel on the anterior thigh. This necessitates two small distal stab incisions – one medial, one lateral – and it is important to ensure that the tunnel does not compress the graft, which can lie without any kinks. Each end of the graft is cut obliquely and anastomosed end-to-side to the artery and vein with 5/0 or 6/0 Prolene, each anastamosis being at least 1 cm in length. Before completing the anastamosis and releasing the vascular clamps, the graft is filled with normal saline. As with a native fistula a thrill should be palpable along the length of the graft. The incision is closed.

Graft Complications

1. *Thrombosis*. Early thrombosis is probably related to technical failure at operation. However most published series (Munda et al. 1983; Bell and

Rosental 1988) demonstrate that patency of graft fistulae at 1 year is 50%–70% compared with 80%–90% for native fistulae (Munda et al. 1983) and in a significant proportion of thrombosed grafts there is evidence of venous stenosis close to the anastomosis. This is caused by venous intimal hyperplasia (Etheredge et al. 1983), possibly resulting from turbulent blood flow in the draining vein. Whilst thrombectomy (Palder et al. 1985) or thrombolytic therapy (Mangiarotti et al. 1984; Zeit 1986) alone may temporarily restore flow through the graft, it is important to identify and correct any stenotic lesion. This may be achieved by surgical intervention but there are also encouraging reports of percutaneous transluminal angioplasty (Schwab et al. 1987).

2. *Infection.* Local infection occurring at the site of graft puncture is a serious complication. Antibiotic therapy, if instituted early enough may be effective but once the infection is established it is extremely difficult to eradicate. By-pass grafting of the infected segment may be possible but there is a strong likelihood that the graft may need to be removed.

3. *Aneurysm formation.* This is more common with the biological grafts than with currently available PTFE grafts.

It has in general been emphasised that many patients with graft fistulae are likely to require surgical intervention to resolve these complications but that this aggressive approach can produce reasonable longterm access using PTFE grafts (Owen 1990).

Access for Dialysis: Conclusions

For a patient with acute renal failure immediate access is probably best provided by a percutaneously placed central venous catheter. However haemofiltration in an intensive care unit may require the arterial flow provided by a shunt. The first choice site for shunt insertion is the forearm, with the leg or brachial vessels being alternatives. Access for a patient with chronic renal failure requires much greater consideration of the long term. Ideally all such patients are seen 3–6 months before dialysis is required and a forearm arteriovenous fistula created at this stage. This can then be used from the initiation of dialysis. However, it is inevitable that a number of patients will not be referred to a dialysis unit until they require dialysis and there are also those in whom the diagnosis is not made before they present in end-stage renal failure or whose disease is so rapidly progressive that they require dialysis within days or weeks of diagnosis. In such patients the choice of acute access is important as every effort must be made to preserve possible fistula sites for subsequent use. Accordingly arm shunts should only be used in a dire emergency. The options are, therefore, to insert a leg shunt or to use central venous dialysis catheters whilst arranging to create a fistula as soon as possible, the temporary acute access being removed as soon as the fistula can be used (usually 6–8 weeks). A problem that has become increasingly recognised recently is the development of thrombosis or stenosis of the subclavian vein following use of a percutaneous subclavian dialysis catheter. This may be clinically insignificant until an AV fistula is created in the ipsilateral arm, at which stage severe oedema of the whole arm becomes evident. This complication is probably related to the duration for which a subclavian line is in situ. Therefore, whilst is may be appropriate to use such a line for dialysis for a few days, it is inadvisable to do so for the full length of time necessary for a fistula to develop. It is the author's practice to insert a Permcath under the same anaesthetic as that used for the fistula formation: the Permcath, being in the internal jugular vein, is not associated with the same problems as the subclavian dialysis catheters.

For those patients without adequate fistula veins a Permcath may provide access for well over a year, and occasionally for longer. However such patients will almost invariably require the insertion of a graft fistula. The PTFE graft described above can be used for dialysis within 10–14 days of surgery. There is some evidence that longterm patency is improved by the use of low-dose aspirin or anti-platelet agents such as dipyridamole, but no convincing benefit has been shown to follow systemic anti-coagulation. All graft fistulae also have a higher incidence than native fistulae of infection and aneurysm formation, and are much more likely to require thrombectomy, local excision and repair, or ligation.

"The Difficult Patient"

Whilst the procedures described so far in this chapter provide reasonable access for most patients there are unfortunately a number in whom multiple procedures are necessary and repeated failures lead to an impending lack of access. In such patients ingenuity and perseverance are needed: for example a Permcath may be placed in the femoral vein or a PTFE graft positioned from the axillary artery to the jugular or subclavian vein (Trout III). There are also specialised external shunts such as the Allen–Brown shunt, the Buselmeir shunt and the Thomas femoral shunt, none of which are used routinely (Owens 1988). Difficult access problems encourage improvisation!

Non-dialysis Access

The two main indications for prolonged intravenous access other than dialysis are parenteral nutrition and the administration of cytotoxic drugs. In both situations the solutions to be given are damaging to peripheral veins and rapidly cause thrombophlebitis or thrombosis. Accordingly they are infused into a larger central vein with a greater blood flow. There are three options:

1. *A tunnelled, percutaneously placed intravenous catheter.* A number of products are available, such as the Nutricath which can be inserted non-surgically and which provide adequate access. They are outside the scope of this chapter.

2. *The Hickman or Broviac catheter.* This is a silastic catheter, 40 cm in length, with a Dacron cuff adherent at its mid-point. Whilst kits are available

that allow this relatively large catheter to be positioned and tunnelled percuta-neously, this technique requires considerable skill and experience and in many centres Hickman catheters are still inserted surgically. The technique is almost identical to that described for Permcath insertion (see above), i.e., the internal jugular vein is exposed through an incision above the medial end of the clavicle, the catheter positioned in a subcutaneous tunnel with the Dacron at the mid-point, and the catheter inserted into the vein using a Prolene purse-string suture. Radiological confirmation that the catheter is correctly positioned is essential.

3. *The Port-a-cath*. The risk of sepsis associated with the Hickman catheter, and the cosmetic disadvantages, led to the development of the Port-a-cath. In this system a silastic catheter identical to that used in a Hickman catheter is inserted in the above manner into the internal jugular vein. However, rather than the catheter being brought through the skin to the exterior it is connected to a chamber which is positioned (and anchored) in a subcutaneous "pocket". On the anterior wall of the chamber is a membrane or diaphragm which can be punctured percutaneously as required for administration of intravenous solu-tions. Whilst this system has a number of practical and theoretical advantages it is considerably more expensive than a standard Hickman catheter and is not widely used.

References

Bell D, Rosental J (1988) Arteriovenous graft life in chronic hemodialysis. Arch Surg 123: 1169–1172

Brescia M, Cimino JE, Appel K et al. (1966) Chronic haemodialysis using venipuncture and a surgically created arteriovenous fistula. N Engl J Med 275:1089–1092

Butler HG, Baker LD, Johnson JM (1977) Vascular access for chronic haemodialysis: Polytetra-fluoroethylene (PTFE) versus bovine heterograft. Am J Surg 134:791–793

Etheredge EE, Haid SD, Maeser MN, Sicard GA, Anderson CB (1983) Salvage operations for malfunctioning polytetrafluoroethylene hemodialysis access grafts. Surgery 94:464–470

Haimov M, Burrows L, Baez A et al. (1974) Alternatives for vascular access for hemodialysis: Experience with autogenous saphenous vein autografts and bovine heterografts. Surgery 75: 447–452

Mangiarotti G, Canavese C, Thea A, Segoloni GP, Stratta P, Salomone M, Vercellone A (1984) Urokinase treatment for arteriovenous fistulae declotting in dialyzed patients. Nephron 36:60–64

Munda R, First MR, Alexander JW, Linnemann CC Jr, Fidler JP, Kittur D (1983) Polytetra-fluoroethylene graft survival in hemodialysis. JAMA 249:219–222

Owen WF Jr (1990) A patient with recurrent thrombosis in polytetrafluoroethylene dialysis grafts. Semin Dial 3:127–131

Owens ML (1988) Specialized External Shunts. In: Wilson SE (ed) Vascular access surgery, 2nd edn. Year Book Medical Publishers Inc, London, pp 185–187

Owens ML, Stabile BE, Gahr JE et al. (1979) Vascular grafts for haemodialysis: An evaluation for site and materials. Dial Transplant 8:521–526

Palder SB, Kirkman RL, Whittemore AD et al. (1985) Vascular access for haemodialysis. Patency rates and results of revision . Ann Surg 202:235–239

Quinton WE, Dillard DH, Scribner BH (1960) Cannulation of blood vessels for prolonged haemo-dialysis. Trans Am Soc Artif Intern Organs 6:104

Schwab SJ, Saeed M, Sussman SK, McCann RL, Stickel DL (1987) Transluminal angioplasty of venous stenoses in polytetrafluoroethylene vascular access grafts. Kidney Int 32:395–398

Tellis VA, Kohlberg WI, Bhat DJ et al. (1979) Expanded polytetrafluoroethylene graft fistula for chronic hemodialysis. Ann Surg 189:101–105

Trout III HH (1988) Unusual access procedures for chronic hemodialysis. In: Wilson SE (ed) Vascular access surgery, 2nd edn. Year Book Medical Publishers Inc, London, pp 273–284

Zeit RM (1986) Arterial and venous embolization: Declotting of dialysis shunts by direct injection of streptokinase. Radiology 159:639–642

Chapter 14

Antibiotic Therapy

W.R. Gransden and P.M. Thompson

Introduction

Infection of the urinary tract is the most common infection to be acquired in hospital and many episodes are associated with instrumentation or manipulation of the urinary tract, usually catheterisation. The development of urinary tract infection during bladder catheterisation has been shown to be associated with an increase in mortality in hospital patients, some as a result of bacteraemia (Platt et al. 1982). Furthermore, the most common localised focus of infection leading to septicaemia in hospital is the urinary tract (Fig. 14.1) (Eykyn et al. 1990; Meers et al. 1980) and outside hospital, in the community, the urinary tract is second in frequency only to the respiratory tract as the focus of infection leading to septicaemia (Eykyn et al. 1990). The infections associated with the use of urinary catheters and endoscopic instruments for transurethral surgery are of particular concern for the urologist. Infection follows the insertion of penile and testicular implants and artificial urinary sphincters less often, but when it occurs the results may be disastrous. In this chapter we shall consider infections associated with urinary catheters and urological prosthetic devices and discuss their pathogenesis, treatment and prevention.

Pathogenesis of Infection

The urinary tract is normally sterile from the kidney to the distal urethra in the healthy individual. There are three potential routes by which bacteria can spread to the urinary tract and establish infection: they may ascend via the urethra, be carried in the bloodstream or arrive by lymphatic spread. By far the most important of these is the first: through the urethra. Bacteria present in the distal urethra, usually derived from perineal and, ultimately, large-bowel flora may be transmitted to the bladder. The shorter urethra in part explains the greater incidence of infection of the urinary tract in women, and sequential

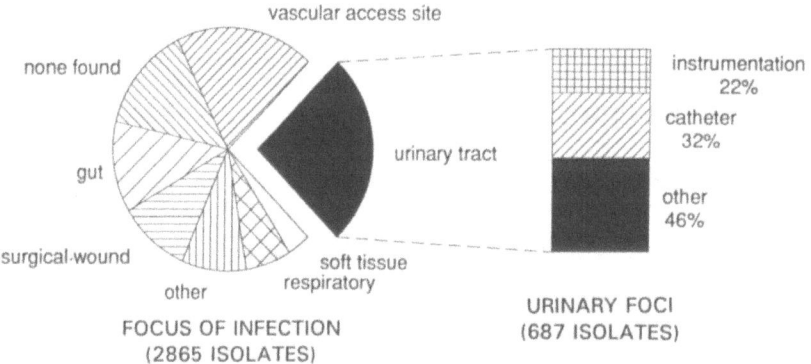

Fig. 14.1. Bacteraemia acquired in hospital. St. Thomas' Hospital 1969–1979.

studies have demonstrated the presence of the same species of bacteria in the periurethral flora, before the onset of infection.

Bacteria may reach the renal tissues by haematogenous spread from infection at a distant site. A relatively common event in bacteraemia caused by *Staphylococcus aureus*, during which micro-abscesses may develop in the renal parenchyma, it is a rare cause of infection of the urinary tract with other organisms.

The suggestion that micro-organisms can spread via the lymphatic route to the urinary tract is based on anatomical evidence. Bacteria may also gain access to the urinary tract by direct spread from local areas of inflammation, through fistulae and during surgery. However ascent via the urethra is the most important route of spread and has particular significance in the context of catheterisation and other manipulations of the urinary tract.

Micro-organisms causing infection of the surgical incision in urological surgery may be derived from several sources, as shown in Table 14.1. The bacteria may be part of the patient's own normal flora, present on the skin at the edge of the wound (e.g., staphylococci), or in the gastrointestinal tract if opened (e.g., *Escherichia coli*). Such infections, derived from the patient's commensal bacteria, are termed *endogenous* infections. Alternatively, the bacteria may be those present in an already infected site; also an endogenous infection. *Exogenous* infections are those derived from sources other than the patient and are probably less common. Sources of exogenous infection include the bacterial flora of the theatre staff, generally skin micro-organisms (e.g., *Staphylococcus*

Table 14.1.   Sources of surgical wound infection

Major group	Example	Type of infection
Animate		
Human	Patient	Endogenous
	Theatre staff peroperatively	Exogenous
	Ward staff post-operatively	Exogenous
Inanimate		
Environment	Dust	Exogenous
Equipment	Instruments	Exogenous
	Infusions	Exogenous

aureus), carried by air or directly inoculated into the wound. The inanimate environment is an unusual source of theatre-acquired surgical wound infection if there is good attention to aseptic technique and satisfactory sterilisation of equipment. Organisms present in dust are often derived from the skin flora of theatre staff.

Following closure of the wound and in the absence of surgical drains, infection becomes less likely and when it occurs post-operatively, is usually the result of a breakdown in aseptic technique during wound care.

Infection of prosthetic devices (device-related or periprosthetic infection) may occur at the time of surgery and may be considered a form of "wound infection". The source is usually the patient's own flora and the septic complication becomes apparent soon after operation. Less commonly infection may occur later, as the consequence of haematogenous spread from a distant site: either infected or supporting a commensal flora (Carson and Robertson 1988).

The virulence factors expressed by *Escherichia coli*, the commonest urinary tract pathogen, have been well studied (Johnson 1991). They include fimbriae, which mediate adherence to the uroepithelium, aerobactin production, serum resistance and K1 capsule production. It is not clear whether certain O-serotypes of *Escherichia coli* possess enhanced "uropathogenicity", however it is likely that the predominance of a small number of O-serotypes in infections of the urinary tract is the result of their predominance in the faecal flora rather than the consequence of particular pathogenicity (Brumfitt 1991).

Host Defences against Urinary Tract Infection

While the chemical constitution of the urine is inhibitory to some microorganisms (because of the pH, osmolarity and oxygen tension) it is an excellent culture medium for many bacteria. The host's first defence mechanism is the flow of urine and the flushing action of micturition, which hinder the invasion of the bladder by bacteria in the distal urethra. Obstruction of the flow of urine or failure to empty the bladder both predispose to infection of the urinary tract. The presence of foreign material not only prevents complete emptying of the bladder but can also provide a site for bacterial persistence and multiplication. Local immune responses and non-specific substances such as mucopolysaccharides and prostatic secretions provide additional protection (Kaufman et al. 1970; Stamey 1981).

Although small numbers of bacteria may be detected in the urine of the bladder of the healthy, bacteriuria is more common in the elderly, in pregnant women and in diabetics.

The factors that predispose to infection of the urinary tract are those that interfere with the normal host defence mechanisms. The urology patient is at particular risk of urinary tract infection, when there are structural or anatomical abnormalities of the urinary tract and when undergoing instrumentation or surgery. In addition there may be other general medical predisposing factors which may reduce the patient's ability to control infection including malignancy elsewhere, state of nutrition and medication.

The mechanisms bacteria employ to evade the host's defence systems in the urinary tract include antiphagocytic capsules and pili which promote adherence to the uroepithelium. In the case of device-related infection, bacteria adhere to the surface of the prosthesis and are maintained there by the production of a mucopolysaccharide matrix, which also acts as a barrier to the activity of host phagocytes and to antibiotics. The role of this biofilm is discussed further in relation to catheter-associated infection.

General Principles of Antimicrobial Chemotherapy

Antibiotics may be administered to treat infection or to prevent it. The former, therapeutic use, may be "empirical", when the antimicrobial sensitivity of the infecting organism is not known, or "definitive" when it is known. The prescriber must be aware of the limitations of antibiotics in treating infection – in order to eradicate infection a relatively intact host immune response must be present, any collection of pus must drain and, where infection involves foreign material, the material must be removed.

In the prevention of infection an antimicrobial is administered before infection has been established. Up to 40% of antibiotic use in hospital is given as "prophylaxis", mainly in surgical patients and much of it inappropriately. Prophylactic use of an antibiotic should be directed at a particular infection: wound infection, bacteraemia, infection of a prosthetic device. The antibiotic should be administered immediately before the procedure likely to result in the particular infection in order to achieve high tissue levels at the time bacteria may have access to the site of infection and should be discontinued soon after the period of exposure is over. These basic principles were established thirty years ago (Burke 1961). Despite this fact there is still much inappropriate use of antimicrobial therapy. In a survey of British urologists in 1983 (Wilson and Lewi 1985) 16% of urological surgeons started antimicrobial "prophylaxis" after the operation; in effect this was early therapy for any infective complication of the operation, rather than prophylaxis.

The choice of antibiotic for empirical treatment of an infection or for prophylaxis requires awareness of the likely pathogens and their anticipated susceptibilities and it is the microbiologist's duty to provide this information. The drug must reach the site of infection in adequate concentration and be active there. Thereafter, matters such as cost and toxicity should be considered. Local purchasing agreements will determine the relative costs or, possibly, availability of different antibiotics. Suitable antibiotics for uncomplicated urinary tract infection include:

Ampicillin or amoxycillin

Co-amoxiclav (amoxycillin + clavulanic acid)

Trimethoprim

Nitrofurantoin

Oral cephalosporins

In the treatment of cystitis caused by sensitive organisms, amoxycillin and pivampicillin offer no significant advantage over ampicillin. An increasing proportion (35%−50%) of strains of *Escherichia coli* are resistant to ampicillin (and hence also amoxycillin and pivampicillin) but many of these organisms are sensitive to the combination co-amoxiclav. Trimethoprim is increasingly being used alone, rather than in the sulphonamide combination co-trimoxazole, since it appears to be as effective as the combination but has fewer side effects, particularly in the elderly. *Proteus* spp are always resistant to nitrofurantoin. Of the oral cephalosporins cefaclor, cephradine, cephalexin and cefadroxil, the latter offers the advantage of a twice-daily regimen.

For acute pyelonephritis and systemic infection with a urinary focus, suitable parenteral antibiotics for sensitive organisms include: ampicillin, co-amoxiclav, cefuroxime and gentamicin. Cephalosporins such as cefotaxime and ceftazidime are active against a wider range of Gram-negative bacteria than cefuroxime but are more expensive. Enterococci are generally resistant to cephalosporins. Of the aminoglycosides gentamicin, tobramycin, netilmicin and amikacin, gentamicin is the least expensive. In view of their potential for renal and oto-toxicity, care must be taken to regulate therapy on the basis of regularly monitored serum levels, particularly in the elderly and those known to have renal impairment. New, once-daily, regimens are less often associated with toxicity and may make these agents more attractive (Kovarik et al. 1989).

The new 4-quinolone antibiotics such as ciprofloxacin, norfloxacin and ofloxacin have the advantage of a twice-daily regimen, oral formulations and a wide range of activity against urinary pathogens, except Enterococci and some Staphylococci. Ciprofloxacin may have a role in oral treatment of simple infection of the urinary tract, but for serious infections the parenteral version is expensive and there are often cheaper alternatives.

Expert advice should be sought before prescribing the new, and expensive, beta-lactam agents aztreonam and imipenem. The former is not active against Gram-positive bacteria and although the latter has an exceptionally wide range of activity, it should not be used as a first-line antibiotic, but rather, reserved for unusually resistant organisms.

It must be emphasized that antimicrobial therapy alone will not eradicate all infections. In the case of a localised focus of infection such as an abscess, drainage will be necessary, and for a foreign body (including a urinary calculus or possibly an encrusted urinary catheter), removal may be indicated. Prosthetic device-related infection once established cannot be cured by antimicrobial therapy; early removal and thorough drainage is required to minimise local damage to tissue that may impede subsequent implantation.

Likely Pathogens

Most organisms infecting the urinary tract are derived from the perineal and, ultimately, the faecal flora. Many factors influence the distribution of organisms encountered in urinary tract infection. Table 14.2 lists the bacteria isolated from the urine in both hospital- and community-acquired infections. By far the most common urinary tract pathogen is *Escherichia coli*. The range of species is greater in nosocomial infection, with more resistant species such as *Pseudomonas*, *Enterobacter*, coagulase-negative Staphylococci and Enterococci

Table 14.2. Bacteria isolated from urine specimens, St. Thomas' Hospital 1985–89

Organism	Hospital isolates					General Practice isolates				
	1985	1986	1987	1988	1989	1985	1986	1987	1988	1989
n =	2889	3018	2746	3599	3248	1070	1216	1806	2455	2501
E. coli	38.4	39.1	41.9	37.3	36.9	72.4	69.5	74.2	65.0	66.1
Proteus mirabilis	10.2	10.3	10.2	10.3	10.4	6.4	7.9	6.4	6.5	6.1
Klebsiella spp	12.8	11.7	8.8	9.8	9.0	6.0	6.7	5.1	6.3	5.3
Staphylococci										
S.saprophyticus	–	–	–	0.5	0.1	–	–	–	4.3	3.7
Other coagulase-negative	6.1	7.5	7.6	5.4	4.2	2.1	2.5	1.6	2.1	1.4
Enterococcus spp	10.9	12.0	9.4	11.3	12.9	3.0	3.6	3.3	4.9	4.7
Non-faecal streptococci	1.6	2.0	1.9	–	–	0.8	0.8	1.4	–	–
Pseudomonas spp	6.6	6.0	7.1	10.2	12.5	1.1	0.8	1.6	3.1	3.8
Enterobacter spp	2.9	2.7	2.9	5.6	4.7	1.3	2.1	2.0	2.2	2.7
Citrobacter spp	2.6	2.0	3.2	2.7	2.6	2.7	1.7	2.1	2.0	2.8
Proteus spp	2.8	2.8	2.4	1.1	1.5	1.8	1.5	1.1	0.4	0.2
Acinetobacter spp and										
unidentified Gram-										
negative bacilli	2.2	1.5	1.9	2.5	2.5	1.5	2.1	0.4	1.9	1.8

From St. Thomas' Hospital, Department of Microbiology.
The columns give the percentages of the urine specimens from which the bacterium was isolated.

Table 14.3. Antimicrobial resistance of hospital-acquired urinary isolates, St. Thomas' Hospital 1989

	E. coli	*P. mirabilis*	*Klebsiella* spp	*Enterococcus* spp
Ampicillin	45.5	19.0	97.7	1.4
Cefadroxil	5.4	6.7	4.8	99.7
Cefuroxime	1.9	0.6	1.8	98.7
Co-amoxiclav	6.8	1.7	3.1	1.5
Gentamicin	0.5	0.3	0.7	100.0
Ciprofloxacin	0.5	0.3	0.0	100.0
Nitrofurantoin	2.8	100.0	15.8	3.4
Trimethoprim	20.3	26.3	10.4	15.0

From St. Thomas' Hospital, Department of Microbiology.
The columns give the percentage of the isolates which were resistant to the antimicrobial agent.

more frequently encountered. Previous exposure to antibiotics will tend to select resistant strains and species and this, in part, may explain the observed difference in the distribution of organisms in community and nosocomial infections of the urinary tract. While selecting empirical ("blind" or initial) therapy for a nosocomial infection, recent cultures from urine from the patient may be available to suggest the likely pathogen and sensitivities will be known. Otherwise a best guess must be made. The sensitivities of individual species vary between geographical areas, between hospitals and even between wards in an individual hospital. Changes in the "typical" resistance patterns vary over time and with the occurrence of epidemics, either local or more general. Typical sensitivity data are given in Tables 14.3 and 14.4 for recent urinary isolates from St. Thomas' Hospital. A local policy for the use of antibiotics

Table 14.4. Antimicrobial resistance of community-acquired urinary isolates. (From St. Thomas' Hospital 1989.)

	E. coli	P. mirabilis	Klebsiella spp	Enterococcus spp
Ampicillin	38.0%*	7.3%	99.3%	0.0%
Cefadroxil	3.5	2.8	3.4	99.1
Cefuroxime	0.5	0.0	1.6	99.1
Co-amoxiclav	3.4	1.4	2.4	10.0
Gentamicin	0.5	0.0	0.0	100.0
Ciprofloxacin	0.0	0.7	0.8	100.0
Nitrofurantoin	2.0	100.0	13.6	100.0
Trimethoprim	17.6	14.0	12.0	10.4

From St. Thomas' Hospital, Department of Microbiology.
The columns give the percentage of the isolates which were resistant to the antimicrobial agent.

should be formulated and agreed between the urologist, microbiologist and pharmacist and should take into account local patterns of pathogens and their sensitivities.

Catheter-Associated Infection

Urinary catheters may promote infection by the introduction of organisms to the bladder during insertion, particularly if there is faulty aseptic technique. In women the route of bacterial spread is from periurethral flora often derived from rectal strains of bacteria. In men intraluminal spread is more common, the organisms ascending from the distal portion of the catheter or the collecting bag, or entering during the disconnection of the catheter from the collecting system. The catheter itself provides a site for colonisation by bacteria, particularly when it remains in place for prolonged periods of time. On the inner surface of the catheter a biofilm forms, derived from glycocalyx and host proteins and containing bacteria (Costerton 1984). Bacteria present in this biofilm may be protected from the effects of antimicrobials (Stickler et al. 1989). Eventually encrustations may form. On the outer surface microcolonies of bacteria develop but contain fewer organisms than biofilms. Microbial adherence to the catheter is influenced by its constituent materials; it is greater for latex than for silicone, silicone-coated, or silastic catheters.

Faults of aseptic technique during emptying of the drainage system may permit cross-infection in hospital. Guidelines for indwelling catheter care and the prevention of catheter-associated infection of the urinary tract have been published (Wong and Hooton 1981).

The risk factors for the development of catheter-associated infection have been shown to include: duration of insertion, female sex, absence of systemic antimicrobial agents and disconnection of the catheter from the collecting system (Shapiro et al. 1984). Generally there is a cumulative risk of infection of 5%–10% each day a closed catheter system is in place (Garibaldi et al. 1974).

Prevention of Catheter-Associated Infection

Knowledge of the pathogenesis of catheter-associated infection has directed methods for prevention. Attempts to reduce the incidence have included improved meatal care to remove one source, the use of catheters coated with silver or silver oxide to impede bacterial adherence (Lundberg 1986) and the administration of systemic antibiotics. The use of various antiseptics, e.g., povidone iodine, simple cleansing, or topical antibiotic preparations applied to the urethral meatus have failed to reduce the incidence of catheter-associated urinary infection (Burke et al. 1981), although the reasons remain unclear, since in at least some patients the infection is derived from bacteria at this site. Conflicting results have been reported from the use of silver-impregnated catheters which aim the reduce the adherence of bacteria although some do suggest that these catheters are associated with a reduced incidence of infection (Johnson et al. 1990) or at least with delayed onset. Systemic antimicrobial agents do delay the onset of bacteriuria but any potential advantage is offset by the cost, the occurrence of side effects and the development of bacterial resistance, particularly in the case of longterm catheterisation. Irrigation with a variety of compounds has not been shown to reduce the incidence of bacteriuria or of febrile episodes. Since this procedure requires the disconnection of the catheter-collecting-system junction, the risk of infection may in fact increase.

Short-term Catheterisation

It is accepted that any role of antibiotics in the prevention of catheter-associated infection of the urinary tract must be secondary to attention to aseptic technique during insertion, closed drainage, minimal manipulation and careful daily maintenance of hygiene with a strict regimen of hand-washing by staff before and after handling the catheter. The administration of systemic antibiotics while a urinary catheter with a closed drainage system is in situ, although delaying the ultimately inevitable onset of bacteriuria, tends to select resistant organisms.

Long-term Catheterisation

When prolonged or permanent urinary catheterisation is required, colonisation of the bladder is unavoidable. The variety of colonising organisms and their sensitivity patterns generally reflects the previous exposure of the patient to antimicrobial agents. Common species include *Proteus* spp, *Pseudomonas* spp, *Morganella* spp and *Providencia stuartii*. Some have noted the prominence of *Providencia stuartii* as a cause of antibiotic-resistant bacteriuria in patients with longterm indwelling catheters and have suggested its ability to persist in the catheterised urinary tract is the result of a particular ability to adhere to the catheter (Warren 1986). Once established, the bacteriuria is characterised by the presence of several bacterial species in a dynamic changing flora within the bladder. They are also resistant to many antimicrobials the patient may receive. While many patients with permanent indwelling urinary catheters live in harmony with their bladder flora, blockage of the catheter and/or a change of catheter or bladder wash-out may precipitate bacteraemia and even septic shock ("catheter fever"). In this instance antimicrobial treatment could be guided by the (usually numerous) previous culture results, although the continuously changing pattern of the colonising organisms should be borne in mind. The use of antimicrobials in an attempt to treat asymptomatic bacteriuria in patients with longterm catheters serves only to select resistant species and strains and must be avoided. Bacteriuria is a constant finding in patients with longterm urinary catheters, and pyuria and haematuria are not uncommon: since the usual symptoms of infection of the lower urinary tract are absent in such patients, a positive urine culture, even with pyuria, should not be taken as an indication to start antimicrobial therapy. While signs and symptoms of upper tract infection or bacteraemia will require systemic antimicrobial therapy, many episodes of low grade fever last less than 24 hours and do not require therapy (Warren et al. 1987). It may be possible to eradicate the organism in the first such episode without removing the catheter, but recurrences are common and usually involve bacteria that are more resistant. Persistence of the bacteria in encrustations and in the biofilm coating the catheter may explain these recurrences.

Transurethral Surgery

An increasing proportion of elderly patients, improvements in anaesthesia and post-operative care and the prevalence of benign prostatic hyperplasia and prostatic cancer have resulted in a growing number of transurethral resections of the prostate (TURP). Infection remains an important preventable cause of morbidity and mortality associated with the procedure. The role of antibiotics in the prevention of these infective complications has received much attention and the medical literature devoted to urological surgery is replete with studies of this topic. The fact that these studies continue to be published may attest to the conflicting results and conclusions from previous work. Many of these investigations have been seriously flawed by poor design, inadequate controls, inappropriate treatment regimens, small numbers and inferior microbiology (Chodak and Plaut 1979). The infective sequelae of TURP related to surgery include:

Bacteraemia

Septicaemia

Post-operative bacteriuria

Pyelonephritis

Epididymitis

In the design of a trial of antimicrobial prophylaxis of "infection" in transurethral surgery, care must be taken to define exactly what infection is to be prevented and there must be recognition of the period the patient is at risk of that infection in order that the timing of administration of the antimicrobial(s) may be appropriate.

Bacteraemia refers to the presence of bacteria in the bloodstream; but the event may be transient and harmless and it may be difficult to rule out the possibility of contamination. Septicaemia is a clinical picture of serious infection accompanied by a systemic response. However, conditions other than infection can mimic septicaemia (Bihari 1990). Septicaemia is more likely to occur as a result of the manipulation of infected urine in the bladder.

Bacteriuria, either before or after the operation, is often defined as 10^5 colony-forming units per ml (cfu/ml) of urine. Although this cut-off value has been useful, it should be recognised that it is an arbitrary figure. Some authors consider, quite inappropriately, that urine with less than 10^5 cfu/ml is "sterile".

Of the infections listed above, septicaemia and bacteriuria receive the most attention: septicaemia because of the associated mortality, and bacteriuria on account of the risk of more serious infection and of secondary haemorrhage. The patient is at greatest risk of bacteraemia or septicaemia for the first 12 hours from the start of the operation. A transient bacteraemia is of little consequence except for the patient with a prosthetic device such as a heart valve or a urological prosthesis who may develop infection involving the foreign material. The risk of septicaemia or transient bacteraemia can be reduced by antimicrobial prophylaxis if it is not possible to eradicate pre-existing urinary infection. The choice of antibiotic will be influenced by the range of usual urinary pathogens for that particular group of patients, but many surgeons prefer to use an aminoglycoside such as gentamicin in combination with amoxycillin.

It is now accepted that the use of prophylactic antimicrobials reduces the incidence of post-operative bacteriuria in patients with pre-existing infection at the time of transurethral operation. Since many patients with a urinary catheter in situ already have bladder colonisation, it is reasonable practice to include them in this group and give prophylaxis. Numerous trials have been, and are still being, performed in order to compare the performance of different antimicrobial agents. What remains to be established is the role, if any, of antimicrobial prophylaxis in transurethral surgery in patients with non-infected urine. It is likely that, in the absence of other risk factors, they need no prophylaxis.

Surgical Wound Infection and its Prevention

The need for antimicrobial prophylaxis to prevent wound infection is related to the risk and consequence of infection. Thus for an operation which carries a high risk of subsequent wound infection the use of antimicrobial prophylaxis is justified. For an operation where the risk is low, prophylaxis is only justified if the subsequent morbidity or mortality related to infection are high. The risk of wound infection in different types of surgery has been well studied and can be related to the nature of the surgery. Table 14.5 shows the findings in a 10-year prospective study of wound infection in Canada. Such a classification has been applied to all forms of surgery and is useful in comparing the rates of infection between centres as similar types of surgery can be assessed. The majority of urological operations involving a skin incision may be classified as "clean"

Table 14.5. Classification of surgical wounds and rate of infection

Classification of surgical wound	Rate of infection (%)	
Clean No infection encountered No hollow muscular organ opened No break in aseptic technique	Very low	1.5
Clean contaminated Hollow muscular organ opened but minimal spillage of contents	Low	7.7
Contaminated Hollow muscular organ opened, with gross spillage of contents Acute inflammation but no pus Traumatic wound less than 4h old Major break in aseptic technique	High	15.2
Dirty Pus encountered Perforated viscus found Traumatic wound more than 4h old	Very high	40.0

From Cruse and Foord (1980).

or "clean/contaminated" (Table 14.5). Examples of clean urological surgery include: scrotal surgery, implantation of prostheses, surgery of the kidney and/or ureter with non-infected urine. However, there are other risk factors which influence the overall risk of wound infection and the value of this simple classification of the type of surgery is now being questioned. Such factors include the underlying state of health of the patient and the duration of surgery. The effect of these factors may be such that given their presence in patients undergoing "clean" surgery the infection rate may be higher than that for patients undergoing clean-contaminated surgery in the absence of the risk factors. Much needs to be learned of these risk factors for all types of surgery in order to identify those patients at risk of infection and so possibly in need of antimicrobial prophylaxis.

Genitourinary Prosthetic Devices

The implantation of penile prostheses and artificial urinary sphincters can be considered "clean" surgery and as such the risk of infection should be low in the uncomplicated case. However the consequences of infection are dire; management of the infected device generally requires removal and the chance of subsequent successful reimplantation is greatly reduced. The use of pro- phylactic antibiotic administration is justified. Infection of the device may present early in the post-operative period in which case it may be assumed that infection occurred during surgery, but a late presentation may reflect haematogenous spread from a distant site of infection or colonisation. The former is more common, should be preventable and the patient is at risk for only a short time (around the time of operation). The risk of late infection, although smaller, is life-long. Some infections acquired at the time of operation do not become manifest for more than a year after surgery and may represent chronic low-grade infection, usually with coagulase-negative Staphylococci (Scott and Fishman 1988).

Non-specific measures to reduce the risk of infection include pre-operative skin disinfection, the use of depilatory cream or "dry shaving" of the operative area immediately before surgery and in the operating theatre, reduction of personnel present in theatre to an absolute minimum and the use of ultra-clean filtered air or devices such as small plastic tents to shield the operative field completely from the theatre atmosphere (Blum 1989).

The prophylactic antibiotic regimen should adhere to the general rules: selection of an agent active against the anticipated pathogens, administered in a dose and at a time guaranteed to deliver good tissue levels when bacteria may enter the wound, with minimal cost and toxicity. Most infection will occur at the time of the operation during implantation of the device and be apparent early. Late infection, generally the result of haematogenous spread (Carson and Robertson 1988; Kabalin and Kessler 1988), is unlikely to be prevented by longterm administration of antibiotics.

The pathogens that have been reported most commonly to cause infection of penile implants include: coagulase-negative Staphylococci (*Staph. epidermidis* and others), most commonly, *Esch. coli*, *Klebsiella* spp and *Pseudomonas* spp. Infection with a single organism is more common but multiple isolates may be found. The incidence of infection increases with each successive reimplantation, the effect being cumulative.

Topical agents applied to the wound by irrigation or aerosol spray or soaking the device in solutions of antimicrobial agents are of doubtful benefit, except for the surgeon's peace of mind.

Late Infection

While some infections acquired during surgery may not become apparent until long after the operation, late infection has been described as a rare event in association with haematogenous spread from a distant focus of infection (Carson and Robertson 1988). Suggestions for the prevention are based on the administration of appropriate prophylactic antibiotics at the time of the manipulation of a focus of infection or of planned surgical manipulation of oropharyngeal, gastro-intestinal or urological surfaces that may result in bacteraemia (Carson and Robertson 1988). Given the paucity of accurate data on the risk of late haematogenous infection and the likely organisms, general recommendations on such prophylaxis cannot yet be made, but expert microbiological advice should be sought and a regimen designed for the individual patient when such a procedure is planned. It should be noted that few of these procedures are performed by urologists and the responsibility to alert the physician, surgeon or dentist will therefore lie with the patient.

Artificial Urinary Sphincters

While slightly higher infection rates have been reported to accompany the insertion of artificial urinary sphincters, the causative organisms, their sources and the means of prevention are the same as for other genitourinary prosthetic devices. However, greater emphasis is placed on the establishment of "sterile" urine pre-operatively.

References

Bihari DJ (1990) Septicaemia – the clinical diagnosis. J Antimicrob Chemother Suppl C, 25:1–7

Blum MD (1989) Infections of genitourinary prostheses. Infect Dis Clin North Am 3:259–274

Brumfitt W (1991) Progress in understanding urinary infections. J Antimicrob Chemother 27:9–22

Burke JF (1961) The effective period of preventive antibiotic action on experimental incisions and dermal lesions. Surgery 50:161–168

Burke JP, Garibaldi RA, Britt MR, Jacobson JA, Conti M, Alling DW (1981) Prevention of catheter-associated urinary tract infections. Efficacy of daily meatal care regimens. Am J Med 70:655–658

Carson C, Robertson CN (1988) Late hematogenous infection of penile prostheses. J Urol 139:50–52

Chodak GW, Plaut ME (1979) Systemic antibiotics for prophylaxis in urologic surgery: A critical review. J Urol 121:695–699

Costerton JW (1984) The etiology and persistance of cryptic bacterial infections: A hypothesis. Rev Infect Dis Suppl 3 6:S608–S616

Cruse PJE, Foord R (1980) The epidemiology of wound infection. A 10-year prospective study of 62,939 wounds. Surg Clin North Am 60:27–40

Eykyn SJ, Gransden WR, Phillips I (1990) The causative organisms of septicaemia and their epidemiology. J Antimicrob Chemother Suppl C 25:41–58

Garibaldi RA, Burke JP, Dickman ML, Smith CB (1974) Factors predisposing to bacteriuria during indwelling urethral catheterisation. N Engl J Med 291:215–219

Johnson JR (1991) Virulence factors in Escherichia coli urinary tract infection. Clin Microbiol Rev 4:80–128

Johnson JR, Roberts PL, Olsen RJ, Moyer KA, Stamm WE (1990) Prevention of catheter-associated urinary tract infection with a silver oxide-coated urinary catheter: clinical and microbiologic correlates. J Infect Dis 162:1145–1150

Kabalin JN, Kessler R (1988) Infectious complications of penile prosthesis surgery. J Urol 139: 953–955

Kaufman DB, Katz R, McIntosh RM (1970) Secretory IgA in urinary tract infections. Br Med J 4:463–465

Kovarik JM, Hoepelman IM, Verhoef J (1989) Once-daily aminoglycoside administration: New strategies for an old drug. Eur J Microbiol Infect Dis 8:761–769

Lundberg T (1986) Prevention of catheter-associated urinary-tract infections by use of silver-impregnated catheters. Lancet 2:1031

Meers PD, Ayliffe GAJ, Emmerson AM et al. (1980) Report on the National Survey of Infection in Hospitals, 1980. J Hosp Inf Supplement 2

Platt R, Polk BF, Murdock B, Rosner B (1982) Mortality associated with nosocomial urinary-tract infection. N Engl J Med 307:637–642

Scott FB, Fishman IJ (1988) Editorial comments. J Urol 139:52

Shapiro M, Simchen E, Izraeli S, Sacks TG (1984) A multivariate analysis of risk factors for acquiring bacteriuria in patients with indwelling catheters for longer than 24 hours. Infect Control 5:525–532

Stamey TA (1981) Prostatitis. J R Soc Med 74:22–40

Stickler D, Dolman J, Rolfe S, Chawla J (1989) Activity of antiseptics against Escherichia coli growing as biofilms on silicone surfaces. Eur J Clin Microbiol Infect Dis 8:974–978

Warren JW (1986) Providencia stuartii: a common cause of antibiotic-resistant bacteriuria in patients with long-term indwelling catheters. Rev Infect Dis 8:61–67

Warren JW, Damron D, Tenney JH, Hoopes JM, Deforge B, Muncie HL Jr (1987) Fever bacteremia and death as complications of bacteriuria in women with long-term urethral catheters. J Infect Dis 155:1151–1158

Wilson NIL, Lewi HJE (1985) Survey of antimicrobial prophylaxis in British urological practice. Br J Urol 57:478–482

Wong ES, Hooton TM (1981) Guideline for prevention of catheter-associated urinary tract infections. Infect Control 2:125–130

Subject Index

Acrylic 39
Acute retention 80
Adhesive plasters 179
Alegra Reusable Underpads 157
Alken telescopic bougie 26
Allen–Brown shunt 266
Alloplastic spermatocele 239–56
    implications of 243
    indications for 239
    results of implantation 243
Amikacin 273
Aminoglycosides 221, 273, 278
Amoxycillin 272, 273, 278
Ampicillin 272, 273
Amplatz sheath 29
AMS 600 penile prosthesis 206–7
AMS 700 multipart inflatable prosthesis
    213–14
Aneurysm formation 263
    as graft complication 265
Antibiotics 269–81
    prophylactic xiv, 100, 221, 250, 272, 280
    therapeutic 272
Antimicrobials 272–3, 277–8
Appliance technicians 182–3
Arterio-venous (AV) fistula 261–3
Arterio-venous (AV) shunt 258–60
Aztreonam 273

Bacteraemia 278
    acquired in hospital 270
    in catheterisation 90, 100–1
Bacteriuria 64, 278
Balloon dilatation xiv, 26
Bedding protection 155–6
Bi-Coude (Roberts) tipped catheter 136
Bilateral ureterohydronephrosis 52
Bladder
    distension 87
    indications for catheterisation 80–8
    innervation 82

irritation 64
    neuropathic 82, 126–7
    outflow 85
    perforation 89
    surgery 87
    transitional cell carcinoma 3
Blood pressure 2
Blood urea nitrogen (BUN) 2
Body-worn pants and pads 157–62
Brantley Scott Artificial Urinary Sphincter
    117–27
    activation and deactivation 122–3
    AS 721 sphincter 118
    AS 742 sphincter 118
    AS 761 sphincter 118
    AS 791 sphincter 120, 128
    AS 792 sphincter 120, 123
    AS 800 sphincter 120, 123
    choice of cuff size and pressure balloon
        121–2
    complications 123–5
    indications for use 125–6
    surgical principles and techniques 120–7
Breast cancer xiv
British Standards Institution (BSI) 191
Broviac catheter 266
Burch colposuspension 129
Buselmeir shunt 266

Calcification in catheterisation 101
Calculous disease 7–10
Cancer, ureteric obstruction in 1
Cardiac failure 262
C-Arm image intensification unit 69
Catheter-associated infection 275–7
Catheter introducers 76–8
Catheters
    complications 88–105
        after withdrawal 103–5
        indwelling 91–102
        insertion 88–90

difficulty in passing 88–9
encrustation 101–2
erratic drainage 95–7
future developments 105
in neuropathic bladder 82
in operative urology 85–8
indwelling 83–4, 91–102
infection 98–101, 275–7
leakage 94
materials 75, 104
percutaneous dialysis 258
permanent indwelling 135–7
Permcath semi-permanent dual-lumen central
      venous 260–1
pressure necrosis 97–8
self-catheterisation 137–9
spasm 94–5
'tumor' 102
tunnelled, percutaneously placed intravenous
      266
types of 75
urinary infections caused by 98–101
withdrawal difficulties 102–3
Cavernosography 199
Cefotaxime 273
Ceftazidime 273
Cefuroxime 273
Cephalosporins 221–3
Cervical cancer 2, 3
Chronic retention 80–1
Ciprofloxacin 273
Clean intermittent self catheterisation (CISC)
      126–7, 137–8
Co-amoxiclav 272, 273
Coated latex 76
Coil-stent 47
Collection devices 78–80
   female 152–5
   male 139–42
Colonic loop urostomy 192
Colostomy 192
Comfie Protector Pants 158
Condom urinals 141–2
Continence cuff, male adult 152
Control of Pollution Act 1974 156
Correctaid 202
Co-trimoxazole 273
Coude catheter 75
Cummings tube 6, 8, 12
Cystitis, treatment of 272–3
Cystofix suprapubic catheter 86
Cystotomy 87

Dacron 169, 172, 223, 250
DDAVP (Desmopressin) 258
Dialysis access 257–8, 265–6
Diaphragm type urinal device 145
Dibbs male drip shield 139–40
Double J stent 44–5
Double pigtail stent 45–6
Dow Corning testicular prosthesis 248

Drainage bags 80, 142–3
   suspensory systems for 143
Dribble bags or pouches, male 139–40
Drip type urinal 147
Drugs in urostomy 193
DuraPhase prosthesis 208
Dynaflex penile prostheses 209

Edwards Female Incontinence Device 154
Elective percutaneous nephrolithotomy
      28–9
Endoscopic access to intra-renal collecting
      system 28–9
Enterobacter 273
Enterococci 273
Enuresis alarms 162–4
Epididymitis 101

Epididymo-orchitis 101
Epispadias 127–8
ErecAid erection device 202
Erectile dysfunction 197
Escherichia coli 99, 270, 271, 273, 280
Exstrophy 127–8
Extracorporeal shock-wave lithotripsy (ESWL)
      9

Fascial dilator set 25
Finney penile prosthesis 205
Flange 178
Flexiflate inflatable prosthesis 210
Foley catheter 8, 26, 73, 88, 135
Forearm fistula 262

Gamete intrafallopian transfer (GIFT) 244
Genitourinary prosthetic devices, infection in
      279–81
Gentamicin 273, 278
Gibbon catheter 75
Gibbons stent 42–3, 63, 68
Gluteal steal syndrome 198
Grafts to create fistulae 263–5
Gram-negative bacteria 273
Gram-positive bacteria 273
Granulomatous hepatitis xiii
Gum elastic 76

Haematoma formation 219
   in testicular prosthesis 255
Haematuria
   in catheterisation 102
   with ureteric stents 65
Haemodialysis
   acute access for 258–61
   chronic access for 261–5
Hand-held urinals 165–6
Helmstein technique 87
Hey–Groves sound 78
Hibitaine 136
Hickman catheter 266, 267
Hospital visitor 183–4

Hydroflex inflatable prosthesis   208–10

Ileal loop urostomy   192
Imipenem   273
Impotence
    diagnosis   197–200
    in organ transplantation   223
    irreversible organic   201
    neurogenic   200
    organic   197–200
    post-priapism   222
    psychogenic factors   200
    psychological   200
    use of term   197
    vasculogenic   198–9
    venogenic   199
Incontinence
    appliances, aids and equipment
        choice of   134–55
        types available   133–66
    implantable devices   109–32
    intermittent male   139
    odour control in   162
    post-prostatectomy   128
    toileting aids in   164–6
Incontinence pads   156
Infection
    as graft complication   265
    endogenous   270
    exogenous   270
    in catheterisation   98–101, 275–7
    in genitourinary prosthetic devices   279–81
    in penile prostheses   219–21
    in testicular prosthesis   255
    pathogenesis of   269–71
    prevention of   xiv
Intermittent clean catheterisation (CIC)   82–3
Internal cannula in vasovasotomy   232
International Ostomy Association   191
International Standards Organisation (ISO)
    191
Intra-urethral stenting   171
Intra-uterine insemination (IUI)   244
Irrigating system via nephrostomy   8

Jock strap appliance   150
Jonas penile prosthesis   205

Kanga pant-and-pad system   157
Kaufman procedure   112–15
Kelâmi–Affeld prosthesis   243
    implantation and aspiration technique
        240–3
Kellett triad   29
Klebsiella spp.   280
Kock continent urostomy   192–3
Kylie Absorbent Bed Sheet   157

Laplace's Law   35
Latex rubber   10, 38, 75
Lofric catheter   138

Lymphadenopathy   xiv
Lyophilised human dura   (LHD)   168

Malignant disease, nephrostomy drainage in
    1–17
Malignant obstruction   52
Manufacturer's agent   183
Mattress protection   155–6
Mentor malleable penile prosthesis   207
Mentor Mark II inflatable penile prosthesis
    212
Mentor multipart inflatable prosthesis   214–15
Metronidazole   221
Microporous tubing   232–5
Microsurgical epididymal sperm aspiration and
    insemination (MESAI)   244
Morganella spp.   276

Neoplasia after insertion of silicone   xiv
Nephrectomy, partial   7
Nephrostent   48–50
Nephrostogram   12
Nephrostomy   1–17
    complications   14–15
    for invasive, incurable cancer   2
    in open renal surgery   6
    in pyonephrosis   3–4
    in ureteric injury   4–6
    irrigating system via   8
    percutaneous palliative   3
    proximal   6
    quality of life following   2
Nephrostomy drainage
    in malignant disease   1–17
    in renal surgery   6
    prognostic indicators for   3
Nephrostomy stents   48–50
Nephrostomy tube   10–12
    connecting to drainage system   12
    placement at open surgery   13
    types of   26–7
Nephrostomy tube connector   13
Nephrostomy tube introducer   14
Netilmicin   273
Neuropathic bladder   126–7
    catheters in   82
Nitrofurantoin   272
Nocturnal enuresis   162–4
Nocturnal penile tumescence (NPT)   200
Norfloxacin   273
Nylon   10, 39

Obstetrical obstruction   52–3
Odour control in incontinence   162
Ofloxacin   273
OmniPhase paired prosthesis   208
Organ transplantation, impotence in   223
Otis urethrotome   223

Pancytopenia   xiii
Paul's (Penrose) tubing   140

Payne Mark 4 lightweight plastic appliance
    150
Payne Mark 7 appliance   148
Payne Mark 8 male incontinence appliance
    148
Penile incontinence clamp   140
Penile oedema   219
Penile prostheses   197–228
    choice of   203–5, 215
    choice of patient for operation   201–3
    complications   218–22
    indications for   198
    infection in   219–21
    inflatable   208–15
    malleable   205–7
    mechanical   208
    multipart inflatable   213–15
    outline of operation   215–17
    patient selection   197–228
    post-operative care   218
    post-operative pain and erosion   221–2
    pre-operative considerations   215
    results   224–5
    special circumstances   222–4
    two-part inflatable   211–13
Percutaneous nephrostomy   19–32
    anaesthesia   21
    anatomical considerations   19–21
    complications   30–1
    continued bleeding following   15
    dilatation methods   25–6
    elective percutaneous nephrolithotomy
        28–9
    endoscopic access to intra-renal collecting
        system   28–9
    experimental methods of access   29–30
    Institute of Urology technique of tube
        placement   27–8
    needle puncture   21–5
    positions for access   19–20
    puncture of obstructed system for temporary
        or long-term drainage   27–8
    site of puncture   20
Pereya-Raz suspension   129
Perforation
    bladder   89
    urethra   89
Permanent nephrostomy   15
Permcath semi-permanent dual-lumen central
        venous catheter   260–1
Peyronie's disease   199, 222
Phalloplasty   224
Pivampicillin   272–3
Plastigel   250
Polyamide   10
Polydimethylsiloxane   10
Polyethylene   10, 39, 43, 65
    in head and neck region   xiii
    prostheses   xiii
Polytetrafluorethylene. See PTFE
Polyurethane   10, 46

Polyvinyl chloride (PVC)   10, 38, 76, 85
Polyvinylpyrrolidone (PVP)   138
Porges Whistle Tip Nephrostomy Catheter   26
Port-a-Cath catheter   267
Potty trainers   164
Pouch covers   178
Pouches   175–8
Pregnancy, urostomy in   193
Pressure plates and belts   179
Priapism   222–3
Prostatectomy   101
    drainage after   85–6
Prostatic cancer   2, 277
Prostatic hyperplasia   277
Protective clothing   155–62
Proteus spp.   273, 276
Providencia stuartii   276
Proximal tubule, techniques for keeping open
        244
Proximal urinary diversion   4
Pseudomonas spp.   273, 276, 280
PTFE (Teflon)   23, 25, 28, 29, 38, 61, 76, 208,
        259, 264, 265
    in urethral prosthetic replacement   169
    injections   109–12
        equipment   110
        indications for   111
    patch substitutes   168, 172
    preparation   110
Pubic pressure device   144
Pyelocalycostomy   7
Pyelonephritis   273
Pyeloplasty   6–7
Pyonephrosis, nephrostomy in   3–4

4-Quinolone antibiotics   273

Radioactive-tritium-labelled thymidine   5
Ramirez winged shunt   259
Red rubber   76
Reflux   64
Renal collecting system
    anatomy of   34
    physiology of   35
Renal failure   84
Renal function   2
Renal surgery, nephrostomy drainage in   6
Residual urine   84–5
Retention
    suprapubic catheters in   81–2
    urethral catheters in   81–2
Retroperitoneal fibrosisia   56
Robert's catheter   75
Rosen device   115–17

Seldinger technique   41, 63
Septicaemia   269, 278
    in catheterisation   100–1
Serum creatinine   2
Sheath type urinal device   145
Shunts   258–60, 266

Silicone   xiii–xiv, 10, 39–40, 76, 170–1, 247
Silicone-tube prosthesis   171
Siliconised Dacron   169, 172
Silitek   48
Siloxan   39–40
Single J stents   56–8
Single pigtail stent   43–4
Siphon effect   66–7
Skin necrosis in testicular prosthesis   255
Skin protectives   179–80
Small-Carrion prosthesis   204, 223
Solvents   180
Sperm reservoirs   239–56
Splint, use of term   33
Staphylococci   273, 280
Staphylococcus epidermidis   280
Staphylococcus epidermiditis (albus)   220
Steal syndrome   263
Stents
   in vasovasotomy   230–2
   use of term   33
Sterile intermittent self-catheterisation   138–9
Sterile pyuria   64
Stint, use of term   33
Stoma appliances   175
Stoma care nurse   181–2, 186–7
Stoma clinics   190
Stone disease   53–4
Stress incontinence   111
   in females   128–9
Super absorbents   161
Suprapubic catheters   78
   history   73
   in retention   81–2
   indications for   81
Surgical wound infection   270, 278–9
Synthetic soft tissue substitutes   xiii–xv
   ideal characteristics of   xiii

Teflon. *See* PTFE
Tenasystem   158
Testicular prosthesis   247–56
   choice of   248–50
   complications   255–6
   development of   248
   haematoma formation in   255
   historical aspects   247
   indications for   247–8
   infection in   255
   psychological studies   248
   skin necrosis in   255
   surgical considerations   250–2
Thomas femoral shunt   266
Thrombosis as graft complication   264
Tiemann catheter   75
Tobramycin   273
Toileting aids in incontinence   164–6
Transitional cell carcinoma of the bladder   3
Transluminal balloon catheters   xiv
Transurethral resections of the prostate
      (TURP)   277

Traumatic paraplegia   223
Trigonal erosion   64
Trimethoprim   272, 273
TUR syndrome   90

Undiversion   128
Uniflate 100 inflatable prosthesis   211–12
Universal stent   48
Ureter
   anatomy of   34
   physiology of   35
Ureteral obstruction   50
Ureteral surgery   55–6
Ureteric catheters, fixation of   87–8
Ureteric damage   5
Ureteric injury
   nephrostomy in   4–6
   potential for   5
Ureteric obstruction   69
   in cancer   1
Ureteric smooth muscle, regeneration of   5
Ureteric stents   33–72
   complications   63–9
   encrustation   65–6
   endoscopic placement   58–9, 63
   flow characteristics   36–7
   history and development   40–2
   in-situ complications   64
   indications for   50–8
   materials   37–40
   migration   65
   modern internal   42–8
   obstruction   65–6
   operative placement   59–60
   percutaneous placement   60–3
   removal problems   67–9
   spontaneous breakage   65
Ureteric strictures   54–5
Ureteropelvic-junction obstruction   56
Ureteroureterostomy   4
Urethra, perforation   89
Urethral catheters   73–108
   history   73
   in retention   81–2
   indications for   81
Urethral prosthetic replacement   167–74
   techniques for   168–71
Urethral strictures   89, 103, 171
Urethral surgery, catheters in   86
Urethral trauma   171
Urinal devices
   body-worn garment incorporation   148
   child-sized male   150
   female body-worn   154
   hand-held   165–6
   male body-worn   144–52
   penis and scrotal type   147
Urinary diversion
   appliances   175–80
   hospital admission   181–2
   indicators for   5

initial patient interview   180–1
Urinary incontinence. *See* Incontinence
Urinary intestinal diversion   56–8
Urinary retention   80–2
   post-operative   219
Urinary sphincters, artificial   280
Urinary tract infection
   host defences against 271–2
   likely pathogens in   272–5
Urine director   166
Urine measurement   84
Urine output assessment   84
Urine specimens   85
Urodynamics   85
Uropass stent   48
Urostomates
   seat belt exemption   194
   training programme   184
   travel abroad   194
Urostomy
   appliances   175–95
      reusable device – two-piece   189–90
   discharge home   187–8
   drugs in   193
   immediate post-operative care   186–7
   in pregnancy   193
   non-surgical considerations   193
   operating theatre procedure   184–6
   patient involvement in changing appliances
      187

patient selection and suitability   192
pouches   175–80
principles of appliance change   188–9
religious considerations   193–4
role of relatives   184
types   192
Urostomy Association   190

Vas deferens prostheses   229–37
   materials for temporary obstruction   235
   valves   236–7
Vascular access   257–68
   non-dialysis   266–7
Vasovasotomy
   internal cannula in   232
   stents in   230–2
Vein grafts   170
Venous hypertension   263
Vitagraft   264
Vitallium testicular prosthesis   247

Wallstent   173
World Congress of Entero-Therapists (WCET)
   191
Woven fabric   38

Zygote intrafallopian transfer (ZIFT)   244